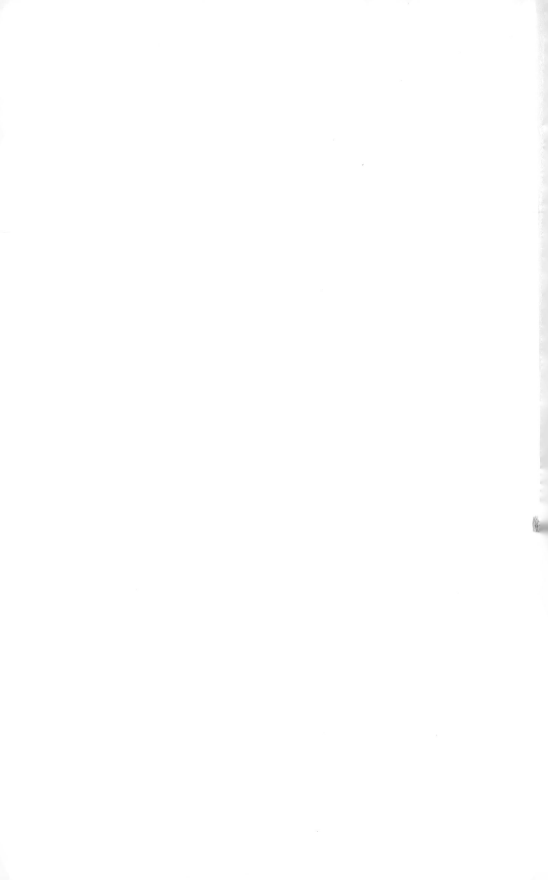

Practical Implementation of an Antibiotic Stewardship Program

Practical Implementation of an Antibiotic Stewardship Program

Edited by

Tamar F. Barlam
Boston University School of Medicine

Melinda M. Neuhauser
Office of Antibiotic Stewardship, Centers for Disease Control and Prevention

Pranita D. Tamma
Johns Hopkins University School of Medicine

Kavita K. Trivedi
Trivedi Consults, LLC

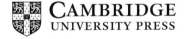
CAMBRIDGE
UNIVERSITY PRESS

CAMBRIDGE
UNIVERSITY PRESS

University Printing House, Cambridge CB2 8BS, United Kingdom

One Liberty Plaza, 20th Floor, New York, NY 10006, USA

477 Williamstown Road, Port Melbourne, VIC 3207, Australia

314–321, 3rd Floor, Plot 3, Splendor Forum, Jasola District Centre, New Delhi – 110025, India

79 Anson Road, #06–04/06, Singapore 079906

Cambridge University Press is part of the University of Cambridge.

It furthers the University's mission by disseminating knowledge in the pursuit of education, learning, and research at the highest international levels of excellence.

www.cambridge.org
Information on this title: www.cambridge.org/9781107166172
DOI: 10.1017/9781316694411

© The Society for Healthcare Epidemiology of America (SHEA) 2018

First published 2018

Printed in the United Kingdom by TJ International Ltd. Padstow Cornwall

A catalogue record for this publication is available from the British Library.

ISBN 978-1-107-16617-2 Hardback

Contents

Contributors

Whitney R. Buckel, PharmD, BCPS-AQ ID
System Antimicrobial Stewardship Pharmacist Manager, Intermountain Healthcare, Murray, UT.

Sara E. Cosgrove, MD, MS
Professor of Medicine, Johns Hopkins University School of Medicine, Baltimore, MD,
Director, Department of Antimicrobial Stewardship, Johns Hopkins Hospital, Baltimore, MD.

Christopher J. Crnich, MD, PhD
Associate Professor, University of Wisconsin School of Medicine and Public Health, Madison, WI,
Chief of Medicine, Hospital Epidemiologist and Director of Antibiotic Stewardship Program, William S. Middleton VA Hospital, Madison, WI.

Stan Deresinski, MD, FACP, FIDSA
Clinical Professor of Medicine, Stanford University School of Medicine, Stanford, CA,
Director, Antimicrobial Stewardship Program, Stanford Health Care, Stanford, CA.

Elizabeth S. Dodds Ashley, PharmD, MHS
Associate Professor of Medicine, Duke University School of Medicine, Durham, NC,
Director of Operations, Duke Antimicrobial Stewardship Outreach Network, Durham, NC.

Richard H. Drew, PharmD, MS, BCPS, FCCP
Associate Professor of Medicine (Infectious Diseases), Duke University School of Medicine, Durham, NC,
Professor and Vice Chair of Research and Scholarship, Campbell University College of Pharmacy and Health Sciences, Buies Creek, NC.

Graeme N. Forrest, MBBS, FIDSA
Associate Professor of Medicine, Veterans Affairs Portland Healthcare System, Portland, OR,
Director, Antimicrobial Stewardship Programs, Oregon Health and Science University, Portland, OR.

B. Joseph Guglielmo, PharmD. FIDSA, FCCP
Professor and Dean, School of Pharmacy, University California San Francisco, San Francisco, CA.

Keith W. Hamilton, MD
Assistant Professor of Clinical Medicine, Perelman School of Medicine at the University of Pennsylvania, Philadelphia, PA,
Director, Antimicrobial Stewardship Program, Hospital of the University of Pennsylvania, Philadelphia, PA.

Emily Heil, PharmD, BCPS-AQ ID
Assistant Professor of Pharmacy, University of Maryland School of Pharmacy, Baltimore, MD,
Pharmacy Director, Antimicrobial Stewardship Program, University of Maryland Medical Center, Baltimore, MD.

Lauri A. Hicks, DO
Director, Office of Antibiotic Stewardship, Division of Healthcare Quality Promotion, Centers for Disease Control and Prevention, Atlanta, GA.

Marisa Holubar, MD, MS
Clinical Assistant Professor of Medicine,
Stanford University School of Medicine,
Stanford, CA,
Associate Director, Antimicrobial
Stewardship Program, Stanford Health
Care, Stanford, CA.

Denise Kirsch, MD
Division of Infectious Diseases, Oregon
Health and Sciences University,
Portland, OR.

Matthew P. Kronman, MD, MSCE
Associate Professor of Pediatrics,
University of Washington School of
Medicine, Seattle, WA,
Associate Medical Director, Infection
Prevention, Seattle Children's Hospital,
Seattle, WA.

Kristi M. Kuper, PharmD, BCPS
Sr. Clinical Manager, Infectious Diseases
Center for Pharmacy Practice Excellence,
Vizient, Irving, TX.

Francesca M. Lee, MD
Assistant Professor, Departments of
Internal Medicine and Pathology,
University of Texas Southwestern Medical
Center, Dallas, TX,
Medical Director, Antimicrobial
Stewardship Program, University of Texas
Southwestern University Hospitals,
Dallas, TX.

Anurag N. Malani, MD
Medical Director, Infection Prevention and
Antimicrobial Stewardship Programs,
St. Joseph Mercy Health System, Ann
Arbor, MI,
Adjunct Clinical Associate Professor of
Internal Medicine, University of Michigan
Medical School, Ann Arbor, MI.

Holly Maples, PharmD
Associate Professor of Pharmacy Practice,
University of Arkansas for Medical

Sciences College of Pharmacy,
Little Rock, AR,
Director, Antimicrobial Stewardship
Program, Arkansas Children's Hospitals,
Little Rock, AR,
Associate Professor and the Jeff and Kathy
Lewis Sanders College of Pharmacy Chair,
Pediatrics, University of Arkansas for
Medical Sciences, Little Rock, AR.

Larissa May, MD, MSPH, MSHS
Professor of Emergency Medicine,
University of California-Davis,
Sacramento, CA,
Director of Emergency Department
Antibiotic Stewardship, University of
California-Davis, Sacramento, CA.

Rebekah W. Moehring, MD, MPH
Assistant Professor of Medicine, Duke
University, Durham, NC,
Medical Director, Duke Antimicrobial
Stewardship and Evaluation Team, Duke
University Hospital, Durham, NC.

George E. Nelson, MD
Assistant Professor of Medicine, Vanderbilt
University, Nashville, TN,
Director, Antimicrobial Stewardship
Program, Vanderbilt University Medical
Center, Nashville, TN.

Whitney J. Nesbitt, PharmD, BCPS
Antimicrobial Stewardship Pharmacist,
Vanderbilt University Medical Center,
Nashville, TN.

Jason G. Newland, MD, Med
Associate Professor of Pediatrics,
Washington University School of
Medicine, St. Louis, MO,
Director, Pediatric Antimicrobial
Stewardship Program, St. Louis Children's
Hospital, St. Louis, MO.

Jason M. Pogue, PharmD
Clinical Pharmacist, Infectious Diseases,
Sinai-Grace Hospital, Detroit, MI,

Clinical Pharmacist, Detroit Medical
Center, Detroit, MI,
Clinical Assistant Professor of Medicine,
Wayne State University School of
Medicine, Detroit, MI.

Emily S. Spivak, MD, MHS
Assistant Professor of Medicine,
University of Utah School of Medicine,
Salt Lake City, UT,
Director, Antimicrobial Stewardship
Program, University of Utah Hospitals and
Clinics, VA Salt Lake City Healthcare
System, Salt Lake City, UT.

Edward Stenehjem, MD, MSc
Associate Professor of Medicine,
Intermountain Healthcare,
Murray, UT,
Director, Antibiotic Stewardship Program,
Intermountain Medical Center,
Murray, UT.

**Marc H. Scheetz, PharmD, MSc, BCPS
AQ-ID**
Associate Professor of Pharmacy Practice,
Chicago College of Pharmacy,
Midwestern University, Chicago, IL,
Infectious Diseases Pharmacist,
Northwestern Medicine,
Chicago, IL.

Trevor C. Van Schooneveld, MD
Associate Professor of Medicine, University
of Nebraska Medical Center, Omaha, NE,
Medical Director, Antimicrobial
Stewardship Program, Nebraska Medicine,
Omaha, NE.

Arjun Srinivasan, MD
Associate Director for Healthcare
Associated Infection Prevention Programs,
Division of Healthcare Quality Promotion,
Centers for Disease Control and
Prevention, Atlanta, GA.

Julia E. Szymczak, PhD
Assistant Professor of Epidemiology,
University of Pennsylvania
Perelman School of Medicine,
Philadelphia, PA.

Annie Wong-Beringer, PharmD, FIDSA
Professor of Clinical Pharmacy,
University of Southern California,
Los Angeles, CA,
Associate Dean for Research and
Graduate
Education, University of Southern
California School of Pharmacy, Los
Angeles, CA, Co-Director, Antimicrobial
Stewardship Program, Huntington
Memorial Hospital, Los Angeles, CA.

The findings and conclusions in this book are those of the authors and editors and do not
necessarily represent the official position of the Centers for Disease Control and Prevention
(CDC) or Department of Veterans Affairs (VA).

Preface

As antibiotic resistance becomes an increasingly urgent public health crisis, there is growing recognition that antibiotic stewardship interventions are of central importance. Government and accreditation agencies are incorporating implementation of antibiotic stewardship programs (ASP) as requirements for quality healthcare. This textbook provides a core curriculum for antibiotic stewardship for both new and experienced stewards. It is designed to be of use across the spectrum of healthcare settings. Chapters discuss how to develop a needs assessment and request resources from administrators, how to leverage the work of the microbiology laboratory and informatics to improve antibiotic use and reduce adverse outcomes, and how to fulfill the basic rules of antibiotic stewardship – prescribing the right drug at the right dose via the right route, and only when indicated.

Most of the chapters of this textbook are coauthored by both a physician and a pharmacist. We believe the physician–pharmacist working relationship is central to the success of an ASP; their roles are complementary and they must work together to lead successful antibiotic stewardship interventions across the healthcare spectrum. Through shared authorship, we have highlighted the importance of a multidisciplinary ASP and captured both the physician and pharmacy perspectives, making each chapter useful for both disciplines.

It is our goal for this textbook to be a valuable resource for any ASP, ranging from those just beginning the process (Chapters 1–4) to established programs looking for new ideas and metrics to measure (Chapters 5–11) or to ensure continued commitment to their program from facility administrators (Chapter 14). There are illustrative examples that should resonate with the reader (Chapter 15) and specific advice for post-acute care and outpatient settings (Chapters 12 and 13). Although there is not a specific chapter focusing on antibiotic stewardship as it relates to the pediatric population, most of the tenets of antibiotic stewardship are identical for children and adults. For scenarios where there may be nuances specific to the pediatric population, they are addressed within relevant chapters (Chapters 6 and 13).

To our authors, thank you for your diligent work on these chapters over the past two years. To our readers, we hope you enjoy this text as much as we enjoyed editing it.

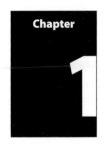

The Need for Antibiotic Stewardship Programs
An Introduction

Emily S. Spivak, Lauri A. Hicks, and Arjun Srinivasan

Access to effective antibiotic therapy is essential to modern medicine. Not only are antibiotics lifesaving for the treatment of many infections, but they also provide the means for preventing and treating life-threatening complications among the growing numbers of patients receiving chemotherapy and stem cell and solid organ transplantation, thus making those therapeutic advances possible. However, antibiotic resistance has developed with each new drug introduced to the market. Although we know the development of resistance is almost certain with exposure to any antibiotic, inappropriate and/or unnecessary antibiotic use is accelerating the process. Realizing antibiotic resistance threatens the achievements of modern medicine, infectious diseases (ID) physicians, pharmacists, and public health officials have warned of the consequences of inappropriate antibiotic use for decades and advocated for preservation of these lifesaving drugs. Halting unnecessary antibiotic use has undoubtedly become one of the leading public health concerns of our time.

An estimated 50% of antibiotic use is inappropriate and/or unnecessary.[1–3] These estimates span inpatient and outpatient settings, various types of providers, and various indications or diagnoses, highlighting the breadth of the problem. Rates of antibiotic resistance have risen dramatically over the last 30 years. In 2013, the Centers for Disease Control and Prevention (CDC) estimated that 2 million people are infected annually in the United States with antibiotic-resistant bacteria, with at least 23,000 resultant deaths.[4] Additionally, roughly 453,000 people contract *Clostridium difficile* infections (CDIs) annually in the United States with nearly 30,000 deaths attributable to this single bacterium. CDI is frequently directly related to antibiotic use.[5]

Antibiotic stewardship programs (ASPs) date back to the 1970s and encompass multidisciplinary efforts to optimize antibiotic use.[6–8] Evidence has shown that effective ASPs not only reduce inappropriate antibiotic use but also improve patient safety and clinical outcomes.[9] Thus, ASPs have expanded across various healthcare settings in an effort to optimize antibiotic use and minimize adverse events and emergence of antibiotic resistance. This chapter focuses mostly on antibiotic stewardship efforts in the United States, although a brief discussion of global strategies is also addressed.

Numerous societies and public health officials have advocated for the expansion of antibiotic stewardship efforts across healthcare. In response to antibiotic overuse, evidence supporting the role of ASPs, and the critical threat antibiotic resistance poses to public health, they have called for mandatory implementation of stewardship through legislative and regulatory mechanisms.[10] These efforts culminated with the release of President Obama's *National Strategy for Combating Antibiotic-Resistant Bacteria* in September 2014, which outlines a framework for implementation of stewardship across the healthcare continuum, improved surveillance of antibiotic use, and national goals for reductions in inappropriate prescribing.[11] These national goals lend new urgency to efforts to implement antibiotic stewardship strategies across healthcare settings and to develop standardized measures for appropriate antibiotic use.

Our goal in this chapter is to highlight the issues surrounding misuse of antibiotics that underscore the importance and need for ASPs, review evidence supporting the role of ASPs in improving patient care and safety, discuss policy initiatives and the evolution of antibiotic stewardship efforts to date, and underline next steps in preserving the precious shared resource of antibiotics.

Rationale for Antibiotic Stewardship Programs

The Scope of the Problem

Hospitals

Antibiotics are among the most frequently prescribed medications. Systematic surveys of inpatients at Boston City Hospital as far back as the 1960s found nearly 30% of patients received antibiotics during their hospitalization, with almost 10% receiving more than one antibiotic.[12, 13] Similar rates of antibiotic use have been reported in a variety of inpatient settings including acute care hospitals based in the community and tertiary care settings, [12, 14] as well as long-term care facilities (LTCFs).[15] Using data from a national administrative database of billing records for patients from a large sample of US hospitals, investigators from the CDC estimated 56% of patients discharged from 323 hospitals in 2010 received an antibiotic during their hospitalization.[3] These rates of antibiotic use have been reported among various patient populations, with the highest prescribing rates often among pediatric and surgical services.[14, 15]

More recent estimates of inpatient antibiotic consumption in the United States come from single or multicenter point-prevalence surveys. Although limited by lack of nationally representative samples and varying sources of data (e.g., pharmacy purchasing data, pharmacy order data, or antibiotic administration data), estimates have repeatedly found that nearly half of hospitalized adults and children receive an antibiotic during their hospitalization.[1, 16] Recognizing limitations of using indirect measurements such as administrative data to delineate the epidemiology of inpatient antibiotic use, CDCs' Emerging Infections Program (EIP) conducted an antibiotic use point-prevalence survey in 183 acute care hospitals across multiple states in one day in 2011.[1] The EIP is a network of ten state health departments and local collaborators representative of the US population. It conducts surveillance and evaluates methods for prevention and control of emerging IDs. Investigators determined not only the prevalence of inpatient antibiotic use across EIP sites, but also the most commonly used drugs and indications. Magill and colleagues found 50% of 11,282 inpatients evaluated received an antibiotic at some point during their hospitalization.[1] The most commonly prescribed drugs included vancomycin (14%), ceftriaxone (11%), piperacillin/tazobactam (10%), and levofloxacin (9%), in total accounting for approximately 45% of all antibiotic therapy.[1] This survey is one of the largest evaluations of inpatient antibiotic use in the United States to date. It confirms previous estimates of inpatient antibiotic use and additionally highlights the common use of broad-spectrum agents even for community-onset infections. The National Healthcare Safety Network (NHSN) recently launched the Antimicrobial Use and Resistance (AUR) Module, facilitating electronic reporting of antibiotic use data that will allow for prospective antibiotic use surveillance and assist with local and national stewardship efforts.[17]

Numerous evaluations of inpatient antibiotic prescribing quality have been conducted to estimate rates of inappropriate and therefore, modifiable antibiotic use. From these evaluations, 25% to 50% of inpatient antibiotic use is deemed inappropriate and/or unnecessary.[1–3] Common reasons for unnecessary or inappropriate antibiotic use include treatment of noninfectious or nonbacterial syndromes, treatment of colonization or contamination, use of overly broad-spectrum antibiotic therapy, and longer than necessary durations of therapy.[18] Most published assessments come from single center evaluations and focus on empiric and definitive drug selection.[14, 19–25] More recent evaluations involve in-depth evaluations of antibiotic prescribing including diagnostic evaluation, drug dosing, and duration of therapy.[26–31] No standard definition of inappropriate antibiotic use exists or is applied across studies, limiting interpretation of results and application to other settings. Most studies rely on expert opinion based on chart review to define appropriate therapy.[22, 23, 26, 28, 30, 32, 33] While more detailed in scope, these evaluations are often labor intensive and difficult to reproduce. Recently, large-scale national and multi-national antibiotic prescribing surveys have been conducted with the use of audit tools developed based on national guidelines and consensus expert opinion. [34–36] These tools are designed for use across various healthcare settings and by professionals of varying clinical expertise. For example, the Australian National Antibiotic Prescribing Survey (NAPS) is conducted annually using a published audit tool. The 2014 results showed a 38% prevalence of antibiotic use among inpatients, with nearly a quarter (23%) considered inappropriate.[37] In the United States, CDC in collaboration with external experts developed audit tools aimed at assessing the appropriateness of inpatient antibiotic use. These tools served as a foundation for the 2011 EIP Antibiotic Use Point Prevalence Survey, which on review of 296 inpatient antibiotic courses found prescribing could be improved in 37% of cases (40% of 111 urinary tract infection [UTI] cases and 36% of 185 vancomycin courses).[3] Standard audit tools are facilitating larger scale qualitative evaluations of antibiotic prescribing. With expanded use of electronic medical records, electronic audits may be possible in the future, making broader evaluations of antibiotic prescribing quality and real-time alerting of patients' charts for ASP review feasible.

Outpatient Settings

While we are gaining a better understanding of the epidemiology of inpatient antibiotic prescribing, the prevalence and various factors affecting antibiotic prescribing patterns have been better characterized for outpatient settings. Data from nearly 50 years ago shows antibiotics are the most commonly prescribed medication in outpatient settings, accounting for 15% of all prescriptions.[38] In 2009, antibiotic expenditures in outpatient settings in the United States totaled $10.7 billion, accounting for over 60% of all antibiotic expenditures across all healthcare settings.[39] Data highlighting the large role outpatient settings play in overall antibiotic use stresses the importance of effective outpatient antibiotic stewardship efforts.

Outpatient antibiotic prescribing rates are highest for children and for adults over the age of 65 years; 50–60% of all antibiotic prescriptions written are for acute respiratory infections (ARIs), which are largely viral in etiology.[40–43] While prescriptions for ARIs in children are declining,[40] data from the Veterans Affairs population and others suggests antibiotic prescriptions for ARIs in adults have remained relatively stable; 69% of Veterans received antibiotics for ARI diagnoses in 2012 as compared to 68% in 2005.[43, 44] Additionally, broad-spectrum agents such as macrolides and fluoroquinolones are commonly used when either an antibiotic is not indicated or a narrower spectrum drug would suffice.[41, 43]

Further characterizations of outpatient antibiotic prescribing patterns have highlighted geographic and provider factors associated with high prescribing rates, potential targets for outpatient stewardship efforts. Higher outpatient antibiotic prescription rates are seen in southern states with family practice physicians prescribing the largest proportion of antibiotic courses.[42, 45] Interestingly, counties with higher proportions of obese patients, children under the age of two years, females, and prescribers per capita have higher antibiotic prescribing rates.[45] Substantial variation in providers' prescribing practices exists, and understanding factors associated with high prescribing is paramount to reducing unnecessary antibiotic use.[43] Interviews of primary care providers indicate providers are knowledgeable about guideline recommendations; however, they often stray from guideline recommendations due to the fear the infection is bacterial, belief that broad-spectrum antibiotics are more likely to cure the infection, and concern for poor patient and parent satisfaction if an antibiotic is not prescribed.[46] Additionally, knowledge of definitions of broad and narrow-spectrum antibiotic agents is poor;[46] therefore, providers may not understand the implications of the antibiotic choice. This information highlights variations in knowledge and attitudes around antibiotic use that may explain variation in practice (see Chapter 3) and should be tackled in order to limit unnecessary antibiotic use.

The Rise of Antibiotic Resistance and Other Adverse Events

Antibiotic resistance has been regarded as a modern phenomenon; however, resistance predates human use of antibiotics and evolving evidence implicates environmental organisms as reservoirs of antibiotic resistance genes. Resistance genes have been detected in 30,000-year-old permafrost sediment and culturable microbiome from a cave isolated from human contact.[47, 48] When populations of bacteria are exposed to antibiotics, susceptible organisms are killed and subpopulations harboring resistance genes may survive resulting in a population of antibiotic-resistant bacteria capable of causing subsequent infection in the host, or spread to others.[49] Additionally, new resistance mutations can develop upon exposure to antibiotics. The more antibiotics are used, the faster these processes happen.

We have seen this repeatedly since the first antibiotics were introduced into clinical practice over 70 years ago. As new antibiotics are released for clinical use, resistance to most is detected within five to ten years.[50] Case-control studies confirm the relationship between antibiotic exposure and subsequent antibiotic-resistant infections. For example, strong associations have been noted with antecedent carbapenem exposure and carbapenem-resistant *Klebsiella pneumoniae* infections. Similarly, receipt of cephalosporins has been identified as a risk factor for subsequent extended-spectrum beta-lactamase (ESBL) producing *Escherichia coli* and *Klebsiella* species infections.[51, 52] In 2013, CDC released a report providing the first overview of antibiotic-resistant organisms and other infections directly related to antibiotic use such as *Clostridium difficile*, and their threat to human health.[4] Carbapenem-resistant *Enterobacteriaceae*, drug-resistant *Neisseria gonorrhoeae* and *C. difficile* are among the most urgent threats. While antibiotic resistance is on the rise, development of new antibiotics has slowed,[53] highlighting the urgent need to curb unnecessary antibiotic prescribing and begin an era of responsible antibiotic use.

Antibiotic use is the single most significant risk factor for CDI.[54] Individual drug risks may vary, but nearly every antibiotic carries a threat of CDI with risk accumulating with increasing numbers of drugs, dose and duration.[55] The epidemiology of *C. difficile* changed in the early 2000s with emergence of the North American pulsed-field gel electrophoresis type 1 (NAP1) strain. The NAP1 strain is associated with higher rates of infection, more severe disease, increased risk of relapse, and increased mortality.[56, 57] Not only has *C. difficile* become the most common cause of healthcare-associated infections in US hospitals, but it is increasingly reported in community settings as well.[58] Based on active population surveillance through CDC's EIP network that encompasses both inpatient and outpatient locations, it is estimated that nearly 500,000 incident CDIs occur annually in the United States, with nearly 30,000 deaths.[5] Although possibly influenced by use of more sensitive testing methods, increasing rates of this largely preventable infection are alarming. CDI has arguably become one of the most difficult infections of our time; antibiotic stewardship is and will continue to be a key component of its prevention.

CDI is one of the most severe adverse side effects resulting from antibiotic use; however, adverse drug events (ADEs) such as allergic reactions, drug toxicities, organ dysfunction, and unintended drug interactions may occur. Data suggest ADEs related to antibiotic use are not uncommon. An estimated 142,505 annual visits are made to emergency departments in the United States for antibiotic-related ADEs.[59] Antibiotics are implicated in 20% of all emergency department visits for ADEs, with the majority related to allergic reactions (78.7%).[59] Antibiotics are the most common drugs implicated in emergency department visits for ADEs in children.[4] Additionally, antibiotic ADEs in inpatients are associated with longer lengths of stay and higher hospital costs.[60] Providers do not always seem to appreciate the harms associated with antibiotic use; perhaps greater awareness of the harms of antibiotic use will bring about more judicious prescribing.

In summary, despite growing awareness of the harms of indiscriminate use, rates of antibiotic use have remained stable, and by some estimates have increased.[1, 43] Inappropriate and/or unnecessary antibiotic use is contributing to alarming rates of antibiotic-resistant infections and potentially life-threatening ADEs.

Evidence to Support Antibiotic Stewardship

Antibiotic stewardship is a multidisciplinary program of activities aimed at optimizing antibiotic use to achieve best clinical outcomes, while minimizing unintended adverse events and limiting selective pressures that drive the emergence of antibiotic-resistant organisms.[10, 61] Stewardship programs promote six principles of appropriate antibiotic use including prescribing: 1) for the right patients (e.g., only in patients with infections for which an antibiotic is indicated); 2) at the right time (e.g., as soon as possible in serious infections like sepsis); 3) with the right drug choice; 4) right route; 5) right dose; and 6) right duration of therapy. Antibiotic stewardship interventions have been shown to decrease antibiotic use, lead to more appropriate antibiotic use, reduce healthcare costs and antibiotic resistance, and most importantly, improve patient outcomes and safety.[62–64]

Impact on Antibiotic Use and Costs

Inpatient stewardship programs have shown significant improvements in antibiotic use in the form of both overall reductions in antibiotic consumption as well as more appropriate therapy, typically defined as improvements in drug selection, adherence to guidelines, and optimization of durations of therapy.[64] As an example, restrictions requiring prior authorization from ID for dispensing of third-generation cephalosporins led to an 86%

decrease in use of target drugs over a ten-year period at a large academic medical center.[65] Similarly, a comprehensive ASP including prior authorization for use of certain antibiotics, a comprehensive educational program, creation of local guidelines, and biannual feedback to providers on prescribing practices led to an overall 35% reduction in antibiotic use.[66] Prospective audit and feedback to hospitalists about prescribing habits for broad-spectrum antibiotics led to higher rates of appropriate antibiotic prescriptions from 43% at baseline to 74% post-intervention.[67] Camins and colleagues conducted a prospective cluster randomized trial assigning medicine teams at a large urban teaching hospital to either prospective audit and feedback focused on use of vancomycin, levofloxacin and piperacillin/tazobactam, or to use of indication-based guidelines for antibiotic use without any feedback.[68] Assessing nearly 800 prescriptions for vancomycin, levofloxacin, and piperacillin/tazobactam, intervention teams were more likely to prescribe antibiotics appropriately, compared with teams that did not receive the intervention, whether for empiric (82% vs. 73%) or definitive therapy (82% vs. 43%).[68]

These improvements in antibiotic use are achieved with the added benefit of reduced hospital costs, without negative impacts on mortality, length of stay, or readmission rates. [64] Reported annual cost savings from ASPs range from $150,000 to $900,000, with varying savings based on facility type and number of stewardship strategies implemented. [69–74] Conversely, Standiford et al. reported that discontinuation of an ASP at their hospital resulted in a 32% increase in antibiotic costs within two years of program discontinuation.[75] Antibiotic-related cost savings often plateau after initial reductions; however, this report underscores the ongoing role ASPs play in controlling antibiotic use and costs.

Antibiotic stewardship interventions aimed at improving outpatient antibiotic prescribing have been shown to reduce antibiotic prescriptions for conditions in which antibiotics are not indicated (e.g., ARIs) and improve choice when antibiotics are indicated.[76–78] Passive educational strategies such as use of printed educational materials alone have little to no impact as compared to active educational interventions including interactive meetings (vs. didactic lectures), individual provider level feedback and in-person education.[76, 77] Although impacts have been modest, clinical decision support (CDS) and care pathways provided either in paper form or integrated into the electronic medical record at the time of prescribing have been shown to reduce antibiotic prescriptions for ARIs and lead to more guideline-concordant management.[79–81] Patient-focused interventions, such as delayed antibiotic prescribing in which a patient is asked to wait a few days before starting an antibiotic to determine if the antibiotic is needed, can lead to reductions in unnecessary antibiotic use without negative impacts on symptom resolution, clinical outcome, or patient satisfaction.[82–84] Posters placed in examination rooms with the clinician's picture, signature, and commitment to use antibiotics appropriately led to a 20% reduction in inappropriate prescribing for respiratory conditions.[85] While several interventions have been shown to improve outpatient antibiotic prescribing, more effort is needed to better understand how to maximize their effect, which combinations of interventions provide the most benefit with available resources and how best to scale up outpatient stewardship interventions in a sustainable manner.

Impact on Antibiotic Resistance

The impact of antibiotic stewardship interventions on antibiotic resistance is difficult to assess given available data is often in the form of antibiograms that aggregate susceptibility data for only initial isolates. This precludes an evaluation of antibiotic resistance that developed over time in hospitalized patients. Additionally, antibiograms- in their traditional form- do not allow for evaluation of multidrug resistance. These limitations combined with the additional factors influencing the development and spread of antibiotic resistance, such as lapses in infection control practices, make measuring the impact of stewardship interventions on antibiotic resistance difficult and results to date have been mixed.[86–88] However, studies have shown associations between antibiotic stewardship interventions and reductions in individual- and population-level antibiotic resistance. In a randomized controlled trial evaluating use of a clinical pulmonary infection score as criteria for antibiotic decision-making, investigators found randomization of patients with low risk of infection to short course empiric therapy as compared to standard of care, not only led to reductions in antibiotic use, but also reduced rates of antibiotic resistance and superinfections among patients receiving short course therapy (15% vs. 35%).[89] Implementation of a requirement for prior authorization of selected broad-spectrum parenteral antibiotics at one institution led to a 32% reduction in antibiotic expenditures coupled with increased activity against Gram-negative organisms for all targeted agents.[69] Interestingly, susceptibilities to both restricted and unrestricted antibiotic agents increased after the intervention, highlighting the selective pressure one class of antibiotics can exert on others.

Impact on CDI and Clinical Outcomes

Arguably one of the most important impacts of ASPs has been their contribution to reducing hospital rates of CDI. Antibiotics are the single most important risk factor for CDI; therefore, stewardship interventions promoting judicious antibiotic use are imperative for prevention. Guidelines recommend implementing an ASP as part of multidisciplinary efforts paired with infection control to prevent CDI in hospital settings.[90, 91] Multiple studies demonstrate the significant impact of ASPs on minimizing CDIs. A comprehensive antibiotic stewardship intervention at a community hospital involving antibiotic detailing with individual provider education as well as automatic stop orders resulted in a 22% decrease in broad-spectrum antibiotic use and a drop in CDI incidence from 2.2 to 1.4 per 1,000 patient days.[74] Decreasing rates of healthcare-associated infections (HAIs) due to resistant *Enterobacteriaceae* were also noted.[74] A combined strategy of restricted use of cephalosporins, a complete ban on fluoroquinolones and infection control measures resulted in termination of a toxigenic NAP1 CDI outbreak in the Netherlands in 2005.[92] After infection control measures were unable to control a hospital outbreak of NAP1 CDI in Quebec, implementation of a nonrestrictive stewardship intervention including dissemination of local guidelines combined with prospective audit and feedback resulted in reductions in antibiotic consumption followed by a marked 60% decrease in CDIs.[93] These studies highlight the significant impact ASPs can have on reducing CDIs. Nearly 30,000 people die annually from CDI in the United States;[5] minimizing unnecessary antibiotic use is critical to preventing this devastating infection and saving lives.

Optimizing antibiotic therapy improves patient outcomes including increased infection cure rates and possible reductions in mortality. Implementation of a guideline to promote effective prescribing for community-acquired pneumonia was associated with decreased 30-day mortality across a large health system.[94] Additionally, growing evidence suggests involvement of ID specialists in the management of patients with *Staphylococcus aureus* bacteremia leads to more appropriate and guideline-concordant management as well as reductions in hospital mortality.[95, 96]

Antibiotic stewardship is a patient safety initiative aimed at preventing antibiotic-associated harms. In addition to CDI, ASPs play an integral role in promoting patient safety through reductions in ADEs,[97] and by working with multidisciplinary teams to improve perioperative surgical prophylaxis in hopes of preventing surgical site infections. Hospitals with pharmacists performing therapeutic drug monitoring of vancomycin and aminoglycosides have lower rates of renal impairment, hearing loss, and overall mortality. [98] In many institutions, therapeutic drug monitoring is performed or supervised by an ASP pharmacist in addition to antibiotic medication reconciliation, evaluation of discharge antibiotics and monitoring drug-drug interactions to avoid adverse reactions. ASPs also play a role in determining the nature of antibiotic allergies, minimizing false labeling of drug allergies that promote use of broad-spectrum therapy, recommending appropriate alternative therapy when necessary and preventing use of drugs to which patient are allergic.[99, 100] Optimizing perioperative antibiotic prophylaxis is associated with reductions in surgical site infections; [101, 102] measures evaluating perioperative prophylaxis are incorporated into The Centers for Medicare and Medicaid Services (CMS) value-based purchasing program. Pharmacist-directed management of perioperative prophylaxis has been associated with improved survival and decreased costs and length of stay.[103] Finally, an evolving body of literature underscores further opportunity to avoid harm by involving ASPs in evaluation of patients for outpatient parenteral antibiotic therapy (OPAT).[104, 105] Use of OPAT is on the rise, adverse events related to antibiotics are frequent, and an estimated 15–30% of use is avoidable or unnecessary.[104–106] ASPs play a pivotal and effective role in not only minimizing unnecessary antibiotic use, but importantly, avoiding unnecessary harm and costs.

Making Antibiotic Stewardship a Reality

Evolution of Antibiotic Stewardship Goals

Despite numerous concerns about misuse of antibiotics and calls for improved prescribing,[7, 8] coordinated efforts to raise awareness, improve prescribing and impact policy did not take hold until the mid-1990s. In response to increased recognition of unnecessary antibiotic prescribing in outpatient settings, the US CDC launched the National Campaign for Appropriate Antibiotic Use in the Community in 1995, which was subsequently renamed Be Antibiotics Aware in 2017.[107] This program focuses on common illnesses that account for the majority of antibiotic prescriptions written in outpatient settings, and works with a wide range of partners to not only raise awareness about the threat of antibiotic-resistant infections and adverse effects of antibiotics, but also provide various clinical and informational resources for providers and patients to improve antibiotic use. The program has expanded to measure and characterize outpatient antibiotic prescribing,[42] evaluate interventions to improve prescribing, [108] and develop policies and guidelines to promote appropriate outpatient antibiotic prescribing.[109, 110] The program also includes Antibiotics Awareness Week, a yearly observance in November to raise awareness about antibiotic resistance and the importance of judicious antibiotic use.[107] During this week, CDC partners with a variety of organizations and over 40 countries to educate clinicians, the public, policymakers, hospital administrators, and the media about the critical issue of antibiotic resistance.

National ID professional societies worked for years to address the rising tide of antibiotic-resistant infections through development of prevention and treatment guidelines, promoting and funding research, and advocating for effective policies to address antibiotic resistance. Recognizing the implications of rising rates of antibiotic-resistant pathogens coupled with dramatic declines in development of new antibiotic agents, the Infectious Diseases Society of America (IDSA) originally published guidelines for improving antibiotic use in hospitals in 1988.[111] This was followed by a joint publication on the topic by IDSA and the Society for Healthcare Epidemiology of America (SHEA) in 1997.[112] These societies more specifically promoted the concept of antibiotic stewardship when they released new guidelines in 2007.[61] This document outlines ideal ASP team members and needed resources as well as core and supplemental strategies for ASPs to improve antibiotic use; yet, it lacked practical details of how to implement an ASP. The 2007 guidelines were followed by an IDSA policy paper titled Combating Antibiotic Resistance: Policy Recommendations to Save Lives that recommended requiring ASPs in all US healthcare facilities.[113] This document recommended new incentives and requirements be established for implementation and maintenance of ASPs across all health care settings as just one part of a multi-faceted approach to address antibiotic resistance.[113] IDSA recommended ASPs be required as a condition of participation in federal CMS programs.[113] A companion policy statement on antibiotic stewardship published the following year by SHEA, IDSA, and the Pediatric Infectious Diseases Society (PIDS) echoed these calls for mandatory implementation of ASPs across health care and additionally outlined minimum program requirements that should be enforced, process and outcome measures to be monitored, and deficiencies in national antibiotic surveillance and research that need to be addressed.[10] SHEA in partnership with other organizations promoting antibiotic stewardship published a guidance document outlining the knowledge and skills necessary for physicians, pharmacists or other healthcare providers to develop and lead an antibiotic stewardship program.[114] Finally, IDSA and SHEA released recommendations for implementation and measurement in antibiotic stewardship in 2016, specifically outlining best approaches and interventions to optimize antibiotic use.[115]

Initial experience with regulation mandating processes to improve antibiotic use in the United States comes from the state of California. California Senate Bill 739, signed into law in 2006, directed the California Department of Public Health to require general acute care hospitals to develop a process for evaluating the judicious use of antibiotics with results jointly monitored by representatives and committees involved in quality improvement. [116] While Senate Bill 739 did not explicitly state ASPs be established, nor outline or require methods for intervening to improve antibiotic use, a preliminary assessment of its impact identified 22% of California hospitals instituting ASPs.[117] While antibiotic stewardship initiatives expanded under this regulation, barriers persisted including staffing constraints and lack of funding. In September 2014, California Senate Bill 1311 [118] expanded previous regulations and required that hospitals adopt and implement an antibiotic stewardship policy adherent with guidelines established by the federal government and professional societies with leadership required by either a physician or pharmacist with training in antibiotic stewardship. California not only learned that legislation is effective in expanding antibiotic stewardship initiatives, but also that the language of such mandates is integral to developing appropriately constructed and funded programs.

Antibiotic resistance is a public health issue and in many ways addressing it falls within the scope of public health services. At a federal level, US CDC has been involved with

Table 1 Core Elements of Hospital Antibiotic Stewardship Programs

1) **Leadership Commitment:** Dedicating necessary human, financial and information technology resources.

2) **Accountability:** Appointing a single leader responsible for program outcomes. Experience with successful programs show that a physician leader is effective.

3) **Drug Expertise:** Appointing a single pharmacist leader responsible for working to improve antibiotic use.

4) **Action:** Implementing at least one recommended action, such as systemic evaluation of ongoing treatment need after a set period of initial treatment (i.e., "antibiotic time out" after 48 hours).

5) **Tracking:** Monitoring antibiotic prescribing and resistance patterns.

6) **Reporting:** Regular reporting information on antibiotic use and resistance to doctors, nurses and relevant staff.

7) **Education:** Educating clinicians about resistance and optimal prescribing.

promoting antibiotic stewardship activities for nearly two decades and has worked to make improving antibiotic use a national priority. CDC has worked to not only provide education about antibiotic stewardship, but also tools and resources to implement effective programs. [107] CDC has worked to describe the human impact of antibiotic resistance in the United States as well as the extent and patterns of our antibiotic use and opportunities for improvement.[1, 3, 4] In 2014, CDC published a report calling for implementation of ASPs in all hospitals and soon after released a document outlining core elements of successful hospital-based ASPs (See Table 1).[3, 119] While acknowledging some flexibility is needed to tailor ASPs to local resources and culture, CDC emphasized success is dependent on leadership and defined multidisciplinary approaches. For the first time, the CDC provided a framework for components of a successful ASP in the Core Elements of Hospital Antibiotic Stewardship Programs [119] and has since outlined core elements of antibiotic stewardship in nursing homes and core elements of outpatient antibiotic stewardship."[120, 121]

In September 2014, President Obama signed Executive Order 13676: *Combating Antibiotic-Resistant Bacteria* which addresses the policy recommendations of the President's Council of Advisors on Science and Technology (PCAST) and identified priorities for combating antibiotic-resistant bacteria further detailed in the *National Strategy on Combating Antibiotic-Resistant Bacteria*.[122, 123] The Executive Order instructed CMS to review regulations and ensure acute care hospitals and LTCFs have ASPs that implement best practices by 2020.[122] Additionally, the national strategy called for reductions in inappropriate prescribing by 20% in inpatient settings and 50% in outpatient settings by 2020 as a key strategy in reducing antibiotic resistance. The subsequent *National Action Plan for Combating Antibiotic-resistant Bacteria* further outlined steps for implementing these goals and the national strategy over the next five years (www.cdc.gov/drugresistance/pdf/national_action_plan_for_combating_antibotic-resistant_bacteria.pdf).[11] In response to these national efforts, the Joint Commission published a new standard for the implementation of ASPs for hospitals, critical access hospitals, and nursing centers for accreditation, which became effective in January 2017.[124]

Similar warnings about the threat of antibiotic resistance and calls for improved antibiotic use have echoed around the world. The World Health Organization (WHO) published a report on global antibiotic resistance in 2014, which describes not only global levels of antibiotic-resistant bacteria, but also highlights the lack of coordinated surveillance efforts.[125] The report declares antibiotic resistance a threat to the achievements of modern medicine that may lead to a post-antibiotic era where common infections cannot be cured. The WHO subsequently published a Global Action Plan on Antimicrobial Resistance in 2015, which was adopted by the World Health Assembly.[126] The action plan outlines five objectives: 1) improve awareness around antibiotic resistance, 2) strengthen knowledge and evidence base through surveillance and research, 3) reduce the incidence of infection, 4) optimize use of antibiotics in humans and animals, and 5) develop the economic case for sustainable investment in new medicines, diagnostic tools, vaccines and other interventions. The action plan calls for coordinated efforts around the globe and the development of multi-sector (i.e., human and veterinary medicine, agriculture, finance, environment and consumer) national action plans by the 2017 World Health Assembly. Finally, in September 2016 Heads of State convened at the United Nations General Assembly signed a commitment to broad, coordinated approaches to addressing antibiotic resistance across human health, veterinary medicine and agriculture, and reaffirmed the blueprint for tackling antibiotic resistance in the WHO global action plan.[127]

The overuse of antibiotics in food animal production and its relationship to antibiotic-resistant bacteria in humans has gained increasing recognition. The first ban on antibiotic use in food animals for growth promotion was enacted in Sweden in 1986, followed by numerous European countries and a European Union ban on all antibiotics in food animals for growth promotion in 2006.[128] The United States has not been so quick to act; however, appreciation of the relationship with antibiotic use in animals and human health motivated reviews of agricultural practices around the world and led the US Food and Drug Administration (FDA) to implement strategies in 2015 to minimize antibiotic overuse by identifying certain antibiotics that require veterinary oversight via the Veterinary Feed Directive.[129] The FDA also worked with drug companies to re-label antibiotics and remove feed efficiency and growth promotion claims. Global initiatives and the push for regulatory requirements have advanced antibiotic stewardship across healthcare, veterinary medicine and agriculture. Work must continue but these efforts have lent new urgency toward efforts to systematically measure antibiotic use and develop standardized measures of appropriate use.

Progress on Measurement and Quality Measures

Quantifying where, when and how antibiotics are used in various healthcare settings is imperative to identifying areas for improvement and implementing change. In conjunction, antibiotic surveillance data is imperative to set and monitor national goals for improvement. In the 1990s, CDC encouraged national reporting of inpatient antibiotic use through the AUR Module of the National Nosocomial Surveillance System, which was transitioned to the NHSN in 2006. Due to difficulties with manual aggregation of data, nearly all reporting to the AUR stopped by 2006.[130] Eliminating the need for manual data entry, CDC released the Antimicrobial Use (AU) option of the AUR Module in 2011 based on electronic medication administration record (eMAR) or bar coding medication administration (BCMA) systems and began receiving antibiotic use data in 2012. Antibiotic use in the AUR Module is measured in days of therapy per 1,000 days present (DOT/1,000 days present) with the short-term goal to provide facilities with local data for quality improvement activities and a means for measuring the effectiveness of stewardship interventions. A forthcoming benefit will be a national database of inpatient antibiotic use with the ability to report risk adjusted facility benchmarks, enabling comparison between facilities. Currently, submission of antibiotic use data is voluntary; however, the national action plan strongly encourages healthcare facilities to submit usage data, and the PCAST report recommends requiring this reporting as part of the Inpatient Quality Reporting Program of CMS.[123]

CDC developed the Standardized Antibiotic Administration Ratio (SAAR) as a risk adjusted quality measure for antibiotic use and a first step toward national antibiotic benchmarking for US hospitals. The SAAR compares observed antibiotic use with expected or predicted use (observed/expected). There are multiple SAARs calculated including those based on adult and pediatric patient location groupings (e.g., ward vs. intensive care unit) and antibiotic groupings [e.g., anti-methicillin resistant *S. aureus* (anti-MRSA) agents, broad-spectrum agents predominantly used for community-acquired infection]. Although questions remain regarding the relationship between the SAAR and appropriate antibiotic prescribing and patient outcomes, it is an initial effort that will inform future benchmarking efforts. While there is no established reference standard with which to measure appropriate antibiotic use, recent efforts by CDC and others have focused on defining quality indicators and developing standardized audit tools for measuring antibiotic prescribing quality based on objective criteria that can be assessed by trained personnel.[34] Future work is needed to validate the SAAR as an inpatient quality measure against these measures of appropriate antibiotic prescribing.

Antibiotic Stewardship Across the Healthcare Continuum

Reported estimates of the prevalence of antibiotic stewardship programs in US hospitals vary, and little is known about the structure and robustness of these programs, number and type of interventions used, and process and outcome measures followed.[117] With increasing recognition of the benefits of antibiotic stewardship as well as recent calls for establishment of ASPs in all acute care hospitals, understanding the national landscape of antibiotic stewardship and current barriers to implementation efforts are imperative.

In order to identify gaps and improve stewardship efforts throughout the State of Michigan, Collins and colleagues in conjunction with the Michigan Society of Health-System Pharmacists (MSHP) conducted a survey of health systems in 2014 to characterize current antibiotic stewardship practices and perceived stewardship-related needs.[131] Of the 47 respondents, 45% were from facilities with less than 150 beds, and the majority of respondents (76%) represented nonteaching facilities. Although response rates were low (26%), 83% of respondents reported having antibiotic stewardship strategies in place.[131] Most stewardship programs were less than two years old (66%), and the majority (63%) reported multidisciplinary ASP teams.[131] Formulary restriction, intravenous to oral conversion, and pharmacist led prospective audit and feedback were the most common interventions used; however, pharmacists in hospitals with fewer than 150 beds were less likely to make interventions related to de-escalation or discontinuation of antibiotics (52% vs. 85%).[131] The most commonly reported barriers to antibiotic stewardship were lack of ASP funding (47%) and other resources (49%, e.g., information technology resources, lack of ID expertise), as well as opposition from physicians and lack of hospital administration support.[131] Interestingly, a low%age of programs (44%) reported following antibiotic utilization patterns, one of the seven core elements for hospital ASPs identified by CDC. Reasons for not monitoring antibiotic use trends were not explored, but highlight the need for further support for program evaluation. This survey underlines significant differences in stewardship practices and resources between large and small hospitals. Most studies evaluating inpatient ASPs come from large academic centers, and there is a limited evidence base with which to guide successful implementation of ASPs in smaller community hospitals. [132] Although resources are often limited in nonacademic settings, successful examples of ASPs in these settings exist,[133] and future efforts are needed to understand how best to implement stewardship in small community hospitals.

The National Veterans Affairs Antimicrobial Stewardship Task Force (ASTF) is a resource for stewardship education and for the development and dissemination of stewardship resources across the VA, the largest integrated healthcare system in the United States. The VA ASTF, in collaboration with the VA Healthcare Analysis and Information Group (HAIG), performed a cross-sectional survey across all VA facilities in 2012 to characterize existing antibiotic stewardship structure and practices.[134] At the time of the survey, 38% of 130 VA facilities reported having an antibiotic stewardship team, defined as an ID physician and a clinical pharmacist who routinely meet to discuss antibiotic stewardship-related issues.[134] Twenty-two% of facilities had a policy establishing an ASP; another 42% reported having a policy under development.[134] The most commonly utilized stewardship activities and processes were formulary restrictions (92%) use of automatic stop orders for antibiotics (75%) and clinical care pathways (74%). Activities that seemed underutilized included systematic review of positive blood cultures, prospective audit and feedback, and group or provider-specific feedback on antibiotic usage.[134] Interestingly, of the 49 facilities with antibiotic stewardship teams, 51% reported working in the outpatient setting and 67% in community living centers, which are VA LTCFs.[134] In January 2014, the VA released a directive establishing a policy for the implementation of ASPs across all VA medical facilities. This policy was significant and affirms the VA's commitment to antibiotic stewardship.

To better characterize inpatient antibiotic stewardship practices across the United States, CDC incorporated antibiotic stewardship questions into the 2015 NHSN facility survey. Questions were aimed at assessing how many hospitals had ASPs meeting the seven core elements of hospital ASPs as outlined by the CDC.[119] In 2014, 39% of US hospitals reported having ASPs meeting all seven core elements.[135] Ninety-four% of hospitals reported compliance with the action core element, meaning they had implemented at least one recommended stewardship intervention, while only 60% of hospitals reported leadership commitment dedicating resources for stewardship. Larger bed size, teaching hospital status and hospital leadership commitment for the ASP were all associated with fulfilling all seven core elements. For example, 56% of hospitals with greater than 200 beds had ASPs meeting all core elements as compared to 22% of hospitals with less than 50 beds. Similarly, 76% of hospitals with dedicated salary support for stewardship resources met all seven core elements, versus only 27% of those without dedicated salary support. While these data suggest a substantial proportion of US hospitals of varying sizes have taken on the antibiotic stewardship charge, more than half of programs do not meet all core elements. Leadership commitment and dedicated resources are clearly associated with more robust ASPs. If we intend to improve antibiotic use in any significant way, garnering hospital leadership support is imperative.

There are over 15,000 nursing homes in the United States with an estimated 1.4 million residents, and these numbers are expected to rise as the US population ages.[136] Between 50% and 80% of LTCF patients receive antibiotics, often coupled with high rates of antibiotic-resistant infections.[137, 138] LTCFs are in great need of antibiotic stewardship given their medically complex patients and care process models, combined with high rates of antibiotic utilization and resistance among their vulnerable patients. Resources and access to ID expertise are often limited in LTCFs and data are limited regarding most effective stewardship practices in this setting. The lack of resources and evidence to guide best practices necessitate creative stewardship approaches to optimize antibiotic use in LTCF settings.[139] Given limited data regarding existing antibiotic stewardship practices coupled with forthcoming regulation requiring ASPs in all LTCFs, the Michigan Department of Health and Human Services conducted a survey of Michigan LTCFs in 2014 to define current stewardship practices and needs.[138] Seventy-five% (60/80) of responding LTCFs reported having ASP policies and procedures, yet only 23% reported having a formal ASP with dedicated staff. Perceived obstacles to ASP implementation included lack of knowledge (54%), absence of an ASP proposal (50%), and staffing constraints (8%). Most commonly involved ASP team members in LTCFs include infection preventionists, medical directors and nurses.[138, 140] Lack of access to ID expertise has been identified as a limitation in other surveys[140]; however, respondents report a strong belief that antibiotics are overused (54%), that an ASP would be beneficial (89%) and a keen interest in pursuing antibiotic stewardship education.[138] These findings are encouraging, but underscore the need for more education of local champions paired with availability of ID and stewardship expertise.

To bolster antibiotic stewardship efforts in long-term care settings, the US CDC released "Core Elements of Antibiotic Stewardship Programs in Nursing Homes" in 2015.[120]. This document outlines the key components and functions of ASPs in nursing homes and will provide a useful foundation as nursing homes work toward implementing stewardship programs (see Chapter 12).

New models for delivering ambulatory care with improved access have grown over the last decade in the form of retail and urgent care clinics and telemedicine. Retail clinics are often located in pharmacies or grocery stores and provide walk-in care for a limited set of low acuity conditions with upper respiratory illnesses, unspecified viral illnesses and UTIs accounting for 88% of visits.[141] Use of retail clinics grew ten-fold between 2007 and 2009; [141] an estimated 3 million patients visited retail clinics in 2008.[142] Use of telemedicine and e-visits where interactions occur virtually over the internet have grown dramatically and these services are now reimbursed by numerous health plans.[143] An evaluation comparing e-visits to office visits at primary care practices within the University of Pittsburgh Health System, found 99% of e-visits for UTIs resulted in an antibiotic prescription as compared to 49% of in-person office visits.[143] Providers were also less likely to order relevant diagnostic tests at e-visits as compared to in-person visits (8% vs. 51%).[143]

Administration of antibiotic infusion therapy in the ambulatory setting, or OPAT, is also increasingly common. It can be safe, efficacious and cost saving with appropriate patient selection.[144] However, there is mounting evidence that as use of OPAT is on the rise so is unnecessary antibiotic use and inadequate follow-up to monitor for antibiotic and central venous catheter-related toxicities.[145] Stewardship interventions to monitor and determine the need for OPAT have been shown to reduce unnecessary use and costs, and improve patient safety and outcomes.[105, 146, 147] While these growing healthcare delivery models have potential advantages including convenience, efficiency and lower costs, evidence suggests they contribute to over-prescribing. They represent the next frontier where we must not only characterize antibiotic prescribing, but also begin to design, implement and evaluate innovative stewardship interventions to reduce overuse.

Where Do We Go from Here?

Next Steps for Antibiotic Stewardship

We are at a pivotal moment for antibiotic stewardship. Previous, smaller efforts to improve antibiotic use have now been galvanized into a formal action plans. Antibiotic stewardship is recognized as a key to combating antibiotic resistance. An unprecedented number of stakeholders have now joined this effort, as evidenced by the White House Forum on Antibiotic Stewardship in 2015, which brought together more than 100 stakeholder groups to discuss ways to expand antibiotic stewardship, and the commitment made by global leaders to coordinate efforts to fight antibiotic resistance at the United Nations General Assembly in September 2016. Regulatory, accreditation and payer organizations are also beginning to explore and implement policies and incentives to promote stewardship. The critical steps lie ahead. The task of harnessing this momentum increasingly rests with the thousands of individual facilities and providers who must now implement stewardship programs in all healthcare settings. Fortunately, there are a large number of groups that stand ready to support providers in their efforts. There is also a great need for more research in antibiotic stewardship to build an evidence base to support even greater change. Stewardship programs must investigate optimal ways to implement interventions known to be effective as well as develop and test new interventions. Federal agencies are helping address the knowledge gap in antibiotic stewardship through increased funding opportunities. There is no doubt ASPs will continue to improve patient care while optimizing healthcare resources.

References

1. Magill SS, Edwards JR, Beldavs ZG, et al. Prevalence of antimicrobial use in US acute care hospitals, May–September 2011. *JAMA* 2014; 312:1438–1446.

2. van de Sande-Bruinsma N, Grundmann H, Verloo D, et al. Antimicrobial drug use and resistance in Europe. *Emerging Infect Dis* 2008; 14:1722–1730.

3. Fridkin S, Baggs J, Fagan R, et al. Vital signs: improving antibiotic use among hospitalized patients. *MMWR Morb Mortal Wkly Rep* 2014; 63:194–200.

4. Centers for Disease Control and Prevention. Antibiotic Resistance Threats. 2013; 1–114. (Accessed Nov 20, 2016, at www.cdc.gov/drugresistance/threat-report-2013/.)

5. Lessa FC, Mu Y, Bamberg WM, et al. Burden of *Clostridium difficile* infection in the United States. *N Engl J Med* 2015; 372:825–834.

6. Kunin CM, Dierks JW. A physician-pharmacist voluntary program to improve prescription practices. *N Engl J Med* 1969; 280:1442–1446.

7. Kunin CM, Tupasi T, Craig WA. Use of antibiotics: a brief exposition of the problem and some tentative solutions. *Ann Intern Med* 1973; 79:555–560.

8. McGowan JE. Antimicrobial resistance in hospital organisms and its relation to antibiotic use. *Rev Infect Dis* 1983; 5:1033–1048.

9. Tamma PD, Holmes A, Ashley ED. Antimicrobial stewardship: another focus for patient safety? *Curr Opin Infect Dis* 2014; 27:348–355.

10. Society for Healthcare Epidemiology of America, Infectious Diseases Society of America, Pediatric Infectious Diseases Society. Policy statement on antimicrobial stewardship by the Society for Healthcare Epidemiology of America (SHEA), the Infectious Diseases Society of America

(IDSA), and the Pediatric Infectious Diseases Society (PIDS). *Infect Control Hosp Epidemiol* 2012; 33:322–327.

11. National Strategy for Combating Antibiotic-Resistant Bacteria. (Accessed Nov 20, 2016, at www.whitehouse.gov/sites/default/files/docs/carb_national_strategy.pdf.)

12. Barrett FF, Casey JI, Finland M. Infections and antibiotic use among patients at Boston City Hospital, February, 1967. *N Engl J Med* 1968; 278:5–9.

13. Kislak JW, Eickhoff TC, Finland M. Hospital-acquired infections and antibiotic usage in the Boston City Hospital–January, 1964. *N Engl J Med* 1964; 271:834–835.

14. Scheckler WE, Bennett JV. Antibiotic usage in seven community hospitals. *JAMA* 1970; 213:264–267.

15. Borda I, Jick H, Slone D, Dinan B, Gilman B, Chalmers TC. Studies of drug usage in five Boston hospitals. *JAMA* 1967; 202:506–510.

16. Kelesidis T, Braykov N, Uslan DZ, et al. Indications and types of antibiotic agents used in 6 acute care hospitals, 2009–2010: A pragmatic retrospective observational study. *Infect Control Hosp Epidemiol* 2016; 37:70–79.

17. Centers for Disease Control and Prevention. National Healthcare Safety Network. (Accessed April 26, 2016, at www.cdc.gov/nhsn/acute-care-hospital/aur/.)

18. Hecker MT, Aron DC, Patel NP, Lehmann MK, Donskey CJ. Unnecessary use of antimicrobials in hospitalized patients: current patterns of misuse with an emphasis on the antianaerobic spectrum of activity. *Arch Intern Med* 2003; 163:972–978.

19. Kollef MH, Sherman G, Ward S, Fraser VJ. Inadequate antimicrobial treatment of infections: a risk factor for hospital mortality among critically ill patients. *Chest* 1999; 115:462–474.

20. Micek ST, Lloyd AE, Ritchie DJ, Reichley RM, Fraser VJ, Kollef MH. Pseudomonas aeruginosa bloodstream infection: importance of appropriate initial antimicrobial treatment. *Antimicrob Agents Chemother* 2005; 49:1306–1311.

21. Fraser A, Paul M, Almanasreh N, et al. Benefit of appropriate empirical antibiotic treatment: thirty-day mortality and duration of hospital stay. *Am J Med* 2006; 119:970–976.

22. Seaton RA, Nathwani D, Burton P, et al. Point prevalence survey of antibiotic use in Scottish hospitals utilising the Glasgow Antimicrobial Audit Tool (GAAT). *Int J Antimicrob Agents* 2007; 29:693–699.

23. Kumar A, Ellis P, Arabi Y, et al. Initiation of inappropriate antimicrobial therapy results in a fivefold reduction of survival in human septic shock. *Chest* 2009; 136:1237–1248.

24. Ciccolini M, Spoorenberg V, Geerlings SE, Prins JM, Grundmann H. Using an index-based approach to assess the population-level appropriateness of empirical antibiotic therapy. *Journal of Antimicrobial Chemotherapy* 2015; 70:286–293.

25. Parta M, Goebel M, Thomas J, Matloobi M, Stager C, Musher DM. Impact of an assay that enables rapid determination of staphylococcus species and their drug susceptibility on the treatment of patients with positive blood culture results. *Infect Control Hosp Epidemiol* 2010; 31:1043–1048.

26. Casaroto E, Marra AR, Camargo TZS, et al. Agreement on the prescription of antimicrobial drugs. *BMC Infect Dis* 2015; 15:248.

27. Vlahovic-Palcevski V, Francetic I, Palcevski G, Novak S, Abram M, Bergman U. Antimicrobial use at a university hospital: appropriate or misused? A qualitative study. *Int J Clin Pharmacol Ther* 2007; 45:169–174.

28. Osowicki J, Gwee A, Noronha J, et al. Australia-wide point prevalence survey of antimicrobial prescribing in neonatal units: How much and how good? *Pediatr Infect Dis J* 2015; 34:e185–90.

29. Osowicki J, Gwee A, Noronha J, et al. Australia-wide point prevalence survey of the use and appropriateness of antimicrobial prescribing for children in hospital. *Med J Aust* 2014; 201:657–662.

30. Peron EP, Hirsch AA, Jury LA, Jump RLP, Donskey CJ. Another setting for stewardship: high rate of unnecessary antimicrobial use in a veterans affairs long-term care facility. *J Am Geriatr Soc* 2013; 61:289–290.

31. van Buul LW, Veenhuizen RB, Achterberg WP, et al. Antibiotic prescribing in Dutch nursing homes: How appropriate is it? *J Am Med Dir Assoc* 2015; 16:229–237.

32. Cooke DM, Salter AJ, Phillips I. The impact of antibiotic policy on prescribing in a London teaching hospital: a one-day prevalence survey as an indicator of antibiotic use. *J Antimicrob Chemother* 1983; 11:447–453.

33. Raveh D, Levy Y, Schlesinger Y, Greenberg A, Rudensky B, Yinnon AM. Longitudinal surveillance of antibiotic use in the hospital. *QJM* 2001; 94:141–152.

34. James RS, McIntosh KA, Luu SB, et al. Antimicrobial stewardship in Victorian hospitals: a statewide survey to identify current gaps. *Med J Aust* 2013; 199:692–695.

35. James R, Upjohn L, Cotta M, et al. Measuring antimicrobial prescribing quality in Australian hospitals: development and evaluation of a national antimicrobial prescribing survey tool. *Journal of Antimicrobial Chemotherapy* 2015; 70:1912–1918.

36. Zarb P, Goossens H. European Surveillance of Antimicrobial Consumption (ESAC): Value of a point-prevalence survey of antimicrobial use across Europe. *Drugs* 2011; 71:745–755.

37. Antimicrobial prescribing practice in Australian hospitals. Sydney: 2015. (Accessed Nov 20, 2016, at www.safetyandquality.gov.au/wp-content/uploads/2015/07/Antimicrobial-prescribing-practice-in-Aust-hospitals-NAPS-2014-Results.pdf.)

38. Stolley PD, Becker MH, McEvilla JD, Lasagna L, Gainor M, Sloane LM. Drug prescribing and use in an American community. *Ann Intern Med* 1972; 76:537–540.

39. Suda KJ, Hicks LA, Roberts RM, Hunkler RJ, Danziger LH. A national evaluation of antibiotic expenditures by healthcare setting in the United States. *J Antimicrob Chemother* 2013; 68(3):715–718.

40. Centers for Disease Control and Prevention (CDC). Office-related antibiotic prescribing for persons aged ≤ 14 years–United States, 1993–1994 to 2007–2008. *MMWR Morb Mortal Wkly Rep* 2011; 60:1153–1156.

41. Shapiro DJ, Hicks LA, Pavia AT, Hersh AL. Antibiotic prescribing for adults in ambulatory care in the USA, 2007–09. *Journal of Antimicrobial Chemotherapy* 2014; 69:234–240.

42. Hicks LA, Taylor TH, Hunkler RJ. U.S. outpatient antibiotic prescribing, 2010. *N Engl J Med* 2013; 368:1461–1462.

43. Jones BE, Sauer B, Jones MM, et al. Variation in outpatient antibiotic prescribing for acute respiratory infections in the veteran population: a cross-sectional study. *Ann Intern Med* 2015; 163:73–80.

44. Barnett ML, Linder JA. Antibiotic prescribing for adults with acute bronchitis in the United States, 1996–2010. *JAMA* 2014; 311:2020–2022.

45. Hicks LA, Bartoces MG, Roberts RM, et al. US outpatient antibiotic prescribing variation according to geography, patient population, and provider specialty in 2011. *Clin Infect Dis* 2015; 60(9):1308-1316.

46. Sanchez GV, Roberts RM, Albert AP, Johnson DD, Hicks LA. Effects of knowledge, attitudes, and practices of primary care providers on antibiotic selection, United States. *Emerging Infect Dis* 2014; 20:2041–2047.

47. D'Costa VM, King CE, Kalan L, et al. Antibiotic resistance is ancient. *Nature* 2011; 477:457–461.

48. Bhullar K, Waglechner N, Pawlowski A, et al. Antibiotic resistance is prevalent in an isolated cave microbiome. *PLoS ONE* 2012; 7:e34953.

49. Mulvey MR, Simor AE. Antimicrobial resistance in hospitals: how concerned should we be? *CMAJ* 2009; 180:408–415.

50. Clatworthy AE, Pierson E, Hung DT. Targeting virulence: a new paradigm for

antimicrobial therapy. *Nat Chem Biol* 2007; 3:541–548.

51. Zaoutis TE, Goyal M, Chu JH, et al. Risk factors for and outcomes of bloodstream infection caused by extended-spectrum beta-lactamase-producing *Escherichia coli* and Klebsiella species in children. *Pediatrics* 2005; 115:942–949.

52. Patel G, Huprikar S, Factor SH, Jenkins SG, Calfee DP. Outcomes of carbapenem-resistant *Klebsiella pneumoniae* infection and the impact of antimicrobial and adjunctive therapies. *Infect Control Hosp Epidemiol* 2008; 29:1099–1106.

53. Spellberg B, Guidos R, Gilbert D, et al. The epidemic of antibiotic-resistant infections: a call to action for the medical community from the Infectious Diseases Society of America. *Clinical Infectious Diseases* 2008; 46:155–164.

54. Thomas C, Stevenson M, Riley TV. Antibiotics and hospital-acquired *Clostridium difficile*-associated diarrhoea: a systematic review. *J Antimicrob Chemother* 2003; 51:1339–1350.

55. Stevens V, Dumyati G, Fine LS, Fisher SG, van Wijngaarden E. Cumulative antibiotic exposures over time and the risk of *Clostridium difficile* infection. *Clinical Infectious Diseases* 2011; 53:42–48.

56. Bartlett JG. Narrative review: the new epidemic of *Clostridium difficile*-associated enteric disease. *Ann Intern Med* 2006; 145:758–764.

57. Redelings MD, Sorvillo F, Mascola L. Increase in *Clostridium difficile*-related mortality rates, United States, 1999–2004. *Emerging Infect Dis* 2007; 13:1417–1419.

58. Khanna S, Pardi DS, Aronson SL, et al. The epidemiology of community-acquired *Clostridium difficile* infection: a population-based study. *Amer J Gastroenterology* 2012; 107:89–95.

59. Shehab N, Patel PR, Srinivasan A, Budnitz DS. Emergency department visits for antibiotic-associated adverse events. *Clinical Infectious Diseases* 2008; 47:735–743.

60. Lin RY, Nuruzzaman F, Shah SN. Incidence and impact of adverse effects to

antibiotics in hospitalized adults with pneumonia. *J Hosp Med* 2009; 4:E7–15.

61. Dellit TH, Owens RC, McGowan JE, et al. Infectious Diseases Society of America and the Society for Healthcare Epidemiology of America guidelines for developing an institutional program to enhance antimicrobial stewardship. *Clinical Infectious Diseases* 2007; 44:159–177.

62. Kaki R, Elligsen M, Walker S, Simor A, Palmay L, Daneman N. Impact of antimicrobial stewardship in critical care: a systematic review. *Journal of Antimicrobial Chemotherapy* 2011; 66:1223–1230.

63. Davey P, Brown E, Charani E, et al. Interventions to improve antibiotic prescribing practices for hospital inpatients. *Cochrane Database Syst Rev* 2013; 4:CD003543.

64. Wagner B, Filice GA, Drekonja D, et al. Antimicrobial stewardship programs in inpatient hospital settings: a systematic review. *Infect Control Hosp Epidemiol* 2014; 35:1209–1228.

65. Lautenbach E, LaRosa LA, Marr AM, Nachamkin I, Bilker WB, Fishman NO. Changes in the prevalence of vancomycin-resistant enterococci in response to antimicrobial formulary interventions: impact of progressive restrictions on use of vancomycin and third-generation cephalosporins. *Clinical Infectious Diseases* 2003; 36:440–446.

66. Rüttimann S, Keck B, Hartmeier C, Maetzel A, Bucher HC. Long-term antibiotic cost savings from a comprehensive intervention program in a medical department of a university-affiliated teaching hospital. *Clinical Infectious Diseases* 2004; 38:348–356.

67. Kisuule F, Wright S, Barreto J, Zenilman J. Improving antibiotic utilization among hospitalists: a pilot academic detailing project with a public health approach. *J Hosp Med* 2008; 3:64–70.

68. Camins BC, King MD, Wells JB, et al. Impact of an antimicrobial utilization program on antimicrobial use at a large teaching hospital: a randomized controlled

trial. *Infect Control Hosp Epidemiol* 2009; 30:931–938.

69. White AC, Atmar RL, Wilson J, Cate TR, Stager CE, Greenberg SB. Effects of requiring prior authorization for selected antimicrobials: expenditures, susceptibilities, and clinical outcomes. *Clinical Infectious Diseases* 1997; 25:230–239.

70. Fishman N. Antimicrobial stewardship. *Am J Med* 2006; 119:S53–61– discussion S62–70.

71. Gentry CA, Greenfield RA, Slater LN, Wack M, Huycke MM. Outcomes of an antimicrobial control program in a teaching hospital. *American Journal of Health-System Pharmacy (AJHP)* 2000; 57:268–274.

72. LaRocco A. Concurrent antibiotic review programs–a role for infectious diseases specialists at small community hospitals. *Clinical Infectious Diseases* 2003; 37:742–743.

73. Bantar C, Sartori B, Vesco E, et al. A hospital wide intervention program to optimize the quality of antibiotic use: impact on prescribing practice, antibiotic consumption, cost savings, and bacterial resistance. *Clinical Infectious Diseases* 2003; 37:180–186.

74. Carling P, Fung T, Killion A, Terrin N, Barza M. Favorable impact of a multidisciplinary antibiotic management program conducted during 7 years. *Infect Control Hosp Epidemiol* 2003; 24:699–706.

75. Standiford HC, Chan S, Tripoli M, Weekes E, Forrest GN. Antimicrobial stewardship at a large tertiary care academic medical center: cost analysis before, during, and after a 7-year program. *Infect Control Hosp Epidemiol* 2012; 33:338–345.

76. Arnold SR, Straus SE. *Interventions to improve antibiotic prescribing practices in ambulatory care.* Chichester, UK: John Wiley & Sons, 1996.

77. Ranji SR, Steinman MA, Shojania KG, Gonzales R. Interventions to reduce unnecessary antibiotic prescribing: a systematic review and quantitative analysis. *Med Care* 2008; 46:847–862.

78. Drekonja DM, Filice GA, Greer N, et al. antimicrobial stewardship in outpatient

settings: a systematic review. *Infect Control Hosp Epidemiol* 2014; 36:142–152.

79. Gonzales R. A cluster randomized trial of decision support strategies for reducing antibiotic use in acute bronchitis. *JAMA Intern Med* 2013; 173:267.

80. Rattinger GB, Mullins CD, Zuckerman IH, et al. A sustainable strategy to prevent misuse of antibiotics for acute respiratory infections. *PLoS ONE* 2012; 7:e51147.

81. Jenkins TC, Irwin A, Coombs L, et al. Effects of clinical pathways for common outpatient infections on antibiotic prescribing. *Am J Med* 2013; 126:327–335.e12.

82. Chao JH, Kunkov S, Reyes LB, Lichten S, Crain EF. Comparison of two approaches to observation therapy for acute otitis media in the emergency department. *Pediatrics* 2008; 121:e1352–6.

83. Little P, Moore MV, Turner S, et al. Effectiveness of five different approaches in management of urinary tract infection: randomised controlled trial. *BMJ* 2010; 340: c199.

84. Little P, Moore M, Kelly J, et al. Delayed antibiotic prescribing strategies for respiratory tract infections in primary care: Pragmatic, factorial, randomised controlled trial. *BMJ* 2014; 348:g1606.

85. Meeker D, Knight TK, Friedberg MW, et al. Nudging guideline-concordant antibiotic prescribing: a randomized clinical trial. *JAMA Intern Med* 2014; 174:425–431.

86. McGowan JE. Antimicrobial stewardship–the state of the art in 2011: focus on outcome and methods. *Infect Control Hosp Epidemiol* 2012; 33:331–337.

87. Schulz LT, Fox BC, Polk RE. Can the antibiogram be used to assess microbiologic outcomes after antimicrobial stewardship interventions? A critical review of the literature. *Pharmacotherapy* 2012; 32:668–676.

88. Schechner V, Temkin E, Harbarth S, Carmeli Y, Schwaber MJ. Epidemiological interpretation of studies examining the effect of antibiotic usage on resistance. *Clin Microbiol Rev* 2013; 26:289–307.

89. Singh N, Rogers P, Atwood CW, Wagener MM, Yu VL. Short-course empiric antibiotic therapy for patients with pulmonary infiltrates in the intensive care unit. A proposed solution for indiscriminate antibiotic prescription. *Am J Respir Crit Care Med* 2000; 162:505–511.

90. Cohen SH, MD, Gerding DN, MD, Johnson S, MD, et al. Clinical practice guidelines for *Clostridium difficile* infection in adults: 2010 update by the Society for Healthcare Epidemiology of America (SHEA) and the Infectious Diseases Society of America (IDSA). *Infect Control Hosp Epidemiol* 2010; 31:431–455.

91. Surawicz CM, Brandt LJ, Binion DG, et al. Guidelines for diagnosis, treatment, and prevention of *Clostridium difficile* infections. *Amer J Gastroenterology* 2013; 108:478–98–quiz 499.

92. Debast SB, Vaessen N, Choudry A, Wiegers-Ligtvoet EAJ, van den Berg RJ, Kuijper EJ. Successful combat of an outbreak due to *Clostridium difficile* PCR ribotype 027 and recognition of specific risk factors. *Clinical Microbiology and Infection* 2009; 15:427–434.

93. Valiquette L, Cossette B, Garant M-P, Diab H, Pépin J. Impact of a reduction in the use of high-risk antibiotics on the course of an epidemic of *Clostridium difficile*-associated disease caused by the hypervirulent NAP1/027 strain. *Clinical Infectious Diseases* 2007; 45 Suppl 2:S112–21.

94. Dean NC, Bateman KA, Donnelly SM, Silver MP, Snow GL, Hale D. Improved clinical outcomes with utilization of a community-acquired pneumonia guideline. *Chest* 2006; 130:794–799.

95. Lahey T, Shah R, Gittzus J, Schwartzman J, Kirkland K. Infectious diseases consultation lowers mortality from *Staphylococcus aureus* Bacteremia. *Medicine* 2009; 88:263–267.

96. Jenkins TC, Price CS, Sabel AL, Mehler PS, Burman WJ. Impact of routine infectious diseases service consultation on the evaluation, management, and outcomes of *Staphylococcus aureus* Bacteremia. *Clinical Infectious Diseases* 2008; 46:1000–1008.

97. Evans RS, Pestotnik SL, Classen DC, et al. A computer-assisted management program for antibiotics and other antiinfective agents. *N Engl J Med* 1998; 338:232–238.

98. Bond CAC, Raehl CL. Clinical and economic outcomes of pharmacist-managed aminoglycoside or vancomycin therapy. *AJHP* 2005; 62:1596–1605.

99. Unger NR, Gauthier TP, Cheung LW. Penicillin skin testing: potential implications for antimicrobial stewardship. *Pharmacotherapy* 2013; 33:856–867.

100. Charneski L, Deshpande G, Smith SW. Impact of an antimicrobial allergy label in the medical record on clinical outcomes in hospitalized patients. *Pharmacotherapy* 2011; 31:742–747.

101. Classen DC, Evans RS, Pestotnik SL, Horn SD, Menlove RL, Burke JP. The timing of prophylactic administration of antibiotics and the risk of surgical-wound infection. *N Engl J Med* 1992; 326:281–286.

102. Bratzler DW, Dellinger EP, Olsen KM, et al. Clinical practice guidelines for antimicrobial prophylaxis in surgery. *Am J Health Syst Pharm* 2013; 70:195–283.

103. Bond CAC, Raehl CL. Clinical and economic outcomes of pharmacist-managed antimicrobial prophylaxis in surgical patients. *Am J Health Syst Pharm* 2007; 64:1935–1942.

104. Spivak ES, Kendall B, Orlando P, et al. Evaluation of outpatient parenteral antimicrobial therapy at a veterans affairs hospital. *Infect Control Hosp Epidemiol* 2015; 36:1103–1105.

105. Gordon SM, Shrestha NK, Rehm SJ. Transitioning antimicrobial stewardship beyond the hospital: the Cleveland Clinic's community-based parenteral anti-infective therapy (CoPAT) program. *J Hosp Med* 2011; 6 Suppl 1:S24–S30.

106. Knackstedt ED, Stockmann C, Davis CR, Thorell EA, Pavia AT, Hersh AL. Outpatient parenteral antimicrobial therapy in pediatrics: An opportunity to expand antimicrobial stewardship. *Infect Control Hosp Epidemiol* 2015; 36:222–224.

107. Centers for Disease Control and Prevention. (Accessed April 26, 2016, at www.cdc.gov/getsmart/.)

108. Sanchez GV, Fleming-Dutra KE, Hicks LA. Minimizing antibiotic misuse through evidence-based management of outpatient acute respiratory infections. *Antimicrob Agents Chemother* 2015; 59:6673.

109. Harris AM, Hicks LA, Qaseem A, High value care task force of the american college of physicians and for the centers for disease control and prevention. appropriate antibiotic use for acute respiratory tract infection in adults: advice for high-value care from the American College of Physicians and the Centers for Disease Control and Prevention. *Ann Intern Med* 2016; 164(6):425-434.

110. Hersh AL, Jackson MA, Hicks LA, American Academy of Pediatrics. Committee on Infectious Diseases. Principles of judicious antibiotic prescribing for upper respiratory tract infections in pediatrics. *Pediatrics* 2013; 132:1146–1154.

111. Marr JJ, Moffet HL, Kunin CM. Guidelines for improving the use of antimicrobial agents in hospitals: a statement by the Infectious Diseases Society of America. *J Infect Dis* 1988; 157:869–876.

112. Shlaes DM, Gerding DN, John JF, et al. Society for Healthcare Epidemiology of America and Infectious Diseases Society of America Joint Committee on the Prevention of Antimicrobial Resistance: guidelines for the prevention of antimicrobial resistance in hospitals. *Clinical Infectious Diseases* 1997; 25:584–599.

113. Infectious Diseases Society of America (IDSA), Spellberg B, Blaser M, et al. Combating antimicrobial resistance: Policy recommendations to save lives. *Clinical Infectious Diseases* 2011; 52 Suppl 5: S397–428.

114. Cosgrove SE, Hermsen ED, Rybak MJ, et al. Guidance for the knowledge and skills required for antimicrobial stewardship leaders. *Infect Control Hosp Epidemiol.* 2014; 35:1444–1451.

115. Barlam TF, Cosgrove SE, Abbo LM, et al. Implementing an antibiotic stewardship program: guidelines by the Infectious Diseases Society of America and the Society for Healthcare Epidemiology of America. *Clin Infect Dis* 2016; 62(10):1197–1202.

116. California Senate Bill No. 739. (Accessed Nov 20, 2016, at www.dhcs.ca.gov/provgovpart/initiatives/nqi/Documents/SB739.pdf.)

117. Trivedi KK, Rosenberg J. The state of antimicrobial stewardship programs in California. *Infect Control Hosp Epidemiol* 2013; 34:379–384.

118. California Senate Bill No. 1311. https://leginfo.legislature.ca.gov/faces/billNavClient.xhtml?bill_id=201320140SB1311.

119. Pollack LA, Srinivasan A. Core elements of hospital antibiotic stewardship programs from the Centers for Disease Control and Prevention. *Clinical Infectious Diseases* 2014; 59 Suppl 3:S97–100.

120. Centers for Disease Control and Prevention. (Accessed April 26, 2016, at www.cdc.gov/longtermcare/pdfs/core-elements-antibiotic-stewardship.pdf.)

121. Sanchez GV, Fleming-Dutra KE, Roberts RM, Hicks LA. Core elements of outpatient antibiotic stewardship. *MMWR Recomm Rep* 2016; 65:1–12.

122. Obama BH. Presidential Executive Order. (Accessed Nov 20, 2016, at www.whitehouse.gov/the-press-office/2014/09/18/executive-order-combating-antibiotic-resistant-bacteria.)

123. Report to the President on Combating Antibiotic Resistance. (Accessed Nov 20, 2016, at www.whitehouse.gov/sites/default/files/microsites/ostp/PCAST/pcast_carb_report_sept2014.pdf.)

124. The Joint Commission. Prepublication Standards – New Antimicrobial Stewardship Standard. (Accessed Nov 20, 2016, at www.jointcommission.org/prepublication_standards_antimicrobial_stewardship_standard/.)

125. The World Health Organization. Antimicrobial resistance: a global report on

surveillance. 2014. (Accessed Nov 20, 2016, at www.who.int/drugresistance/documents/surveillancereport/en/.)

126. The World Health Organization. Global action plan on antimicrobial resistance. (Accessed Nov 20, 2016, at www.who.int/antimicrobial-resistance/publications/global-action-plan/en/.)

127. The United Nations General Assembly. Draft political declaration of the high-level meeting of the General Assembly on antimicrobial resistance. (Accessed Nov 20, 2016, at www.un.org/pga/71/wp-content/uploads/sites/40/2016/09/DGACM_GAEAD_ESCAB-AMR-Draft-Political-Declaration-1616108E.pdf.)

128. MaronDF, Smith TJ, Nachman KE. Restrictions on antimicrobial use in food animal production: an international regulatory and economic survey. *Global Health* 2013; 9: 48.

129. The Food and Drug Administration. Veterinary Feed Directive. (Accessed Nov 20, 2016, at www.federalregister.gov/documents/2015/06/03/2015–13393/veterinary-feed-directive.)

130. Fridkin SK, Srinivasan A. Implementing a strategy for monitoring inpatient antimicrobial use among hospitals in the United States. *Clinical Infectious Diseases* 2014; 58(3): 401–406.

131. Collins CD, Miller DE, Kenney RM, et al. The state of antimicrobial stewardship in Michigan: Results of a statewide survey on antimicrobial stewardship efforts in acute care hospitals. *Hospital Pharmacy* 2015; 50:180–184.

132. Stenehjem E, Hersh AL, Sheng X, et al. Antibiotic use in small community hospitals. *Clinical Infectious Diseases* 2016; 63:1273–1280.

133. Trivedi KK, Kuper K. Hospital antimicrobial stewardship in the non university setting. *Infect Dis Clin North Am* 2014; 28:281–289.

134. Chou AF, Graber CJ, Jones M, et al. Characteristics of antimicrobial stewardship programs at veterans affairs hospitals: results of a nationwide survey.

Infect Control Hosp Epidemiol 2016; 37 (6):647–654.

135. Pollack LA, van Santen KL, Weiner LM, Dudeck MA, Edwards JR, Srinivasan A. Antibiotic stewardship programs in U.S. acute care hospitals: findings from the 2014 National Healthcare Safety Network (NHSN) Annual Hospital Survey. *Clinical Infectious Diseases* 2016; 63(4):443–449.

136. Centers for Disease Control and Prevention. (Accessed Apr 26, 2016, at www.cdc.gov/nchs/fastats/nursing-home-care.htm.)

137. Rhee SM, Stone ND. Antimicrobial stewardship in long-term care facilities. *Infect Dis Clin North Am* 2014; 28:237–246.

138. Malani AN, Brennan BM, Collins CD, Finks J, Pogue JM, Kaye KS. Antimicrobial stewardship practices in Michigan long-term care facilities. *Infect Control Hosp Epidemiol* 2016; 37:236–237.

139. Doernberg SB, Dudas V, Trivedi KK. Implementation of an antimicrobial stewardship program targeting residents with urinary tract infections in three community long-term care facilities: a quasi-experimental study using time-series analysis. *Antimicrob Resist Infect Control* 2015; 4:54.

140. Van Schooneveld T, Miller H, Sayles H, Watkins K, Smith PW. Survey of antimicrobial stewardship practices in Nebraska long-term care facilities. *Infect Control Hosp Epidemiol* 2011; 32:732–734.

141. Ashwood JS, Reid RO, Setodji CM, Weber E, Gaynor M, Mehrotra A. Trends in retail clinic use among the commercially insured. *Am J Manag Care* 2011; 17:e443–448.

142. Laws M, Scott MK. The emergence of retail-based clinics in the United States: Early observations. *Health Aff (Millwood)* 2008; 27:1293–1298.

143. Mehrotra A, Paone S, Martich GD, Albert SM, Shevchik GJ. A comparison of care at e-visits and physician office visits for sinusitis and urinary tract infection. *JAMA Intern Med* 2013; 173:72–74.

144. Tice AD, Rehm SJ, Dalovisio JR, et al. Practice guidelines for outpatient

parenteral antimicrobial therapy. IDSA guidelines. Clinical Infectious Diseases 2004; 38:1651–1672.

145. Lane MA, Marschall J, Beekmann SE, et al. Outpatient parenteral antimicrobial therapy practices among adult infectious disease physicians. *Infect Control Hosp Epidemiol* 2014; 35:839–844.

146. Shrestha NK, Bhaskaran A, Scalera NM, Schmitt SK, Rehm SJ, Gordon SM. Contribution of infectious disease consultation toward the care of inpatients being considered for community-based parenteral anti-infective therapy. *J Hosp Med* 2012; 7:365–369.

147. Madigan T, Banerjee R. Characteristics and outcomes of outpatient parenteral antimicrobial therapy at an academic children's hospital. *Pediatr Infect Dis J* 2013; 32:346–349.

Structure of an Antibiotic Stewardship Team and Core Competencies

Whitney R. Buckel and Sara E. Cosgrove

The first step in developing any antibiotic stewardship program (ASP) is to determine the members of the core ASP team, which consists of, at a minimum, the physician and pharmacist who will be performing the work of stewardship; the extended ASP team, which consists of departments with which the core ASP team must closely interact; and the members and structure of the ASP committee, which consists of the key personnel who will support the functions and activity of the core team and take messages back to the constituents that they represent.

According to the Harvard Business Review, a team is "a small number of people with complementary skills who are committed to a common purpose, set of performance goals, and approach for which they hold themselves mutually accountable."[1] To be successful, each team member must embody specific key competencies. This chapter will identify key members to include on an ASP team and committee, discuss how to tailor the structure of the program to different settings and practices, and define important competencies of each core team member.

Core ASP Team Members

The two essential team members for any ASP team are a physician and a pharmacist. Physician leadership is critical, as most interactions of the ASP are with clinicians regarding medical care of patients. Physicians have skills in diagnosis, management, and treatment of the syndromes that are common targets of ASPs. The physician champion is key in determining ASP goals; educating physicians, physician assistants, and nurse practitioners about improving antibiotic use; and settling disagreements that might arise between the ASP and clinicians. Pharmacist leadership of ASPs is also important; the ASP pharmacist often performs the majority of interventions of an ASP, has expertise in the dosing and monitoring of therapeutic drugs, and provides an important link to the pharmacy department. While successful ASPs have been founded without both a physician and a pharmacist, [2] the synergy between these two positions in the process of developing and executing interventions augments the reach of the ASP and is strongly preferred.

Physician The ASP physician lead must be someone who is well-respected in the institution, ideally by all clinical disciplines, as they will serve as the "face" of the program and will impact the ASP's credibility. The ideal physician to co-lead an ASP team has formal training in infectious diseases (ID), a strong interest in antibiotic stewardship and patient safety, and the ability to interact diplomatically and collegially with other clinicians. An estimated 42% of US hospitals lack on-site ID specialists; many of those hospitals have fewer than 300 beds.[3] Smaller hospitals may lack the financial resources to employ ID physicians on staff who can be involved in their ASPs.[4, 5] Fewer ID physicians are available in nonurban areas. As more small community hospitals (SCH) develop ASPs, non-ID physician champions may be engaged in antibiotic stewardship (AS) initiatives.[6] Innovative strategies such as ID hotlines [3] or telemedicine [7] may help to increase access to ID physicians across all settings. Physicians not trained in ID who are leading ASPs should seek out AS-specific training as offered through multiple professional societies such as the Infectious Diseases Society of America (IDSA) and Society for Healthcare Epidemiology of America (SHEA) and some public health departments.[8]

Pharmacist The pivotal role of pharmacists in the development, implementation, and maintenance of ASPs is well established. The ideal pharmacist to co-lead an ASP has residency or fellowship training in ID, a strong interest in AS and patient safety, and is comfortable advising physicians and other providers on treatment choices. The pharmacist should be competent in pharmacokinetics and pharmacodynamics and use this knowledge to optimize antibiotic therapies and patient outcomes (see Chapter 8). The American Society of Health-System Pharmacists (ASHP), IDSA, SHEA, and the Society of Infectious Diseases Pharmacists (SIDP) recommend pharmacists with ID training when available. [9,10] One study suggested that ASPs staffed by ID pharmacists had greater adherence to local treatment guidelines compared to ASPs staffed by ward pharmacists.[11] However, as more SCHs develop ASPs, non-ID trained clinical pharmacists will be called upon to lead AS initiatives.[2] Several national organizations offer programs targeting pharmacists without formal ID training who need training in AS, including Making a Difference in Infectious Diseases (MAD-ID), SIDP, SHEA and others. Another strategy is to have ID-trained pharmacists serve remotely as mentors to front-line clinical pharmacists who are leading ASPs.[12, 13]

The stewardship pharmacist is the key liaison between the ASP and the pharmacy department. The relationship with the pharmacy department is critical in enforcement of restriction policies, providing data on antibiotic use, optimizing antibiotic dosing, limiting serious adverse events, and identifying prescribing trends. In addition, clinical specialists and decentralized pharmacists, if available, can be engaged in ASP activities on the units and medical teams that they serve.[12, 14] In many institutions, two or more ID pharmacists may be required to organize a comprehensive ASP, especially when the hospital has many licensed beds and ASP team members have other obligations, such as to an ID consultation service or to a school or college of pharmacy.

Extended Stewardship Team Members

Clearly defined roles are essential for a successful team. Research demonstrates that "collaboration improves when the roles of individual team members are clearly defined and well understood."[1] These clearly defined roles will also help each team member understand the duties of each member, understand ways to assist one another, and share information. The following are departments that should provide membership to the extended ASP team; examples of competencies for each team member are included. The list is not exhaustive. When identifying these members, consider expertise, credibility, and leadership [15] as well as the informational, social, and personal resources these members could provide.[16] As defined by Cross et al, informational resources are the knowledge and skills we commonly attribute to each job description, social resources "involve one's awareness, access, and position in a network," and personal resources refer to personal time and energy.[16]

Administration Examples of administration to involve include chief medical officers, patient safety and quality officers, departmental heads, and directors of pharmacy. It may be important to include administrators who are responsible for different departments, as most initiatives require collaboration between multiple disciplines. All ASP teams should identify administrative support and ideally these representatives should regularly attend AS committee meetings. At a minimum, administration should be involved by receiving regular updated reports of programmatic progress, barriers, and resource needs. Representative(s) from administration would be expected to support the program and its mission, to secure resources for the program, and provide leadership expertise to the committee. For example, they can provide counsel on how to leverage resources for new projects or to sustain current projects, connect the committee with key stakeholders, assist the ASP to get on upper management committee agendas, and ensure AS goals are aligned with institutional goals. In addition, administrators can serve as mentors and support for core ASP members if they encounter difficult prescribers when implementing practice changes.[17]

Information Technology (IT) Examples of IT partners include data analysts, data managers, and programmers. IT personnel responsible for updating and maintaining the electronic medical record (EMR) are particularly valuable. IT representatives can be key to effectively operationalizing AS initiatives. The IT team member is primarily responsible for assisting with collating antibiotic, microbiological, and clinical data from several sources to facilitate identification of cases for intervention and track antibiotic use. As this may represent a broad scope of expertise, multiple representatives from IT may be necessary. Not all institutions have on-site informatics support and some institutions may not have a fully integrated EMR. In these settings, the ASP should find an IT representative who is adept at using hospital-specific computer programs to query needed data.

For larger institutions, a dedicated analyst should be part of the core stewardship team and is an important position for which to advocate for funding and staffing. An analyst is important in providing data on antibiotic use, antibiotic resistance and other metrics such as those recommended for monitoring by the Centers for Disease Control and Prevention (CDC), The Joint Commission (TJC), and Centers for Medicare and Medicaid Services (CMS); thus, this person should be trained to understand these metrics. With most institutions investing in EMRs, IT members can help creatively utilize technology to solve safety and workflow problems.[18] In addition, the ASP team may be asked to help with electronic order sets which can establish a working relationship with the IT department. More information regarding the role of informatics within antibiotic stewardship can be found in Chapter 10.

Microbiology Examples of microbiology partners include medical microbiology directors, microbiology laboratory managers, and lead microbiology technologists/technicians. Involvement of microbiology team members is especially important when implementing laboratory-centric AS initiatives, such as a rapid diagnostic test to improve prescribing. ASP and microbiology discussions of turn-around time and application of results is crucial to the ability of these tests to improve prescribing. Many institutions do not have on-site microbiology resources in which case a key contact person or resource at the off-site microbiology laboratory should be identified for the ASP. The core ASP team members should serve as the contacts for the microbiology laboratory. Representative(s) from microbiology should be adept in the standard operating procedures of the microbiology lab as well as play a key role in implementing microbiology lab process changes. Because microbiology lab personnel educate providers when new breakpoints are implemented, which impact antibiotic use and AS initiatives, they should be up to date on Clinical

Laboratory Standards Institute (CLSI) breakpoints and guidelines as well as Federal Drug Administration (FDA) approvals and recommendations.[19] Having a microbiology representative can also facilitate a collegial relationship between ASP pharmacists/physicians, who call frequently, and laboratory personnel.

Implementation of rapid diagnostics to improve patient care and antibiotic use should be a collaborative approach between the microbiology department and the ASP to optimize impact. Discussion should include appropriate indications for the tests, timing of batching, language for reporting test results, education of providers on the new tests available, and contacting providers in real time with test results to ensure appropriate action is taken.[20] The microbiology lab should also collaborate with the ASP committee to assist with the development of institutional and unit-based antibiograms, define selective reporting of susceptibility testing, and edit comments on laboratory reports for multidrug-resistant organisms such as extended-spectrum beta-lactamase (ESBL)-producing bacteria and carbapenem-resistant *Enterobacteriaceae* (CRE). Microbiology comments can guide appropriate treatment and note situations for which ID consultation is recommended. The ASP committee can also work with the microbiology lab to develop innovative communication strategies for results. For example, the lab can provide minimum inhibitory concentration (MIC) data to the ASP pharmacist and/or physician that is hidden to others, or can contact ASP members with test results in addition to the standard notification processes. More information regarding the role of microbiology personnel within antibiotic stewardship can be found in Chapter 9.

Infection Prevention Infection prevention and control programs and ASPs have several common goals, such as preventing the emergence and spread of resistant organisms and *C. difficile* infections. A relationship with the infection prevention and control department (the healthcare epidemiologist and infection preventionists) will augment success with all ASP initiatives and allow for optimal collaboration on joint projects. In addition, infection prevention and control programs and ASPs can often share resources, such as data management expertise and project management. Healthcare epidemiologists and infection preventionists help reduce antibiotic resistance by improving hand hygiene compliance and implementing precautions to prevent transmission. These experts have in-depth knowledge of hospital antibiotic resistance patterns, infection control policies and procedures, and the CDC's National Healthcare Safety Network (NHSN). Representative(s) from infection control can assist with the education of clinicians, especially nurses, when new initiatives are implemented; report and analyze data submitted to NHSN; and collaborate on important reporting measures, such as rates of *C. difficile* infections, that are relevant to the ASP. [21] Representatives from Infection Control can also assist with acquiring, tabulating, and disseminating data given their familiarity with this process.

Nursing Directors of nursing, nurse educators, and bedside nurses can add value to the ASP's initiatives. There is growing discussion of how to integrate nursing into AS. As the nation's largest healthcare profession, practicing in a wide diversity of practice areas, nurses can be key advocates for AS. Because formal inclusion of nursing is in its infancy, it would be best to include a nurse with either administrative or educational responsibilities. Nurses are already actively involved in processes key to antibiotic stewardship success, including obtaining accurate allergy histories, collecting cultures prior to antibiotics, monitoring patient response to therapy, and assessing antibiotic adverse events (Box 1).[22] Nurse leaders, such as administrators or educators, can help strategize how to leverage the expertise of their discipline. AS interventions, such as the conversion of intravenous to oral antibiotics [23] or guidelines for appropriate *C. difficile* testing, can either involve nurses or be supported by nurse education.[24]

Box 1 Examples of Nursing Role in Antibiotic Stewardship

1. Antibiotic administration (e.g., extended infusion, timing after blood cultures are drawn)
2. Antibiotic time outs (e.g., checking culture results prior to hanging an antibiotic to encourage de-escalation, prompting clinicians about daily antibiotic reviews)
3. Antibiotic duration of therapy reminders (e.g., antibiotic prophylaxis)
4. Appropriate documentation (e.g., antibiotic allergy reactions)
5. Appropriate testing (e.g., not testing for *Clostridium difficile* after recent laxatives, not culturing urine just because it is foul smelling)
6. Appropriate culture obtainment technique (e.g., not culturing urine from bed pans, not swabbing wound cultures)
7. Infection prevention (e.g., appropriate duration of urinary catheters and central lines)
8. Order review (e.g., ensuring all antibiotics have an indication)
9. Monitoring therapy for effectiveness and toxicity (e.g., coordinating timing of therapeutic drug monitoring for vancomycin and aminoglycosides; monitoring temperature curve; monitoring for *C. difficile*, skin rashes, and other adverse events)
10. Patient education (e.g., antibiotic indication, potential side effects)

Key Stakeholders These individuals will vary in different institutions. Key stakeholders are people from multiple disciplines with an interest in antibiotic stewardship and who are thought leaders within their divisions, departments, or practice groups. In general, they should be well known and trusted by their colleagues and willing to collaborate with the ASP in the development of guidelines related to their expertise, implementation of interventions within their groups, and two-way transmission of information and concerns between their colleagues and the ASP. These stakeholders should be members of the AS committee. Representatives should be knowledgeable about ID literature within their discipline. These members from other disciplines help to provide significant social collaborative resources, such as awareness, access, and influence within the institution, which can be used to help facilitate collaboration across the organization. They can be advocates for change and quality improvement and provide leadership.[25] These members may be involved on a routine basis, or on an *ad hoc* basis when discipline-specific issues arise. In addition, when developing institution-specific guidelines it is important to obtain input and agreement from thought leaders from other relevant services.

Quality Improvement and Patient Safety The development and measurement of interventions to improve antibiotic use are critical components of ASPs. Such interventions should optimally be developed using approaches from implementation science to enhance their impact and success. In some institutions, quality and patient safety groups may have expertise that complements that of ASPs in the areas of executing interventions and obtaining relevant data for measurement. In addition, these groups are often involved in implementation and assessment of performance measures such as the Centers for Medicare and Medicaid Services (CMS) Sepsis Core Measure. As implementation of such a measure involves antibiotic selection and timing, the ASP must be involved in work developed to satisfy the measure.

Regulatory Affairs As regulations regarding antibiotic stewardship emerge from The Joint Commission and CMS, partnering with an institution's Department of Regulatory

Affairs or similar department has gained importance. The Joint Commission Antimicrobial Stewardship Standard requires hospitals to have an antibiotic stewardship program.[26] The Standard has eight elements of performance that include requiring the institution to establish AS as an organizational priority, educating healthcare workers about antibiotic stewardship, developing an AS team, following the ASP principles outlined in the CDC's *Core Elements of Hospital Antibiotic Stewardship Programs*,[27] performing AS according to institutional policies and procedures, collecting and reporting data on antibiotic use and resistance, and performing interventions to improve antibiotic use. The ASP must work proactively with experts in regulatory affairs to assess strengths and weaknesses of stewardship infrastructure and activities to ensure that expected requirements are met. Concerns regarding institutional risk of not meeting requirements can be an important driver to enhance staffing and access to data in an ASP.

Project Manager Institutions with adequate resources may benefit from an AS project manager. This position can help keep the ASP productive by serving as the primary communicator – organizing team projects and meetings, assisting in interdisciplinary coordination across departments, and holding colleagues accountable – while allowing physicians and pharmacists to focus more on patient care activities.[28] This position may also require formalized process improvement training to assist in the systematic development and maintenance of AS initiatives.

Structures in Unique Settings

Large Teaching Hospitals A central duty of academic hospitals is the education of students, residents, and fellows. ASP initiatives can be more far-reaching by incorporating medical house staff and fellows as well as pharmacy students and residents into the ASP. In addition, because new trainees frequently enter and exit academic facilities, unique strategies for AS education need to be considered. For programs with ID fellows and/or pharmacists, it is especially important to involve these trainees, as they will likely have AS responsibilities in the future. Front-line physicians, clinical pharmacists, and nurses are also important AS advocates in these institutions and should be included on AS initiatives and used as content experts for specific interventions.

Resource Limited Settings In resource-limited settings, such as critical access hospitals, long-term care facilities, and ambulatory settings, it may not be feasible to incorporate all of the extended AS team members previously discussed. Most important in these settings is to focus on the core AS team and their integration into existing structures and processes.

It may not be realistic in small community and critical access hospitals to have a separate committee for AS, particularly in hospitals with less than 100 beds. An alternative approach would be to integrate the AS committee objectives within an existing committee, as a standing agenda item for evaluation and discussion. As it is more likely that small hospitals have private physicians with independent practices, it may be more challenging to recruit physician leads for AS. However, there likely are still physicians interested in AS and having a well-respected physician champion is important. These settings may be prime opportunities for AS education for the ASP champions and/or creative involvement of ID-trained physicians and pharmacists through telemedicine, telephone hotlines, and/or remote mentoring programs.[13] Front-line physicians, clinical pharmacists, and nurses are also important AS advocates in these institutions and should be included on AS initiatives and used as content experts for specific interventions.

Long-Term Care Facilities Currently, there are a low number of ASPs in long-term care facilities, although their numbers should increase due to new CMS regulations requiring their implementation.[29] Physicians and pharmacists are often only available on-site intermittently. However, they may help serve as content experts in the development of procedures and protocols executed and evaluated by nurses. In addition, family members are often heavily involved in residents' care; thus, different interventional strategies may be employed to include those community stakeholders. More information is available in Chapter 12.

Ambulatory Setting A significant portion of antibiotic prescribing takes place in the outpatient setting and represents a ripe area for AS interventions. The CDC recently developed the *Core Elements of Outpatient Antibiotic Stewardship* [30] that recommend having a written, publicly displayed commitment to antibiotic stewardship; developing policy and practice recommendations for diagnosis and treatment of one or more conditions; tracking and reporting antibiotic prescribing practices; and providing educational resources on antibiotic stewardship to patients and clinicians. Clinics should identify one or more high-priority condition for intervention, identify barriers that lead to deviation from best practices for the condition(s), and establish standards for antibiotic prescribing. While ID-trained clinicians can be content experts in the development and assessment of AS initiatives for outpatient facilities, on-site physicians, pharmacists, and nurses must co-lead these efforts.[31] A systematic review found that the public's knowledge and beliefs about antibiotic resistance is incomplete and sometimes inaccurate;[32] thus, ongoing education of the public is also of value in this setting. More detailed information is available in Chapter 13.

Antibiotic Stewardship Committee

Establishing an AS Committee is important to provide a structure for accountability, progress, and discussion on key issues with important stakeholders; to combine different disciplines and skills for more effective intervention implementation; to help ensure that AS messages are unified and consistent; and to facilitate the opportunity to develop relationships for better communication and collaboration. The ASP should have committee meetings, similar to an infection control committee, rather than a list of people who are resources to the stewards as they implement or develop ASP interventions and clinical guidelines. An example of members to consider for the team can be found in Box 2. The frequency of committee meetings is variable. Some institutions have successfully implemented committees that meet once monthly with a core group of team members, and then quarterly with a larger group of team members and service-line stakeholders. The purpose of having a standing meeting, rather than an *ad hoc* group that only communicates electronically, is to formalize the ASP and establish a systematic process to disseminate information throughout the institution. Work groups formed to tackle specific problems (e.g., to develop guidelines) can report at this standing meeting, but this should not be the sole focus. Rather, the committee should meet to identify and reevaluate program objectives, provide updates on current projects, discuss data trends, and approve new protocols, procedures, and guidelines, with the majority of the work done outside of the meeting.

Box 2 Potential Antibiotic Stewardship Team Members

1. Representatives from the Adult Antibiotic Stewardship Program including the Director, Associate Director, and infectious diseases pharmacists
2. Representatives from the Pediatric Antibiotic Stewardship Program including the Director, Associate Director, and infectious diseases pharmacists
3. Prescriber (including physicians, nurse practitioners, and physician assistants) representatives from Adult and Pediatrics, Infectious Diseases, Anesthesiology and Critical Care Medicine, Emergency Medicine, Medicine, Obstetrics/Gynecology, Oncology, Pediatrics, and Surgery
4. Representatives from the Department of Pharmacy
5. Representative from Clinical Microbiology
6. Representative from Hospital Epidemiology and Infection Control
7. Representatives from Adult and Pediatric Nursing
8. Representative from Hospital Administration
9. Representative from Quality Improvement
10. Representative from Patient Safety
11. Representative from the Pharmacy and Therapeutics Committee
12. Data Manager
13. Patient Representative

Basic Structure

Reporting Structure The reporting structure of the committee is important. ASP committees should report to the institutional administration not only for better accountability and clarity, but also to engage the administration in the value and impact of AS. Examples of different approaches include having the ASP committee report to the Pharmacy and Therapeutics Committee, Quality and Patient Safety Committees, and/or directly to the Chief Medical or Operations Officer. It is best to report as an independent committee rather than as part of the infection control committee given the different personnel and activities associated with AS relative to infection control. Where the ASP committee reports depends on the institution. At its core, AS seeks to influence how physicians and licensed independent practitioners prescribe antibiotics; thus, reporting to committees and individuals that oversee the work and concerns of these groups is strongly recommended. No matter to whom the ASP committee reports, it is important to develop solid collaborative relationships within each of the aforementioned committees. For example, it is important for the ASP committee to provide expertise on the development of the formulary to the Pharmacy and Therapeutics Committee. In turn, it can support restrictions and endorse protocols, procedures, and guidelines associated with antibiotic use.

Ground Rules and Charter Successful teams exhibit a number of key team values that "encourage listening and responding constructively to views expressed by others, giving others the benefit of the doubt, providing support, and recognizing the interests and achievements of others."[1] Teams all need to be adept at "appreciating others, being able to engage in purposeful conversations, productively and creatively resolving conflicts, and program management."[1] It is important to have a common approach, often put in writing through a committee charter. Examples of key items to include in such a charter are how schedules will be set and adhered to, what skills need to be developed, how responsibility for specific jobs is determined, how continuing membership in the team is earned, and how the group will make and modify decisions.[1]

Meeting Agendas A productive committee should have efficiently managed meetings. This includes setting agendas, energizing team members, managing conflict during the meeting, and staying on time.[33] Each meeting should have an agenda developed and distributed in advance and meeting minutes recorded for approval at the next meeting. A standing meeting agenda should include: evaluation of data and antibiotic usage reports; review of guidelines, policies, procedures, and upcoming Pharmacy and Therapeutics Committee agenda items (such as new agents to be added to the formulary); review of ASP approaches to antibiotic shortages; and review of data on new or select ongoing antibiotic stewardship initiatives. Additional agenda items can include approaches and materials for patient and healthcare worker education relating to antibiotic use; issues related to the microbiology lab including approaches for obtaining microbiology cultures, reporting microbiologic data, implementation of new rapid diagnostic tests, and evaluation of the antibiogram; and/or implementation problems with antibiotic clinical decision support systems and/or electronic medical record tools.

Setting Goals "The combination of purpose and specific goals is essential to performance."[1] Goal setting and the ability to prioritize goals are important first steps for the ASP leaders, in conjunction with their team members, as well as an essential ongoing activity. Important types of goals include improving patient safety, reducing lengths of stay, increasing compliance with regulations, standardizing patient care (within one facility, across facilities in one health-system, or in comparison to competing hospitals), and decreasing or controlling costs. Additional examples of goals are available throughout this textbook (e.g., see Chapters 1 and 14).

Physician and Pharmacist Competencies

The specific competencies of ASP team members have been delineated by the Society for Healthcare Epidemiology of America into nine categories: general principles of antibiotic stewardship; approaches to antibiotic stewardship interventions; antibiotics; microbiology and laboratory diagnostics; common infectious syndromes; measurement and analysis; informatics; program building and leadership; and infection control.[34] In this chapter, these categories have been further divided into beginning and advanced competencies to provide a starting place for new antibiotic stewards (Table 1). Practitioners who are new to antibiotic stewardship should first focus on the beginning knowledge and skills and progress from there. Much of the rationale for these competencies has been described previously in this chapter. Below, additional information is provided regarding program building and leadership.

Program Building and Leadership To prevent fatigue, it is best to view the approach to AS as a marathon rather than a sprint – this requires prioritization of time and the appreciation of small wins.

Ronald Heifetz has noted, "The most common cause of failure in leadership is to treat adaptive challenges as technical problems."[35] The challenge of AS for physicians and pharmacists most often involves adaptive challenges – problems that require changes in priorities, beliefs, habits, loyalties, roles, or ways of thinking regarding how they use antibiotics.[35] However, ASPs often respond to these challenges with technical solutions such as developing guidelines and giving didactic lectures. While such activities are components of AS, when used alone without concomitant approaches to engage prescribers in

Table 1 Knowledge and Skills for Implementation of an Antibiotic Stewardship Program

Category	Knowledge	Basic or Advanced
General Principles of Antibiotic Stewardship		
	Understand the mission and goals of antibiotic stewardship	Basic
	Understand the linkage between antibiotic use and resistance, selection of pathogenic organisms (e.g., *Clostridium difficile*), and other adverse patient outcomes	Basic
	Understand the roles and responsibilities of stakeholders in antibiotic stewardship – physician, pharmacist, infection preventionist, microbiologist, and hospital administrators	Basic
Approaches to Stewardship Interventions		
	Describe the common methods for antibiotic stewardship and approaches for their implementation, including • Restriction with approval required before the first dose or after a certain time period (e.g., 24 hours) • Post-prescription prospective audit and feedback, including discontinuation of antibiotics when unwarranted, de-escalation of antibiotic therapy, correction of mismatch between antibiotic therapy and microbiology results, and recommendation regarding duration of therapy • Formulary management • Education • Algorithm/order set development • Guideline development • Intravenous (IV) to oral (PO) switch	Basic
	Understand how to assess an antibiotic formulary for redundant agents	Basic
	Understand the role and limitations of education regarding appropriate antibiotic use	Basic
	Understand approaches for IV to PO conversion, including both switches to the oral form of the same agent and substitution of oral agents that provide the same coverage as an IV regimen for the purpose of earlier discharge and avoidance of IV access	Basic
	Understand the pros and cons of restriction of antibiotic therapy	Basic

Table 1 (*cont.*)

Category	Knowledge	Basic or Advanced
	Understand the pros and cons of post-prescription prospective audit and feedback regarding antibiotic therapy including specific interventions such as discontinuation of antibiotics when unwarranted, de-escalation of antibiotic therapy, correction of mismatch between antibiotic therapy and microbiology results, and recommendations regarding duration of therapy	Basic
	Recognize situations in which an intervention is required	Advanced
	Understand how to develop institutional algorithms and guidelines for antibiotic use	Advanced
Antibiotics		
	Understand different classes of antibiotics, including antibiotics, antifungals, and antivirals	Basic
	Understand common side effects/adverse events associated with different antibiotics, including adverse reactions that mimic infectious syndromes	Basic
	Assess and respond to antibiotic shortages	Basic
	Understand the different types of allergic reactions to antibiotics and how they may be prevented or minimized	Basic
	Understand common drug interactions between antibiotics, between antibiotic and other therapeutic agents, and between antibiotics and food including their clinical significance and strategies to avoid them	Basic
	Understand approaches to therapeutic monitoring of antibiotics, such as vancomycin and aminoglycosides	Basic
	Understand associations between use of specific antibiotic agents and development of resistance or *C. difficile*	Basic/Advanced
	Understand pharmacokinetic (PK) and pharmacodynamic (PD) properties of different antibiotic agents and their application to selection of appropriate dosing based on patient, pathogen, and syndrome characteristics	Advanced

Table 1 (cont.)

Category	Knowledge	Basic or Advanced
	Understand common mechanisms of resistance for different antibiotic/organism combinations and their impact on resistance to other antibiotics	Advanced
	Understand antibiotic therapy options for highly resistant organisms	Advanced
Microbiology and Laboratory Diagnostics		
	Describe microbiologic characteristics of bacteria that cause clinical disease in humans including appearance on Gram stain and other stains (e.g., acid fast, modified acid fast) and state expected antibiotic susceptibilities	Basic
	Understand how to appropriately obtain cultures and other samples for microbiology testing and interpret results	Basic
	Describe laboratory approaches to testing for C. difficile disease and interpret results	Basic
	Understand approaches to detecting and reporting antibiotic susceptibilities	Basic
	Understand the strengths and weaknesses of using an antibiogram to assist with decisions on recommendations for empiric therapy	Basic
	Understand minimal inhibitory concentrations (MIC) and breakpoints including both their role in determining appropriate antibiotic therapy and the impact of CLSI breakpoint changes on microbiology reporting	Basic/Advanced
	Understand options for rapid diagnostic testing in the microbiology lab	Advanced
	Describe laboratory approaches to testing for common viral pathogens in humans and interpret results	Advanced
	Understand when MIC data should be requested at institutions that do not routinely provide such data	Advanced
	Understand the basic principles of testing antibiotic combinations for synergy and antagonism	Advanced
	Describe microbiologic characteristics of fungi that cause clinical disease in humans including	Advanced

Table 1 *(cont.)*

Category	Knowledge	Basic or Advanced
	appearance on relevant stains and state expected antifungal susceptibilities	
	Understand CLSI recommendations for constructing institutional antibiograms	Basic
	Understand the uses of inflammatory biomarkers (e.g., procalcitonin) in antibiotic stewardship	Advanced
	Understand the strengths, weaknesses, and diagnostic accuracy of testing performed in the microbiology lab	Advanced
Common Infectious Syndromes		
	Critically read national guidelines for infectious diseases relevant to antibiotic stewardship	Basic
	Describe the recommended durations of antibiotic therapy for common infectious diseases including those based on sound evidence versus those based on tradition	Basic
	Critically read recent literature on infectious disease issues relevant to antibiotic stewardship	Basic
	Understand presentation, diagnosis, management, and appropriate antibiotic use including appropriate duration of therapy associated with common infectious syndromes: • Upper and lower respiratory tract infection • Urinary tract infection • Intra-abdominal/pelvic infection • Skin, soft tissue, bone and joint infection, diabetic foot infection • Central nervous system infection • Bloodstream, catheter and endovascular infection • Infections involving prosthetic materials and devices other than catheters • Gastrointestinal infection, including *C. difficile* infection • Methicillin-resistant *S. aureus* infection • Sepsis • Febrile neutropenia • Fungal infections • Viral infections	Basic

Table 1 (cont.)

Category	Knowledge	Basic or Advanced
	Understand the infectious and noninfectious differential for certain common conditions (e.g., infiltrates on chest x-ray)	Basic
	Recognize clinical syndromes and infections where combination therapy is recommended	Basic/Advanced
Measurement and Analysis		
	Understand methods, data needs and interpretation of data on antibiotic use	Basic
	Understand and compare standard methods of measuring antibiotic use including metrics such as defined daily doses (DDD), days of therapy (DOT), and length of therapy (LOT)	Basic
	Discuss approaches to measure the impact of a stewardship program or stewardship intervention including <ul><li>Reductions in antibiotic use</li><li>Reductions in inappropriate antibiotic use</li><li>Improved patient outcomes (e.g., decreased length of hospitalization, mortality, readmissions)</li><li>Changes in rates or proportions of resistant organisms</li><li>Decreases in rates of *C. difficile*</li><li>Decrease in adverse events (e.g., renal dysfunction)</li><li>Adherence to institutional pathways/protocols</li><li>Decrease in time to appropriate therapy</li><li>Decrease in antibiotic costs and costs of care</li></ul>	Basic
	Understand how to display and report data regarding process and outcome measures in internal and external presentations and reports/manuscripts	Basic/Advanced
	Understand processes and definitions associated with the NHSN Antibiotic Use and Resistance (AUR) module	Advanced
	Understand approaches to benchmarking antibiotic use within and across institutions	Advanced
	Understand appropriate types of study design (e.g., before-after, cluster randomized) and	Advanced

Table 1 (cont.)

Category	Knowledge	Basic or Advanced
	analysis (e.g., time-series analysis) for stewardship interventions	
Informatics/IT		
	Assess IT resources available at an institution for performing antibiotic stewardship activities	Basic
	Determine order sets that may be useful for an institution	Basic
	Assess external proprietary antibiotic stewardship IT software programs	Advanced
Program Building and Leadership		
	Understand how your antibiotic stewardship program intersects with the institution's strategic plan	Basic
	Understand how to obtain physician/ prescriber buy-in for a program or intervention	Basic
	Understand how to obtain pharmacy/ pharmacist buy in for a program or intervention	Basic
	Understand the medical-legal implications of a stewardship program at your institution	Basic
	Understand reporting requirements and regulatory mandates related to antibiotic use (e.g., SCIP, core measures, *US News and World Report* rankings for pediatric hospitals)	Basic
	Understand the complex interpersonal and interprofessional needs to best develop and sustain an ASP	Basic
	Understand how to write and present a strategic plan and business case to institutional leadership for stewardship programs for initial establishment of a program	Basic/Advanced
	Understand how to write and present a business case to institutional leadership for stewardship programs for maintenance of a program	Basic/Advanced
	Understand basic theories regarding patient safety, quality science, implementation science, and organizational change	Advanced
	Understand unique challenges and strategies for implementing and managing antibiotic	Advanced

Table 1 (cont.)

Category	Knowledge	Basic or Advanced
	stewardship across multiple institutions or within a health system	
Infection Control		
	Discuss basic infection prevention principles and processes and the interrelationship with ASP	Basic
	Understand current recommendations for use of antibiotics for surgical prophylaxis	Basic
	Understand the differences between surveillance definitions and clinical definitions for healthcare associated infections (HAI)	Advanced
Special Populations and Non-Acute Hospital Settings		
	Understand how to apply and modify stewardship approaches for special populations (e.g., immunocompromised, oncologic, neonatal and other intensive care unit, transplant, geriatric)	Facility-Specific
	Understand how to apply and modify stewardship approaches in non-acute hospital settings (e.g., long-term acute care, ambulatory surgery center), the emergency department, and the operating room	Facility-Specific
	Understand the approaches to implementing stewardship activity when resources are limited	Facility-Specific

understanding their behavior, they are unlikely to yield long-term changes in prescribing. Both the physician and pharmacist should be respected as agents of change, and to do this, a better understanding of the social determinants of antibiotic prescribing is key (see Chapter 3). The three key skills the physician and pharmacist antibiotic stewardship champions must possess are leadership skills in quality improvement and managing change, effective communication, and in-depth infectious diseases knowledge. Research skills may also be useful, depending on the setting.

A comprehensive survey of 14 hospitals identified four key behaviors of leaders who successfully implemented hospital-associated infection prevention practices;[36] these leadership behaviors are also relevant for antibiotic stewardship and include nurturing a culture of clinical excellence and effectively communicating it to staff; overcoming barriers of resistance from people or processes that prevent effectiveness; acting as inspirational role models; and thinking strategically while acting locally. Framing leadership behaviors in this manner may help to identify strengths and weaknesses among team members and may help with implementing various AS initiatives.

Another important skill is fostering constructive conflict, i.e. conflict that leads to improved team decision-making while mitigating interpersonal discord.[1] Eisenhardt, Kawhwajy, and Borgeois found "teams unable to foster substantive conflict ultimately achieve, on average, lower performance."[1] Strategies to promote productive conflict include focusing on facts, discussing alternatives, emphasizing common goals, using humor, balancing the power structure, and seeking a fair decision-making process through "consensus with qualification."[1] Consensus with qualifications focuses on establishing a fair decision-making process in which decisions are made by consensus when possible, and if not possible, the most senior team member makes the decision after receiving input from all team members.

Interventions are the cornerstone of AS, thus it is important not to just monitor antibiotic use and resistance trends, but to make changes to improve appropriate use and decrease the development of resistance. Central to this mission is continuous quality improvement that recognizes areas for improvement, understands the context of the issue, sets realistic goals and the appropriate strategy to accomplish each goal, assesses the risks and benefits of different change approaches, executes changes as well as measures their impact, and adjusts course as needed.[37] Change is not easy, but it is a key part of any steward's role. There are strategies to help approach change in a productive manner. One framework is Kotter's Steps for Managing Change.[38] These eight steps are:

1. Create a sense of urgency.
2. Form a powerful guiding coalition.
3. Create a compelling vision for change.
4. Communicate the vision effectively.
5. Empower others to act on the vision.
6. Plan for and create short-term wins.
7. Consolidate improvements and create still more change.
8. Institutionalize new approaches.

Morris and colleagues reported how they successfully used this framework to establish two fully funded ASPs.[15] First, they presented safety and cost data to hospital administrators that demonstrated the urgent need to implement an ASP. Next, they organized an operational team (including an ID physician, ID pharmacist, data analyst, and project manager) and an oversight team (including a hospital senior executive, critical care leader, ID leader, and pharmacy leader) that met on a regular basis, along with an advisory committee (including infection control personnel, an internist, a microbiologist, a surgeon, nurses, and others). A simple and memorable vision was created – "Helping patients receive the right antibiotics, when they need them" – and communicated extensively to empower others.

Another framework for quality improvement is provided by Pronovost and colleagues:[39]

1. Summarize the evidence.
2. Identify local barriers to implementation.
3. Measure performance.
4. Ensure all patients receive the intervention.
   a. Engage
   b. Educate

   c. Execute

   d. Evaluate

   e. Repeat

An example of how to use this framework for an ASP is provided by Jenkins and colleagues.[40] After the investigators reviewed the evaluation and treatment of inpatient cellulitis and cutaneous abscess at their institution for areas for improvement, they developed a clinical practice guideline using expertise from a multidisciplinary working group. This guideline was disseminated physically, via email, and incorporated into the electronic order entry system. The investigators conducted an educational campaign, and measured performance via audit and feedback quarterly, which was communicated to front-line staff through designated key attending physician peer champions.

There are two types of ASP implementation: development of the program structure itself, which is the focus of this chapter, and implementation of the interventions to improve antibiotic use. Although much effort is often expended on initiating and maintaining a program, it is very important to also place equal or greater weight on implementing facility-specific interventions. The quality improvement approaches previously outlined can help to determine the best intervention with available time and resources. To choose between intervention strategies, leaders of the ASP need to understand options and expectations (see Chapters 4 and 5). A key component of both quality improvement and implementation science is the understanding of various metrics used to evaluate the results of an intervention (see Chapter 7).

It is important to recognize that there are different approaches to developing and maintaining ASP activities in a healthcare setting. The ASP should consider the models discussed earlier in the chapter for change and implementation or others in the literature. To be most successful, stewards must be open to new strategic approaches and cognizant of team dynamics and behavior.

Communication Skills Antibiotic stewardship requires expert skills in both formal and informal written and verbal communication. These communication skills are important to successfully promote behavioral change among health professionals. Antibiotic stewardship leaders must be able to successfully communicate in crucial conversations and conflict resolution.[41, 42] AS core team members must be able to communicate their recommendations with positivity, clarity and confidence but also know when to back down. It is also important to identify the most appropriate and effective method of communication – whether to address the issue in the moment or proactively later; whether in person, over the phone, or through email.[43] It is generally expected that the physician and pharmacist ASP leaders will make numerous presentations to a variety of audiences; thus, formal communication skills are of great importance in addition to informal communication.

Another area in which communication skills are important is in running a problem-solving meeting; below are proposed steps for the chair(s) of the antibiotic stewardship committee to follow based on Harvard Business School Press:[33]

1. Find out participants' perceptions of the problem.
2. Get agreement on the definition of the problem.
3. Discuss the duration of the problem and current status.
4. Determine potential causes of the problem perceived by the group.
5. Outline the future consequences of the problem if it is not solved.

6. Brainstorm options for solving the problem. Clarify the advantages and disadvantages of each option.
7. Choose the most effective method. Consider the key factors, such as time, resource, financials, values, and so forth, involved in the choice.
8. Gain full agreement, or at least a consensus, on an option for problem resolution or management.

Conclusion

The key to a successful ASP team is to identify and engage key members and partners. These members should have clearly defined roles and meet basic competencies. This multidisciplinary team can identify common goals and strategies to achieve those goals.

References

1. Harvard Business Review. *HBR's 10 Must Reads on Teams*. Boston, MA: Harvard Business Review Press, 2013.

2. Waters CD. Pharmacist-driven antimicrobial stewardship program in an institution without infectious diseases physician support. *Am J Health Syst Pharm* 2015; 72:466–468.

3. Septimus EJ, Owens RC, Jr. Need and potential of antimicrobial stewardship in community hospitals. *Clin Infect Dis* 2011; 53 Suppl 1:S8–S14.

4. Reese SM, Gilmartin H, Rich KL, Price CS. Infection prevention needs assessment in Colorado hospitals: rural and urban settings. *Am J Infect Control* 2014; 42:597–601.

5. Sunenshine RH, Liedtke LA, Jernigan DB, Strausbaugh LJ. Role of infectious diseases consultants in management of antimicrobial use in hospitals. *Clin Infect Dis* 2004; 38:934–938.

6. Rohde JM, Jacobsen D, Rosenberg DJ. Role of the hospitalist in antimicrobial stewardship: a review of work completed and description of a multisite collaborative. *Clin Therap* 2013; 35:751–757.

7. Parmar P, Mackie D, Varghese S, Cooper C. Use of telemedicine technologies in the management of infectious diseases: a review. *Clin Infect Dis* 2015; 60:1084–1094.

8. Trivedi KK, Pollack LA. The role of public health in antimicrobial stewardship in healthcare. *Clin Infect Dis* 2014; 59 Suppl 3: S101–S103.

9. Heil EL, Kuti JL, Bearden DT, Gallagher JC. The essential role of pharmacists in antimicrobial stewardship. *Infect Control Hosp Epidemiol* 2016;37 (7):753–754.

10. Drew RH, White R, MacDougall C, Hermsen ED, Owens RC, Jr. Insights from the Society of Infectious Diseases Pharmacists on antimicrobial stewardship guidelines from the Infectious Diseases Society of America and the Society for Healthcare Epidemiology of America. *Pharmacotherapy* 2009; 29:593–607.

11. Bessesen MT, Ma A, Clegg D, et al. Antimicrobial stewardship programs: comparison of a program with infectious diseases pharmacist support to a program with a geographic pharmacist staffing model. *Hosp Pharm* 2015; 50:477–483.

12. DiazGranados CA, Abd TT. Participation of clinical pharmacists without specialized infectious diseases training in antimicrobial stewardship. *Am J Hosp Pharm* 2011; 68:1691–1692.

13. Michaels KMM, Krug A, Kuper K. Implementation of an antimicrobial stewardship program in a community hospital: results of a three-year analysis. *Hosp Pharm* 2012; 8:608–616.

14. Smith T, Philmon CL, Johnson GD, et al. Antimicrobial stewardship in a community hospital: attacking the more difficult problems. *Hosp Pharm* 2014; 49:839–846.

15. Morris AM, Stewart TE, Shandling M, McIntaggart S, Liles WC. Establishing an antimicrobial stewardship program. *Health Q (Toronto, Ont)* 2010; 13:64–70.

16. Cross RRR, Grant A. Collaborative overload. *Harvard Business Review* 2016; Jan.–Feb:74–79.

17. Gaffin N. Reflections from an antimicrobial stewardship program. *Clin Infect Dis* 2015; 60:1588–1589.

18. Evans RS, Olson JA, Stenehjem E, et al. Use of computer decision support in an antimicrobial stewardship program (ASP). *App Clin Inform* 2015; 6:120–135.

19. Kim J, Craft DW, Katzman M. Building an antimicrobial stewardship program: cooperative roles for pharmacists, infectious diseases specialists, and clinical microbiologists. *Lab Med* 2015; 46:e65–71.

20. Avdic E, Carroll KC. The role of the microbiology laboratory in antimicrobial stewardship programs. *Infect Dis Clin NA* 2014; 28:215–235.

21. Moody J, Cosgrove SE, Olmsted R, et al. Antimicrobial stewardship: a collaborative partnership between infection preventionists and healthcare epidemiologists. *Infect Control Hosp Epidemiol* 2012; 33:328–330.

22. Olans RN, Olans RD, DeMaria A, Jr. The critical role of the staff nurse in antimicrobial stewardship–unrecognized, but already there. *Clin Infect Dis* 2016; 62:84–89.

23. Gillespie E, Rodrigues A, Wright L, Williams N, Stuart RL. Improving antibiotic stewardship by involving nurses. *Am J Infect Control* 2013; 41:365–367.

24. Buckel WR, Avdic E, Carroll KC, Gunaseelan V, Hadhazy E, Cosgrove SE. Gut check: *Clostridium difficile* testing and treatment in the molecular testing era. *Infect Control and Hosp Epidemiol* 2015; 36:217–221.

25. May L, Cosgrove S, L'Archeveque M, et al. A call to action for antimicrobial stewardship in the emergency department: approaches and strategies. *Ann Emerg Med* 2013; 62:69–77.

26. The Joint Commission. Approved: New Antimicrobial Stewardship Standard. *Joint Commission Perspectives* 2016; 36(7):1, 3–4, 8.

27. Centers for Disease Control and Prevention. Core elements of hospital antibiotic stewardship programs. (Accessed March 14, 2017, at www.cdc.gov/getsmart/healthcare/implementation/core-elements.html.)

28. Bryant B, Curello J, Uslan D, Humphries R, Kanatani M, Kassamali Z. Antimicrobial stewardship programs: engaging project managers to increase productivity. *Infect Control Hosp Epidemiol* 2016; 37:739–740.

29. Dyar OJ, Pagani L, Pulcini C. Strategies and challenges of antimicrobial stewardship in long-term care facilities. *Clin Microb Infect* 2015; 21:10–19.

30. Sanchez GV, Fleming-Dutra KD, Roberts RM, Hicks LA. Core elements of outpatient antibiotic stewardship. *MMWR Recomm Rep* 2016; 65:1–12.

31. Gerber JS, Prasad PA, Fiks AG, et al. Effect of an outpatient antimicrobial stewardship intervention on broad-spectrum antibiotic prescribing by primary care pediatricians: a randomized trial. *JAMA* 2013; 309:2345–2352.

32. McCullough AR, Parekh S, Rathbone J, Del Mar CB, Hoffmann TC. A systematic review of the public's knowledge and beliefs about antibiotic resistance. *J Antimicrob Chemother* 2016; 71:27–33.

33. Harvard Business Review. *Running Meetings: Expert Solutions to Everyday Challenges*. Boston, MA: Harvard Business School Press, 2006.

34. Cosgrove SE, Hermsen ED, Rybak MJ, File TM, Jr., Parker SK, Barlam TF. Guidance for the knowledge and skills required for antimicrobial stewardship leaders. *Infect Control Hosp Epidemiol* 2014; 35:1444–1451.

35. Heifetz RA, Grashow A, Linsky M. *The Practice of Adaptive Leadership: Tools and Tactics for Changing Your Organization and the World*. Boston, MA: Harvard Business School Press, 2009.

36. Saint S, Kowalski CP, Banaszak-Holl J, Forman J, Damschroder L, Krein SL. The importance of leadership in preventing healthcare-associated infection: results of a

multisite qualitative study. *Infect Control Hosp Epidemiol* 2010; 31:901–907.

37. Batalden P, Davidoff F. Teaching quality improvement: the devil is in the details. *JAMA* 2007; 298:1059–1061.

38. Kotter JP. *Leading Change*. Boston, MA: Harvard Business Review Press, 2012.

39. Pronovost PJ, Berenholtz SM, Needham DM. Translating evidence into practice: a model for large scale knowledge translation. *BMJ* 2008; 337:a1714.

40. Jenkins TC, Knepper BC, Sabel AL, et al. Decreased antibiotic utilization after implementation of a guideline for inpatient cellulitis and cutaneous abscess. *Arch Intern Med* 2011; 171:1072–1079.

41. Patterson KGJ, McMillan R, Switzler A. *Crucial Conversations: Tools for Talking When Stakes Are High*. San Francisco, CA: Hill Companies, 2012.

42. Gallo A. *HBR Guide to Managing Conflict at Work*. Boston, MA: Harvard Business Review Press, 2015.

43. Goldstein EJ, Goff DA, Reeve W, et al. Approaches to modifying the behavior of clinicians who are noncompliant with antimicrobial stewardship program guidelines. *Clin Infect Dis* 2016; 63:532–538.

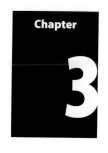

Chapter

3

The Social Determinants of Antibiotic Prescribing
Implications for the Development and Implementation of Stewardship Interventions

Julia E. Szymczak and Jason G. Newland

Introduction

Antibiotic stewardship programs (ASPs) use a number of strategies to improve antibiotic use. Davey and colleagues characterize stewardship interventions as persuasive, restrictive, or structural.[1] Persuasive interventions include education, audit and feedback to clinicians on the appropriateness of their prescriptions, and written or verbal reminders. Restrictive interventions include prior approval for certain medications by infectious diseases physicians or pharmacists as a requirement, restrictive antibiotic formularies, selective reporting of laboratory susceptibilities, and automatic stop orders. Structural interventions include computerized decision support systems, rapid laboratory testing, and quality monitoring. Available evidence suggests that restrictive interventions have a greater impact on decreasing the use of targeted antibiotics than persuasive or structural interventions,[1, 2] although a combination of approaches might be most effective.[3]

At the core of all stewardship interventions is an effort to change clinician behavior, a notoriously difficult task in any domain.[4, 5] Prescribing behavior is a complex decision-making process whose intricacies are not yet fully understood.[6] There are likely multiple "drivers" of the decision to use an antibiotic in any one clinical situation. Figure 1, a conceptual framework for antibiotic use adapted from Fishman, illustrates the complexity.[7]

Figure 1 depicts four key domains of drivers that shape antibiotic use: knowledge, resources, attitudes, and social dynamics. The **knowledge** that a prescribing clinician has about the treatment of infectious diseases and how to use antibiotics as well as their level of familiarity with the patient shape their decisions. The **resources** available to a prescribing clinician, including ease of access to diagnostic testing systems and the organization's antibiotic formulary, shape the decision. The **social dynamics** that characterize the delivery of healthcare, including organizational context, face-to-face interaction among groups of clinicians and between clinicians and patients, and the cultural beliefs that both groups bring to the clinical encounter shape the decision. The **attitudes and perceptions** that clinicians and patients hold about infectious diseases and antibiotics also shape the decision. In this chapter, we are chiefly concerned with elaborating the latter two domains and making the case for why they need to be considered in the design and implementation of antibiotic stewardship interventions in both inpatient and outpatient clinical settings.

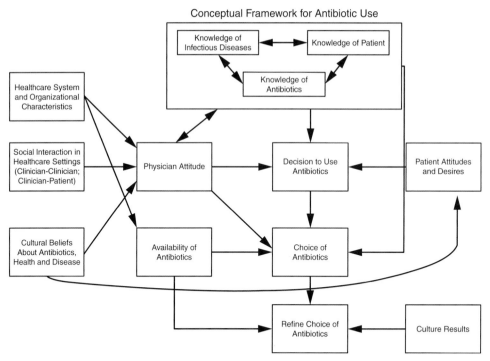

Figure 1

Defining a "Social Determinant" of Antibiotic Prescribing

If I see a patient a week after surgery, and there's still a little redness, and Mom's nervous I am inclined to just put the kid on the antibiotic. It just makes everyone comfortable, and then a week later, the redness is gone. Did I treat an infection or was there just some redness? Some inflammatory post-operative discharge? I don't know. I'm more careful about how I give antibiotics than I used to be in the past. You don't want to be part of the societal issue of creating superbugs, but it is surprisingly difficult to look Mom in the face when she is convinced it's infected and you're trying to say "look, it's not infected," when you don't even know for sure yourself and a week later it could pus out and Mom's like "See? Should have put her on antibiotics. I can't believe you did this to my kid!" That is what you imagine the scenario being if you don't do something. It's so much easier to say "look, we'll put her on a little antibiotic" (Interview with a Pediatric General Surgeon).[8]

Social scientists have long-recognized that prescribing a drug is a highly social as well as clinical act.[9] A prescription has latent cultural, psychological, and communicative functions.[10] Prescribing a medicine symbolizes the clinician's concern for the patient; legitimizes the patient's suffering which signals that the patient is indeed sick and therefore entitled to the societal privileges reserved for the sick;[11, 12] and bolsters the clinician's authority and claim to specialized knowledge.[13] Giving a prescription can help the clinician avoid lengthy conversations with patients about the meaning of symptoms in a time-pressured clinical setting that prioritizes efficiency [14] and can be a major source of satisfaction for the clinician in moments of uncertainty about the cause and cure of sickness since it may be the only action he or she can take to help the patient.[15] Emotions, expectations, obligations, the management of uncertainty, identity, and social relationships are at stake when a clinician prescribes a medication.

An emerging literature identifies the factors that drive antibiotic prescribing beyond clinician knowledge of appropriate practice or medical need.[16, 17] This literature suggests that knowledge about biomedical principles, evidence-based guidelines, or concern for clinical outcomes only partially determines the choice to use an antibiotic. There is a growing recognition that the social and behavioral dynamics that shape antibiotic use must be better understood and incorporated into the design of antibiotic stewardship interventions.[6, 18]

We use the term "social determinant of antibiotic prescribing" to refer broadly to nonmedical factors arising out of the social environment that influence the choice to prescribe. We adopt a sociological lens, with a focus on understanding how the dynamic social relationships that make up everyday life in healthcare settings where people are working together to care for patients/families shape medical decision-making.[19–22] Diagnosis and treatment are not simply problems of cognition or information processing – of clinicians gathering patient data as objectively as possible and matching them to a given disease category and then selecting a therapeutic approach. These decisions are also highly social in nature, which involves the way that clinicians decide, via interaction with each other and with patients/families, how to label what is wrong, what *can* be done to remedy it, and what *should* be done.[23]

Medical sociologists have long shown that daily life in healthcare settings is strongly ordered by cultural logics that guide behavior in ways that may have more to do with maintaining social norms than with achieving a particular medical outcome.[24] We take seriously, as Charani et al. suggest, that antibiotic prescribing occurs within the context of a large, dynamic social environment with multiple "agents" who continuously interact, including physicians, nurse practitioners, nurses, pharmacists, hospital/healthcare system executives, payors, patients, and family members.[25] Our approach complements, but is distinct from, a growing literature drawing from the cognitive and behavioral sciences that focus on the thinking styles of individual clinicians to reduce inappropriate antibiotic use in the outpatient setting.[26, 27] We refer to this work later in the chapter as a model for how to leverage behavioral theory to shape the design of interventions.

In the following section, we review four social determinants of antibiotic prescribing that have been identified in the literature to date. Many of these studies employ qualitative methodology, which is particularly well suited to identifying the social mechanisms that underpin certain phenomena.[22] Throughout this chapter, we will present excerpts of qualitative data, from published studies and studies by one of this chapter's authors (Szymczak), to illustrate key points.

Four Social Determinants of Antibiotic Prescribing

Relationships between Clinicians

Numerous studies have demonstrated that the choice to use an antibiotic is shaped, in part, by the relationships and social interactions between clinicians within healthcare organizations.[28–30] Most of this research focuses on the prescribing behavior of teams of physicians working in the inpatient setting. A key finding is that prescribing behavior is strongly influenced by local social norms that emerge out of professional, unit-based, and organizational subcultures. These social norms, known as "prescribing etiquette," are a set of unwritten but widely accepted cultural rules that exist in healthcare organizations about what is considered appropriate or inappropriate when making decisions about antibiotics. [25, 31] Although social norms are likely to be specific to particular organizations or groups of clinicians, investigators have found similar themes across medical work settings: (1) deference to hierarchy and (2) a norm of noninterference.

Hierarchy

In hospital settings especially, antibiotic prescribing has been found to be sensitive to the hierarchical relationships between clinicians. Multiple studies have found that the prescribing behavior of junior clinicians and trainees is strongly influenced by clinicians who are located higher in the social hierarchy.[29, 30, 32] Junior clinicians report that even when they recognize that a prescribing decision made by a superior deviates from best practice, they defer to what the attending physician wants.[25, 28] Given that in most academic medical settings junior clinicians are the ones writing the orders for antibiotics, this social norm can obstruct opportunities to improve prescribing. Additionally, this dynamic has long-term consequences as trainees internalize this social norm and, when they rise in the hospital hierarchy, perpetuate the dynamic. As one infectious diseases physician and ASP director explains,

> Physicians don't like being told what to do, especially by pharmacists or fellows or someone lower on the totem pole than them. And I understand where they are coming from. They are thinking "I went to medical school. I did a residency. I am a doctor." Yes, the structure of medicine has changed over time and we're trying to be more open-minded. But in training it is still you are a plebe, a plebe, a plebe, a plebe, and then you become a boss. And you are told what to do, told what to do, told what to do and then you tell the plebes what to do. You've earned that. So I get that accepting stewardship restrictions can be really hard for doctors to swallow.[33]

Despite efforts to "flatten" the traditional medical hierarchy to improve patient safety,[34] multidisciplinary efforts to change physician antibiotic prescribing behavior must consider and contend with hierarchy. This is especially true given that pharmacists play a major role in delivering stewardship interventions. Pharmacists, who possess expert knowledge about antibiotics, do not have the authority to prescribe them. Yet frequently, pharmacists act as gatekeepers to physicians. This has led to, as a number of studies have found, tension between pharmacists and physicians around the implementation of antibiotic stewardship interventions.[35, 36]

Norm of Noninterference

Multiple studies have described a very strong norm of noninterference, where clinicians report going to great lengths to avoid providing feedback on or altering other prescribers' decisions.[28, 31, 37] When clinicians describe this norm in qualitative studies, they frequently use terms like "uncomfortable"[31] or "awkward"[28] to describe how they perceive the act of interfering with someone else's prescribing decisions. In clinical settings where care is provided by teams of clinicians, prescribers consider overall team dynamics in deciding whether to challenge a prescribing decision. Clinicians have a strong motivation to avoid making an "enemy" of one's colleagues [38] by calling out a prescribing decision and causing the prescriber to "lose face."[36] That the people who deliver antibiotic stewardship recommendations have to contend with the reputation of being seen as "antibiotic police" is further evidence of the norm of noninterference – a stigma surrounds the person charged with delivering feedback. Additionally, providing constructive feedback on antibiotics is particularly fraught because the decision is rarely clear-cut. We know from research on speaking up to prevent safety risks from reaching patients that clinicians feel it is acceptable to intervene on prescribing decisions that are immediately harmful (e.g., an overdose) but not for those that are apparently inappropriate.[39]

The norm of noninterference is exacerbated by the fact that, given the way that medical care happens in complex, busy inpatient settings, opportunities to have conversations or deliver face-to-face feedback about antibiotic prescribing decisions are limited.[40, 41] As one attending physician describes in Livorsi et al.[28] qualitative study of antibiotic prescribers in two Midwest US academic hospitals,

> Part of it is convenience ... I think if you ran into that person and you were talking about it, [feedback would be okay] ... but in the way that we practice, they rotate off service for weeks at a time and then by the time you [see them again] ... you have forgotten all about that.
>
> (p. 1068)

The norm of noninterference is especially consequential in inpatient settings where multiple teams of clinicians may care for the same patient over the course of a hospitalization. Without the active intervention of an antibiotic steward, it is easy to see how inappropriate antibiotic decisions can be made and persist because clinicians do not feel comfortable speaking up to each other to modify them.

Relationships between Clinicians and Patients

Patient pressure or demand is a social factor that is repeatedly invoked when prescribing clinicians working in outpatient settings are asked about the reasons why they use antibiotics inappropriately.[41–45] Although this factor has predominantly been identified in ambulatory settings and emergency departments, patient and family pressure for antibiotics occurs in long-term care facility settings as well.[46, 47] Clinicians explain that they capitulate to patient pressure because they want to please the patient and to provide them with something tangible so they do not go home "empty handed."[48] In a healthcare system that increasingly frames patients as consumers, the dynamics of a buyer-seller relationship can take over, with clinicians in private practices fearful that a patient who leaves a clinic visit dissatisfied will take their business elsewhere and/or post their "negative" experience on the internet. As one primary care pediatrician explained in an interview study about the overuse of antibiotics in children:

> There was a new mother in our community who I knew from somewhere else and she had her first baby recently and I thought she would become a patient at our practice. But she said to me "oh, we are going to this other practice because we know that if we walk in there, we can get an antibiotic right away." I was surprised that she didn't want to come to our practice, but she said "I will know when my kid is sick. So if I know my kid is sick, I don't want to wait it out."[45]

Additionally, the growing emphasis by health system administrators on measures of patient satisfaction may also serve as a barrier to judicious antibiotic prescribing when what the patient desires is at odds with what the prescribing clinician knows is the best course of action.[41]

While prescribing clinicians may want to engage patients in a conversation about why an antibiotic is not necessary, the time pressures that characterize most clinical work environments make this difficult. As one primary care pediatrician explained in an interview study about the overuse of antibiotics for children, "honestly, I think some patients do get antibiotics that they don't need them just because we are running behind when we don't have time to explain to parents why they aren't necessary."[45] A clinician's resolve to have these difficult conversations with patients can erode over the course of a busy clinic day as they become fatigued, as Linder et al. demonstrated in a study showing that primary care clinicians' likelihood of prescribing unnecessary antibiotics increased later in a clinic day.[49]

While patient expectation for antibiotics may be acutely felt by prescribing clinicians, there is evidence to suggest that clinicians actually over-estimate patient demand.[50, 51] When a clinician perceives that a patient is expecting an antibiotic, they are more likely to inappropriately prescribe them.[52] However, patient-reported expectations do not often correlate with prescribing clinician perceptions.[51] Even when a patient does not make a verbal request for antibiotics in a clinical encounter, prescribing clinicians still perceive an expectation for antibiotics.[53] As the public becomes more aware of antibiotic resistance over time, some patients are becoming more aware and wary of overuse.[54, 55] Clinicians may be prescribing on the basis of perceived rather than actual patient expectations for antibiotics in cases where they are not necessary.[52, 56] Despite their best intentions or knowledge of the appropriate course of action, the social dynamics that characterize the way that clinicians interact with patients, form impressions, and interpret expectations coupled with the environmental context in which medical work happens can push clinicians to make suboptimal decisions about antibiotics.

Risk, Fear, Uncertainty, Identity, and Emotion

One of the defining social dilemmas of medical work is the management of uncertainty[57, 58] and the navigation of risk.[59] Clinicians are frequently faced with diagnostic and therapeutic dilemmas in which the best course of action is not completely clear while the risk of a poor outcome weighs heavily. Despite this uncertainty, clinicians must act, and they must do so in the best interest of the patient while also maintaining their professional identity and sense of self.[60] Emotional dynamics shape this medical decision-making, especially when the stakes are high (patient morbidity and mortality). The ways that clinicians perceive risk and feel about fulfilling their social obligations to patients influence their choice to use antibiotics or not. Clinicians may prescribe antibiotics based on their anxiety surrounding and fear of the worst-case scenario [28, 61] and the corresponding desire to avoid medicolegal consequences. As one infectious diseases physician explained in an interview study of the barriers to judicious antibiotic use in critical care settings:

> They do it [overprescribe] because they don't want the patient to do badly … As a physician, you feel really bad when you do something and you could have done something differently and the patient does badly. That is what haunts you. I can't remember a time where I clearly did too much and I was bothered by that later. I'm not haunted by those. I'm haunted by the ones I missed and I could have done more.[33]

The use of the term "haunted" by this physician conveys the emotional footprint that decisions about antibiotics can leave on a prescribing clinician's memory. These past experiences or stories about other clinicians undertreating an infection can shape prescribing behavior in ways that might be contrary to evidence-based practice.

Risk-aversive antibiotic prescribing is reflected in a qualitative study investigating the knowledge, attitudes, and practices of medical residents toward broad-spectrum antibiotics. [32] In this study, Laake et al. found that residents perceive overly dire consequences for initiating antibiotic coverage that is too narrow and describe broad-spectrum drugs as "safe" and "comfortable." These trainees describe that the overarching goal that shapes their orientation to clinical decision-making around antibiotics is to prevent disaster from occurring in the short term. Other studies have shown that clinicians perceive the risk of undertreating a patient as greater than the individual patient risk from receiving unnecessary antibiotics.[41, 62] Additionally, the potential adverse effects of antibiotics are not appreciated and have limited impact on decision-making in busy clinical settings.[28]

Studies have found that clinicians have an emotional desire to provide all immediate therapeutic options to an individual patient, regardless of wider population consequences. [63] These emotional responses are shaped by the face-to-face interactions that prescribing clinicians have with patients and their families. As one pediatric surgeon describes in a qualitative study about the barriers to getting surgeons to use antibiotics more judiciously:

> I would say surgeons are very much focused on the trees and not on the forest simply because – I mean, a mom gives me her baby. She just met me. She gives me her newborn baby and says "I trust you." I mean, it makes me want to throw up. Really, it does. Or like a case I recently did, it was this family's only child. They had been trying for 15 years to have this kid. They did IVF six times. It's a baby. In that moment that is all that motivates me. And I know there's this big grand epidemiological scheme we should be worrying about, but I just don't see it at that moment.[33]

The emotional dynamics that arise from the repeated interactions that occur between clinicians and patients at the bedside can be more motivating in terms of decision-making than evidence-based guidelines or the apparently far off threat of antibiotic resistance at the hospital or population level. As one clinician suggests, in a qualitative study of the prescribing experiences of hospital physicians, "my relationship with my patient is much stronger than my relationship with the hospital inpatient population and the microbial ether that we live in. You've got an emotional bond with that patient."[63] The "pull" of social relationships is stronger than the "push" of knowledge, guidelines, or awareness of the global threat of antibiotic resistance at the moment in which a prescribing decision is to be made.

(Mis)perception of the Problem

The final social determinant of antibiotic use stems from the way that prescribing clinicians perceive the problem of antibiotic overuse, resistance, adverse drug reactions, their own and others' prescribing habits, and the role of guidelines in driving practice. From a sociological perspective, understanding perceptions is of critical importance in making sense of why people behave the way that they do. As the Thomas theorem states "if men define situations as real, they are real in their consequences."[64] The way a person interprets a situation shapes their action within that situation. It is crucial to take perceptions seriously, regardless of accuracy, because they strongly influence behavior.

A robust literature has demonstrated how clinicians perceive the problem of antibiotic overuse, resistance, and stewardship interventions.[45, 65–69] Although attitudes may be changing as antibiotic resistant organisms infect more patients,[70] previous survey research has shown that clinicians often frame the problem of antibiotic resistance as a public health issue far removed from the everyday choices they make for their patients.[65, 71, 72] Qualitative work on the perceptions surrounding resistance finds clinicians describing it as a "theoretical" or "intellectual" concern, not a practical one.[62, 63] The mis- or overuse of antibiotics is not always tightly coupled to its negative consequences – clinicians cannot "see" directly how their behavior contributes to antibiotic resistance. This loose coupling impacts a clinician's motivation and risk perception surrounding the downsides of antibiotic use.[73] Adverse drug reactions and antibiotic-associated diarrhea are more proximal to the decision to use antibiotics unnecessarily or excessively; however, evidence suggests that these adverse consequences fail to shape physician decision-making and are not discussed with patients.[28] A resident in this qualitative study by Livorsi et al. suggests: "I think there is more pressure toward you are going to look bad if you missed something and did not treat it appropriately versus … giving people C. difficile and diarrhea, [which] is a little more anonymous." (p. 1069). Clinicians feel a more urgent sense of accountability for bad outcomes that directly reflect their decision-making.

Another repeated finding in this literature is that clinicians perceive that antibiotic overuse is a problem generally, but not locally at their own institutions.[65, 69] Clinicians also do not perceive that they overuse antibiotics themselves, even when presented with data to the contrary.[45, 69] When asked to locate responsibility for antibiotic overuse, clinicians frequently point to other medical specialties or clinical contexts as the biggest culprits, not their own. As one primary care pediatrician who had participated in an outpatient antibiotic stewardship intervention reasoned, "antibiotic overuse is a big problem, but pediatricians are probably the least offenders. Family practitioners, internists, ER doctors and the staff at urgent care or minute clinics, those are the greatest offenders."[45] This perception is crucially important because if a prescriber does not perceive that their actions contribute to antibiotic overuse, they may lack the motivation needed to change and be less responsive to improvement efforts aimed at changing their behavior.

Finally, investigators have found perceptions of exceptionalism, or the sense that one is unusual or unique in some way and therefore does not need to conform to normal rules or principles, to surround antibiotic use.[25] This is particularly true surrounding antibiotic prescribing guidelines, which clinicians may express skepticism about, thinking that guidelines do not apply to their patient population, believing that their own past experience and expertise trump the application of guidelines in everyday clinical practice,[74] or thinking about guidelines as "academic" and not always practical in application.[45]

Leveraging Social Determinants to Design Antibiotic Stewardship Interventions

Although antibiotic stewardship interventions have been modestly successful,[75] there is considerable room for improvement in the magnitude of their impact. We know that direct educational approaches generally do not result in sustained improvement,[76] which makes sense when we consider the complex factors that shape prescribing summarized in Figure 1 and in the preceding text. While restrictive stewardship interventions have been shown to result in a greater median change in antibiotic prescribing compared to persuasive interventions,[1, 2] this approach can be circumvented. A handful of studies have described dysfunctional behavioral reactions or work-arounds used by prescribing clinicians when restrictive interventions are implemented such as "stealth dosing," where prescribers wait until the prior approval period has ended for the day to order off-guideline or unnecessary restricted antibiotics.[77] Other studies have documented prescribing clinicians misrepresenting clinical information in order to get approval to prescribe the antibiotics that they believe are appropriate.[66, 78] These dysfunctional behavioral reactions limit the impact that stewardship interventions have and suggest that prescribing clinicians do not embrace the principles of judicious prescribing.

To achieve lasting change in the way that antibiotics are used, prescribing clinicians and patients need to internalize new social norms surrounding these drugs.[79] By this, we mean a shift in prescribing etiquette, the definition of prudent use, perceptions, and expectations surrounding antibiotics. In a sense, antibiotics have an image problem – despite the fact that they are critical, life-saving medications they do not stoke the same level of societal attention as chemotherapeutic, narcotic, or psychiatric drugs. This, coupled with the fact that their adverse effects are underappreciated and they are seen to be relatively "benign" in comparison with other medications, have put them at a perceptual disadvantage. We have to engage with the social determinants of antibiotic prescribing as described above to make change on a broad scale.

On a more local, immediate level, these social determinants must be incorporated into the design and implementation of antibiotic stewardship interventions. As the large literature in patient safety and quality improvement in health care attests, when developing any kind of intervention, it is crucial to understand the attitudes, motivations, and intentions of those whose behavior is the target of change[80] as well as the features of the local social and environmental context that may shape the successful uptake of the intervention.[81] The design of antibiotic stewardship interventions is in its infancy surrounding the incorporation of social determinants.

Two recent review articles argued that it is vitally important to understand the social, contextual, and behavioral factors that influence antibiotic prescribing before or in concert with the implementation of stewardship interventions.[6, 18] In one systematic review, Charani and colleagues found that, despite evidence to suggest the overwhelming importance of social and behavioral factors in influencing antibiotic prescribing, these factors are frequently overlooked in the design and implementation of stewardship interventions.[18] As a result they state, "when designing new interventions in antibiotic prescribing, it is paramount that primary research into prescribing behavioral intention of individuals is performed and that interventions are tailored to the target audience in whom behavior change is desired." This information can be used to develop interventions that are sensitive to local social context, a strategy that has been shown to be crucial for successful implementation of other patient safety and quality improvement initiatives in healthcare.[81–83] In the field of healthcare epidemiology and infectious diseases, researchers in infection prevention[84–86] have achieved success by incorporating sociobehavioral theory, methods, and approaches to identify barriers and facilitators to changing healthcare worker behavior to improve patient outcomes.

Application of behavioral economics theory to the design of antibiotic stewardship interventions has been successfully done by Meeker and colleagues.[27, 87] In one randomized controlled trial of a stewardship intervention, they investigated the use of a behavioral "nudge" based on the principle of public commitment on the judicious use of antibiotics for acute respiratory tract infections in outpatient primary care clinics in California. The intervention was simple and included placing a large, poster-sized commitment letter in the clinic's exam rooms for 12 weeks. The letter stated clearly that the practice was committed to only using antibiotics when necessary. The letter included photographs of clinicians working at the practice, as well as their signatures. This simple intervention was effective at improving guideline-concordant antibiotic prescribing. Controlling for baseline prescribing rates, they found that the posted commitment letter resulted in an almost 20 percent reduction in the rate of inappropriate prescribing relative to control.

Table 1 Tips for Designing Antibiotic Stewardship Interventions Using Sociobehavioral Research*

Sociobehavioral Principle	Strategy
Giving provider tools to mitigate patient pressure	• Pop up box in the electronic medical record (EMR) appears at the moment a provider selects an antibiotic for an unwarranted diagnosis with a list of suggested alternatives (over the counter symptom remedies) and tools to address patient concerns (letter templates to excuse the patient from work)
Holding providers publicly accountable for their prescribing behavior	• Free text pop up box in the EMR appears at the moment a provider selects an antibiotic for an unwarranted diagnosis with a requirement that the provider document the reasons for using an antibiotic; If provider chooses not to leave written justification this is noted in the patient's chart
Leveraging peer competition to motivate improved performance	• Providers emailed monthly about their performance relative to peers
Making a public commitment to a community to improve performance	• Hang poster-sized letters in clinic waiting rooms that state "the providers at this practice are committed to only using antibiotics when necessary" complete with photos of the prescriber and a signature

* The tips in this table are derived from research described in citations 26, 27, and 28

In a second study, this group conducted a large clustered randomized controlled trial among 47 adult primary care practices comparing the impact of three techniques based on behavioral science: suggested alternatives (electronic order set provides nonantibiotic alternative), accountable justification (clinician provides reason for prescribing antibiotic when not indicated), and peer comparisons (clinicians receive reports comparing an assessment of their prescribing behaviors with others).[87] The study randomized the practices to receive zero, one, two, or three of the interventions. Antibiotic prescribing was reduced significantly in the practices utilizing accountable justification (18 percent reduction) and peer comparisons (16 percent reduction). Other investigations have utilized peer comparisons to significantly improve antibiotic prescribing in ambulatory settings, such as the cluster randomized trial by Gerber and colleagues that provided prescribing report cards to individual clinicians depicting their own rates of broad-spectrum antibiotic use versus those of their colleagues.[88] These studies are an excellent model of a fruitful way to integrate sociobehavioral principles into the design of stewardship interventions. Table 1 summarizes some practical strategies for utilizing sociobehaviorally informed interventions to design stewardship interventions.

Thinking Sociologically about Stewardship Implementation

Resistant Clinicians

Despite the urgency surrounding antibiotic resistance and growing regulatory pressures, fewer than 50 percent of healthcare facilities in the United States perform regular stewardship activities.[89] A frequently cited barrier to the implementation of stewardship interventions, in addition to lack of resources and poor information technology infrastructure, is resistance from prescribing clinicians.[38, 90] As described above, some prescribing clinicians engage in dysfunctional behavioral reactions when exposed to antibiotic stewardship interventions, especially if they are restrictive, indicating the lack of full support for the principles of judicious prescribing. Resistance toward stewardship can be expressed along a continuum of slight frustration to more intense antagonism.[66] As one neonatologist at a hospital with restrictive stewardship describes, in a qualitative study about the perceptions of prescribing clinicians toward ASPs:

> Rarely do I have satisfying experiences with ID anymore. Where we have an interesting case and we work collaboratively to treat it. Now it's mostly "I'm not smart enough to pick an antibiotic." We've empowered ID at this hospital to build a wall and there is never humility for the other side. There is no "well I have great respect for your experience as a neonatologist and what it looks like to have a baby that might or might not be infected. And I don't see this as an infection but I support you and if you think you need to treat here is how I would do it." It's "nope, you're not allowed."[33]

Resistance toward stewardship interventions not only limits their impact on prescribing, but it also stokes antagonism between antibiotic stewards and prescribing clinicians, which is not productive, may lead to further conflict in other domains, and undermines the teamwork that has been shown to improve patient outcomes in an increasingly complex healthcare system.[91]

Dealing with resistant clinicians is part and parcel of any effort to change practice to improve healthcare safety and quality.[80, 84] It is important for those leading antibiotic stewardship efforts to recognize that addressing clinician resistance will require time, attention, and *social* solutions. Pronovost usefully distinguishes between "technical" and "adaptive" challenges that arise when trying to improve care delivery processes.[80] Technical challenges are logistical in nature whereas adaptive challenges are social, political, cultural, and emotional. Adaptive challenges are harder to address because they require changes in people's priorities, beliefs, habits, and loyalties.

While it may be tempting to discount actively resistant clinicians as stubborn or to attribute their objections to a difficult personality, to bring about lasting change, these individuals must be taken seriously. One way to do this is to identify and better understand the motivations of the resistant individual. Antibiotic stewards need to engage clinicians in recognizing a change is needed, but they also must accept that there are some aspects of practice that clinicians want to preserve.[80] Whether it a desire to maintain a sense of autonomy or a fear that an intervention will threaten the efficiency of their workflow, antibiotic stewards need to identify and address these adaptive threats to stewardship interventions. It is a mistake to treat an adaptive problem as a technical one.[79] Table 2 includes a series of strategies to use in understanding and engaging the resistant clinician.

Changing Social Norms about Antibiotics

While behavioral economic principles offer one route to changing clinician antibiotic prescribing behavior by manipulating the work environment to "nudge" better choices, sociological theory offers insights that can be leveraged to facilitate lasting change. The distinct contribution of sociology to the design of patient safety and quality improvement interventions is that we must not ignore the dynamics that characterize groups of people in healthcare settings and the interactions among them. As we have previously argued, there is

Table 2 Strategies for Understanding and Engaging the "Resistant" Clinician

Strategy	Example Actions
Investigate motivations of resistant clinician	• Host face-to-face meeting with clinician, some of their stewardship-friendly colleagues and the stewardship team to discuss contentious situations • Ask what the clinicians are concerned about and brainstorm solutions • Follow through on changes promised to resistant clinician
Engage stewardship-friendly clinical community members	• Enlist colleagues in the resistant clinician's department or specialty to act as a change agent by providing support for them in exchange for giving lectures to the department and championing stewardship interventions at administrative meetings • Start a special stewardship working group for the resistant clinician's department or specialty
Build trust between stewardship team and resistant clinicians	• Stewardship team members go on rounds with resistant clinicians to better understand his or her point of view • Be available and visible on the resistant clinician's unit to answer questions, understand the challenges of their patient population, and build credibility

an urgent need to fundamentally change the social norms surrounding antibiotics. Because norms exist at the level of the social group, we need to think about collective change and adapting our stewardship interventions to the different "agents" that exist in complex healthcare organizations.

One way to do this is to investigate whether there is variation in attitudes, social norms, and beliefs about antibiotics among prescribing clinicians from different specialties, a topic on which there is currently no research. Most stewardship interventions approach improving the use of antibiotics with a "one size fits all" strategy to changing prescriber behavior. These strategies do not take into account the distinct subcultures that influence how prescribers in different specialties approach their work or the "prescribing etiquette" that may shape intraspecialty relations.[25] Medical sociologists have long demonstrated that, far from being a monolithic whole, the profession of medicine is instead characterized by a number of groups that have distinctive identities that shape how clinicians orient to the delivery of clinical care,[92] hierarchical divisions with some subspecialties allotted greater prestige and status than others,[93–95] and efforts by medical specialties to maintain intra-professional boundaries and power via rejection of efforts to limit autonomy.[96] Given that antibiotics are used across all medical specialties, it is an important empirical question whether the attitudes, social norms, and beliefs about antibiotic use and stewardship vary by professional subculture. Future research should investigate this and use the results to inform the design of stewardship interventions to improve their impact and sustainability.

Instead of a "top-down" approach to stewardship, in which rules are imposed onto a group from outside, changing social norms about antibiotics will lead to "ground-up" stewardship, where frontline prescribing clinicians steward themselves and their peers.

Of course, changing norms takes time and effort directed at multiple domains of social life. Again, the infection prevention improvement literature provides a useful model. In their analysis of the Michigan Intensive Care Unit (ICU) Project, which successfully reduced rates of central venous catheter bloodstream infections (CVC-BSIs) in over 100 ICUs,[97] Dixon-Woods et al. trace the complex social factors that enabled the project to achieve its effects.[98] The project generated peer pressures for ICUs to join the program and act in accordance with its requirements. It also reframed CVC-BSIs as a social problem to be fixed via a grassroots professional movement using interventions to foster a culture of commitment to doing better in practice, harnessing data on infection rates as a disciplinary force, and using "hard edges" to promote accountability. While the public narrative about the Michigan ICU project is that a simple central line insertion checklist was the cause of the intervention's success, this analysis illustrates that it was far more complex and social in nature.[79] Antibiotic stewardship could be bolstered by considering interventions within networked communities of hospitals, wards, or particular groups of professions to leverage social support and peer pressure to improve performance.

Conclusion

In this chapter, we have demonstrated that the use of antibiotics is shaped by social, behavioral, and contextual factors. Antibiotic prescribing does not happen in a vacuum and is instead sensitive to the relationships that characterize everyday clinical practice, including the interactions between clinicians and those that clinicians have with patients. Treating suspected infections can sometimes be an uncertain task with serious consequences. Risk, fear, anxiety, and emotion are bound up in this task and may strongly shape the decision to use an antibiotic. The problem of antibiotic resistance suffers perceptually since it is difficult to link the behavior of any one person to the development of resistant organisms. These features of antibiotic prescribing suggest that we need to design stewardship interventions and generate implementation strategies that are informed by social and behavioral theory to achieve sustainable change. The threat of antibiotic resistance is urgent, frightening, and fundamentally social in nature. Mitigating this threat will require creative, multilevel solutions that draw from multiple disciplines.

References

1. Davey P, Brown E, Charani E, et al. Interventions to improve antibiotic prescribing practices for hospital inpatients. *Cochrane Database Syst Rev* 2013; 4: CD003543.

2. Mehta JM, Haynes K, Wileyto EP, et al. Comparison of prior authorization and prospective audit with feedback for antimicrobial stewardship. *Infect Control Hosp Epidemiol* 2014; 35(9):1092–1099.

3. Cosgrove SE, Seo SK, Bolon MK, et al. Evaluation of postprescription review and feedback as a method of promoting rational antimicrobial use: a multicenter intervention. *Infect Control Hosp Epidemiol* 2012; 33(4):374–380.

4. Cabana MD, Rand CS, Powe NR, et al. Why don't physicians follow clinical practice guidelines? A framework for improvement. *JAMA* 1999; 282(15):1458–1465.

5. Armstrong D. Clinical autonomy, individual and collective: the problem of changing doctors' behaviour. *Soc Sci Med* 2002; 55(10):1771–1777.

6. Hulscher ME, Grol RP, van der Meer JW. Antibiotic prescribing in hospitals: a social and behavioural scientific approach.

The Lancet Infectious Diseases. 2010; 10(3):167–175.

7. Fishman N. Antimicrobial stewardship. *Am J Med* 2006; 119(6 Suppl 1):S53–61; discussion S62–70.

8. Szymczak JE. 2013. "The Complexity of Simple Things: An Ethnographic Study of the Challenge of Preventing Hospital-Acquired Infections." PhD diss., University of Pennsylvania. ProQuest.

9. van der Geest S, Whyte S, Hardon A. The anthropology of pharmaceuticals: A biographical approach. *Annual Review of Anthropology* 1996; 25:25.

10. Smith M. The relationship between pharmacy and medicine. In: Mapes R, ed. *Prescribing Practice and Drug Usage*. London: Croom Helm, 1980:157–200.

11. Parsons T. *The Social System*. New York, NY: Free Press, 1951.

12. Conrad P. *The Medicalization of Society: On the Transformation of Human Conditions into Treatable Disorders*. Baltimore, MD: Johns Hopkins University Press, 2007.

13. Freidson E. *Profession of Medicine: A Study of the Sociology of Applied Knowledge*. New York, NY: Dodd Mead, 1970.

14. Szymczak JE, Bosk CL. Training for efficiency: work, time, and systems-based practice in medical residency. *J Health Soc Behav* 2012; 53(3):344–358.

15. Pellegrino E. Prescribing and drug ingestion: symbols and substances. *Drug Intell Clin Pharm* 1976; 10:6.

16. Charani E, Castro-Sanchez E, Holmes A. The role of behavior change in antimicrobial stewardship. *Infect Dis Clin North Am* 2014; 28(2):169–175.

17. Teixeira Rodrigues A, Roque F, Falcao A, Figueiras A, Herdeiro MT. Understanding physician antibiotic prescribing behaviour: a systematic review of qualitative studies. *Int J Antimicrob Agents* 2013; 41(3):203–212.

18. Charani E, Edwards R, Sevdalis N, et al. Behavior change strategies to influence antimicrobial prescribing in acute care: a systematic review. *Clin Infect Dis* 2011; 53(7):651–662.

19. Timmermans S. *Postmortem: How Medical Examiners Explain Suspicious Deaths*. Chicago, IL: University of Chicago Press, 2006.

20. Leidner R. *Fast Food, Fast Talk: Service Work and the Routinization of Everyday Life*. Berkeley, CA: University of California Press, 1993.

21. Bosk CL. *Forgive and Remember: Managing Medical Failure*. 2nd ed. Chicago, IL: University of Chicago Press, 2003.

22. Timmermans S. Seven warrants for qualitative health sociology. *Soc Sci Med* 2013; 77:1–8.

23. Bosk CL. Occupational rituals in patient management. *N Engl J Med* 1980; 303(2):71–76.

24. Dixon-Woods M, Suokas A, Pitchforth E, Tarrant C. An ethnographic study of classifying and accounting for risk at the sharp end of medical wards. *Soc Sci Med* 2009; 69(3):362–369.

25. Charani E, Castro-Sanchez E, Sevdalis N, et al. Understanding the determinants of antimicrobial prescribing within hospitals: the role of "prescribing etiquette." *Clin Infect Dis* 2013; 57(2):188–196.

26. Meeker D, Linder JA, Fox CR, et al. Effect of behavioral interventions on inappropriate antibiotic prescribing among primary care practices: a randomized clinical trial. *JAMA* 2016; 315(6):562–570.

27. Meeker D, Knight TK, Friedberg MW, et al. Nudging guideline-concordant antibiotic prescribing: a randomized clinical trial. *JAMA Intern Med* 2014; 174(3):425–431.

28. Livorsi D, Comer A, Matthias MS, Perencevich EN, Bair MJ. Factors influencing antibiotic-prescribing decisions among inpatient physicians: a qualitative investigation. *Infect Control Hosp Epidemiol* 2015; 36(9):1065–1072.

29. Cortoos PJ, De Witte K, Peetermans WE, Simoens S, Laekeman G. Opposing

expectations and suboptimal use of a local antibiotic hospital guideline: a qualitative study. *J Antimicrob Chemother* 2008; 62(1):189–195.

30. De Souza V, MacFarlane A, Murphy AW, Hanahoe B, Barber A, Cormican M. A qualitative study of factors influencing antimicrobial prescribing by non-consultant hospital doctors. *J Antimicrob Chemother* 2006; 58(4):840–843.

31. Lewis PJ, Tully MP. Uncomfortable prescribing decisions in hospitals: the impact of teamwork. *J R Soc Med* 2009; 102(11):481–488.

32. Laake AM, Yoon B, Bernabe KG, Adenew AB, Peterson J, Liappis AP. Prescribing habits of housestaff: an important component to effective antibiotic stewardship. IDWeek; 2013; San Francisco, CA. https://idsa.confex.com/idsa/2013/webprogram/Paper40704.html.

33. Szymczak JE, Gerber JS, Hamilton K. Barriers and facilitators to implementing antimicrobial stewardship in Philadelphia-area hospitals. Paper presented at the Society for Healthcare Epidemiology of America annual meeting; 2016; Atlanta, GA.

34. Walton M. Hierarchies: the Berlin Wall of patient safety. *Quality and Safety in Healthcare.* 2006; 15:2.

35. Minooee A, Rickman L. Expanding the role of the infection control professional in the cost-effective use of antibiotics. *American Journal of Infection Control* 2000; 28:8.

36. Broom A, Broom J, Kirby E, Plage S, Adams J. What role do pharmacists play in mediating antibiotic use in hospitals? A qualitative study. *BMJ Open* 2015; 5(e008326).

37. Armstrong D, Ogden J. The role of etiquette and experimentation in explaining how doctors change behaviour: a qualitative study. *Sociol Health Illn* 2006; 28(7):951–968.

38. Pakyz AL, Moczygemba LR, VanderWielen LM, Edmond MB, Stevens MP, Kuzel AJ. Facilitators and barriers to implementing antimicrobial stewardship strategies: results from a qualitative study. *American Journal of Infection Control* 2014; 42(10 Suppl): S257–263.

39. Schwappach D, Gehring K. "Saying it without words": a qualitative study of oncology staff's experiences with speaking up about safety concerns. *BMJ Open* 2014; 4(e004740).

40. Avorn J, Solomon DH. Cultural and economic factors that (mis)shape antibiotic use: the nonpharmacologic basis of therapeutics. *Ann Intern Med* 2000; 133(2):128–135.

41. May L, Gudger G, Armstrong P, et al. Multisite exploration of clinical decision making for antibiotic use by emergency medicine providers using quantitative and qualitative methods. *Infect Control Hosp Epidemiol* 2014; 35(9):1114–1125.

42. Bauchner H, Pelton S, Klein J. Parents, physicians, and antibiotic use. *Pediatrics* 1999; 103(2):6.

43. Brookes-Howell L, Hood K, Cooper L, et al. Understanding variation in primary medical care: a nine-country qualitative study of clinicians' accounts of the non-clinical factors that shape antibiotic prescribing decisions for lower respiratory tract infection. *BMJ Open* 2012; 2(4): e000796.

44. Vazquez-Lago JM, Lopez-Vazquez P, Lopez-Duran A, Taracido-Trunk M, Figueiras A. Attitudes of primary care physicians to the prescribing of antibiotics and antimicrobial resistance: a qualitative study from Spain. *Fam Pract* 2012; 29(3):352–360.

45. Szymczak JE, Feemster KA, Zaoutis TE, Gerber JS. Pediatrician perceptions of an outpatient antimicrobial stewardship intervention. *Infect Control Hosp Epidemiol* 2014; 35 Suppl 3:S69–78.

46. van Buul L, van der Steen J, Doncker S, et al. Factors influencing antibiotic prescribing in long-term care facilities: a qualitative in-depth study. *BMC Geriatrics* 2014; 14(136).

47. Fleming A, Bradley C, Cullinan S, Byrne S. Antibiotic prescribing in long-term care facilities: a qualitative, multidisciplinary

investigation. *BMJ Open* 2014; 4(11): e006442.

48. Butler CC, Rollnick S, Pill R, Maggs-Rapport F, Stott N. Understanding the culture of prescribing: qualitative study of general practitioners' and patients' perceptions of antibiotics for sore throats. *BMJ* 1998; 317(7159):637–642.

49. Linder JA, Doctor JN, Friedberg MW, et al. Time of day and the decision to prescribe antibiotics. *JAMA Intern Med* 2014; 174(12):2029–2031.

50. Mangione-Smith R, McGlynn E, Elliott M, Krogstad P, Brook R. The relationship between perceived parental expectations and pediatrician antimicrobial prescribing behavior. *Pediatrics* 1999; 103(4 Pt 1):7.

51. Stivers T, Mangione-Smith R, Elliott M, McDonald L, Heritage J. Why do physicians think parents expect antibiotics? What parents report vs what physicians believe. *Journal of Family Practice* 2003; 52(2):8.

52. Mangione-Smith R, Elliott M, Stivers T, McDonald L, Heritage J. Ruling out the need for antibiotics: are we sending the right message? *Arch Pediatr Adolesc Med* 2006; 160(9):7.

53. Mangione-Smith R, McGlynn E, Elliott M, McDonald L, Franz C, Kravitz R. Parent expectations for antibiotics, physician-parent communication, and satisfaction. *Arch Pediatr Adolesc Med* 2001; 155(7):6.

54. Finkelstein J, Dutta-Linn M, Meyer R, Goldman R. Childhood infections, antibiotics, and resistance: what are parents saying now? *Clinical Pediatrics (Philadelphia)* 2014; 53:5.

55. Szymczak JE, Klieger S, Vendetti N, Miller M, Fiks AG, Gerber JS. What parents think about antibiotics for their child's acute respiratory tract infection. IDWeek 2015; San Diego, CA.

56. Ong S, Nakase J, Moran GJ, et al. Antibiotic use for emergency department patient wiht upper respiratory infections: Prescribing practices, patient expectations and patient satisfaction. *Ann Emerg Med.* 2007; 50(3):7.

57. Fox RC. Training for uncertainty. In *The Student-Physician: Introductory Studies in the Sociology of Medical Education.* Edited by Robert K. Merton, George Reader, and Patricia L. Kendall, 207–241. Cambridge, MA: Harvard University Press, 1957.

58. Light Jr D. Uncertainty and control in professional training. *J Health Soc Behav* 1979; 20(4):310–322.

59. Aronowitz R. *Risky Medicine: Our Quest to Cure Fear and Uncertainty.* Chicago, IL: University of Chicago Press, 2015.

60. Fox RC. The evolution of medical uncertainty. *The Milbank Memorial Fund Quarterly, Health and Society* 1980:1–49.

61. Flanders SA, Saint S. Enhancing the safety of hospitalized patients: who is minding the antimicrobials? Comment on overtreatment of enterococcal bacteriuria. *Arch Inter Med* 2012; 172(1):38–40.

62. Bjorkman I, Berg J, Roing M, Erntell M, Lundborg CS. Perceptions among Swedish hospital physicians on prescribing of antibiotics and antibiotic resistance. *Qual Saf Health Care* 2010; 19(6):e8.

63. Broom A, Broom J, Kirby E. Cultures of resistance? A Bourdieusian analysis of doctors' antibiotic prescribing. *Soc Sci Med* 2014; 110:81–88.

64. Thomas W, Thomas D. *The Children in America: Behavior Problems and Programs.* New York: Knopf; 1928.

65. Giblin TB, Sinkowitz-Cochran RL, Harris PL, et al. Clinicians' perceptions of the problem of antimicrobial resistance in health care facilities. *Arch Intern Med* 2004; 164(15):1662–1668.

66. Seemungal IA, Bruno CJ. Attitudes of housestaff toward a prior-authorization-based antibiotic stewardship program. *Infect Control Hosp Epidemiol* 2012; 33(4):429–431.

67. Wood F, Phillips C, Brookes-Howell L, et al. Primary care clinicians' perceptions of antibiotic resistance: a multi-country qualitative interview study. *J Antimicrob Chemother* 2013; 68(1):237–243.

68. Stach LM, Hedican EB, Herigon JC, Jackson MA, Newland JG. Clinicians' attitudes towards an antimicrobial stewardship program at a children's

hospital. *J Pediatric Infect Dis Soc* 2012; 1(3):190–197.

69. Abbo L, Sinkowitz-Cochran R, Smith L, et al. Faculty and resident physicians' attitudes, perceptions, and knowledge about antimicrobial use and resistance. *Infect Control Hosp Epidemiol* 2011; 32(7):714–718.

70. CDC. *Antibiotic Resistance Threats in the United States.* Atlanta, GA: CDC, 2013.

71. Brinsley KJ, Sinkowitz-Cochran RL, Cardo DM, Team CDCCtPAR. Assessing motivation for physicians to prevent antimicrobial resistance in hospitalized children using the Health Belief Model as a framework. *Am J Infect Control* 2005; 33(3):175–181.

72. Wester CW, Durairaj L, Evans AT, Schwartz DN, Husain S, Martinez E. Antibiotic resistance: a survey of physician perceptions. *Arch Intern Med* 2002; 162(19):2210–2216.

73. Dixon-Woods M, Suokas A, Pitchforth E, Tarrant C. An ethnographic study of classifying and accounting for risk at the sharp end of medical wards. *Soc Sci Med* 2009; 69(3):362–369.

74. Grant A, Sullivan F, Dowell J. An ethnographic exploration of influences on prescribing in general practice: why is there variation in prescribing practices? *Implementation Science* 2013; 8:72.

75. Wagner B, Filice GA, Drekonja D, et al. Antimicrobial stewardship programs in inpatient hospital settings: a systematic review. *Infect Control Hosp Epidemiol* 2014; 35(10):1209–1228.

76. Arnold SR, Straus SE. Interventions to improve antibiotic prescribing practices in ambulatory care. *Cochrane Database Syst Rev* 2005; 4:CD003539.

77. LaRosa LA, Fishman NO, Lautenbach E, Koppel RJ, Morales KH, Linkin DR. Evaluation of antimicrobial therapy orders circumventing an antimicrobial stewardship program: investigating the strategy of "stealth dosing." *Infect Control Hosp Epidemiol* 2007; 28(5):551–556.

78. Calfee DP, Brooks J, Zirk NM, Giannetta ET, Scheld WM, Farr BM.

A pseudo-outbreak of nosocomial infections associated with the introduction of an antibiotic management programme. *J Hosp Infect* 2003; 55(1):26–32.

79. Bosk CL, Dixon-Woods M, Goeschel CA, Pronovost PJ. Reality check for checklists. *Lancet* 2009; 374(9688):444–445.

80. Pronovost PJ. Navigating adaptive challenges in quality improvement. *BMJ Quality & Safety* 2011; 20(7):560–563.

81. Aveling EL, Martin G, Armstrong N, Banerjee J, Dixon-Woods M. Quality improvement through clinical communities: eight lessons for practice. *JHOM* 2012; 26(2):158–174.

82. Sawyer M, Weeks K, Goeschel CA, et al. Using evidence, rigorous measurement, and collaboration to eliminate central catheter-associated bloodstream infections. *Crit Care Med* 2010; 38(8 Suppl):S292–298.

83. Anthierens S, Tonkin-Crine S, Douglas E, et al. General practitioners' views on the acceptability and applicability of a web-based intervention to reduce antibiotic prescribing for acute cough in multiple European countries: a qualitative study prior to a randomised trial. *BMC Fam Pract* 2012; 13:101.

84. Saint S, Kowalski CP, Banaszak-Holl J, Forman J, Damschroder L, Krein SL. How active resisters and organizational constipators affect health care-acquired infection prevention efforts. *Jt Comm J Qual Patient Saf* 2009; 35(5):239–246.

85. Saint S, Kowalski CP, Banaszak-Holl J, Forman J, Damschroder L, Krein SL. The importance of leadership in preventing healthcare-associated infection: results of a multisite qualitative study. *Infect Control Hosp Epidemiol* 2010; 31(9):901–907.

86. Greene MT, Saint S. Followership characteristics among infection preventionists in U.S. hospitals: results of a national survey. *Am J Infect Control* 2016; 44(3):343-345.

87. Meeker D, Linder JA, Fox CR, et al. Effect of behavioral interventions on inappropriate antibiotic prescribing among primary care practices: a randomized clinical trial. *JAMA* 2016; 315(6):562–570.

88. Gerber JS, Prasad PA, Fiks AG, et al. Effect of an outpatient antimicrobial stewardship intervention on broad-spectrum antibiotic prescribing by primary care pediatricians: a randomized trial. *JAMA* 2013; 309(22):2345–2352.

89. Septimus EJ, Owens RC, Jr. Need and potential of antimicrobial stewardship in community hospitals. *Clin Infect Dis* 2011; 53 Suppl 1:S8-S14.

90. Pope SD, Dellit TH, Owens RC, Hooton TM. Results of survey on implementation of Infectious Diseases Society of America and Society for Healthcare Epidemiology of America guidelines for developing an institutional program to enhance antimicrobial stewardship. *Infect Control Hosp Epidemiol* 2009; 30(1):97–98.

91. Wells R, Jinnett K, Alexander J, Lichtenstein R, Liu D, Zazzali JL. Team leadership and patient outcomes in US psychiatric treatment settings. *Soc Sci Med* 2006; 62(8):1840–1852.

92. Bucher R, Strauss A. Professions in process. *American Journal of Sociology*. 1961; 22(2):6.

93. Abbott A. Status and status strain in the professions. *American Journal of Sociology* 1981; 86(4):16.

94. Nancarrow S, Borthwick A. Dynamic professional boundaries in the helathcare workforce. *Sociol Health Illn* 2005; 27(7):22.

95. Sanders T, Harrison S. Professional legitimacy claims in the mulitidisciplinary workplace: the case of heart failure care. *Sociol Health Illn* 2008; 30(2):19.

96. Oh H. Hospital consultations and jurisdiction over patients: consequences for the medical profession. *Sociol Health Illn* 2014; 36(4):15.

97. Pronovost P, Needham D, Berenholtz S, et al. An intervention to decrease catheter-related bloodstream infections in the ICU. *N Engl J Med* 2006; 355 (26):2725–2732.

98. Dixon-Woods M, Bosk CL, Aveling EL, Goeschel CA, Pronovost PJ. Explaining Michigan: developing an ex post theory of a quality improvement program. *Milbank Q.* 2011; 89(2):167–205.

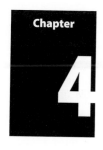

Chapter 4

Selecting and Applying Antibiotic Stewardship Strategies

Rebekah W. Moehring and Whitney J. Nesbitt

The practice of antibiotic stewardship (AS) is complex with many possible strategies. Guidelines stress the importance of tailoring stewardship strategies to the needs and infrastructure of each institution.[1, 2] There is no "one size fits all" mix of initiatives, policies, and daily work duties for an antibiotic stewardship program (ASP). Outcomes data comparing different antibiotic stewardship strategies to each other are lacking. Most studies compare an ASP intervention to a standard of care without that intervention.[1, 3] As a result, there is large variation in how ASPs are designed and how AS is practiced even among well-established programs. Thus, it is challenging to predict which strategies are most likely to be successful and fit best with local institutional culture. More evidence-based research is needed to guide these program design decisions. ASP design must also address current and future regulatory requirements.[4, 5]

The goals of this chapter are to 1) provide an overview of the process of selecting strategies for antibiotic stewardship and 2) discuss successful antibiotic stewardship strategies including strategies recommended in guidelines as well as other targeted strategies for specific clinical disease states and patient scenarios.[1] Readers are encouraged to review the Infectious Diseases Society of America (IDSA)/Society for Healthcare Epidemiology of America (SHEA) guidelines for Implementing an Antibiotic Stewardship Program,[1] the CDC's Core Elements of Hospital and Outpatient Antibiotic Stewardship Programs, [6, 7] and The Joint Commission Antimicrobial Stewardship Standard.[8]

Overview of the Process for Selecting Antibiotic Stewardship Strategies

Selection of strategies for an ASP should be based on a clear understanding of institutional needs and available resources. We recommend that a program evaluation and needs assessment be completed at least annually to maintain a focused direction for the ASP and to highlight and celebrate past achievements (**Table 1**). This evaluation should then be used to develop a written annual plan that can be presented to relevant hospital committees and discussed with leadership. The annual ASP plan should define the strategic approach and establish expectations and timelines for the coming year. The plan may also include longer, three- to five-year goals for the program and define the necessary incremental steps to achieve them.

Needs should be assessed by asking questions and gathering information to better define areas for improvement and program development. Targeted areas for intervention may include specific prescribing practices (e.g., double anaerobe coverage), treatment of certain clinical syndromes or scenarios (e.g., treatment of community-acquired pneumonia),

Table 1 Items to Define during Antibiotic Stewardship Strategic Planning

Needs	Prescribing practices to target for intervention
	Clinical syndromes or clinical scenarios to target for intervention
	Practice settings to target for intervention
	Patient populations to target for intervention
	"Problem" pathogens
	Cost savings
	Regulatory requirements
	Personnel or other resource deficits
	Expectations from hospital leadership
Resources	Personnel for daily ASP interventions
	Multidisciplinary champions (e.g., microbiology, infection prevention, hospital medicine, surgery, pediatrics, nursing)
	Champion(s) within hospital leadership
	Data and informatics resources (e.g., electronic medical record (EMR), CPOE, surveillance software, data analysts)
	Existing educational avenues
Accomplishments	Successful ASP initiatives and ongoing activities
Planned Assessments	Medication use evaluations (MUE)
	Infectious syndrome-based clinical management assessments
	Monitoring the impact of ongoing activities
	Monitoring the impact of new initiatives

specific practice settings or patient populations, targeted drug-resistant pathogens (e.g., carbapenem-resistant *Enterobacteriaceae*), and/or requirements for cost-saving initiatives. Needs may also include seeking additional support for program personnel and data resources. These resources may include dedicated funding for ASP team personnel or funds to facilitate stewardship-focused training. Data resource needs may include dedicated effort to establish a standardized tracking system for antibiotic use, such as reporting to the National Healthcare Safety Network Antimicrobial Use and Resistance Module.[9] At a minimum, data resource needs should include access to quarterly antibiotic utilization data such as days of antibiotic therapy per 1,000 patient days.

ASP leaders should seek to gain a practical understanding of expectations from hospital leadership. For example, hospital leadership may expect that the ASP will achieve impact in high-priority areas (e.g., reductions in rates of *C. difficile* infection), cost savings, adherence with reporting requirements, and/or compliance with regulatory requirements (see Chapter 14). ASP leaders must also gain a sense of institutional "culture" when planning their strategy. The culture of an institution is a complex concept that may include provider attitudes, perceptions, and a qualitative understanding of institutional history, authority, and politics. Provider perceptions of the ASP can be assessed with a qualitative survey performed as a part of the needs assessment process. The aim of the survey may be to identify common misconceptions about ASP practices, how much providers feel resistance is a problem on which they have influence, and awareness and "satisfaction" with the ASP, as well as methods in which they would like to receive feedback concerning their antibiotic use. [10] No standardized guides or checklists for assessing ASP needs have been widely adopted. CDC provides *The Core Elements of Hospital Antibiotic Stewardship Programs*

Checklist as well as a gap analysis example, which may provide good starting points.[11, 12] In our opinion, ASP leaders must gather a broader, qualitative understanding of stakeholders, expectations, institution-specific practice, and attitudes than can be captured with a simple checklist.

In-depth analyses, such as medication use evaluations or syndrome-based antibiotic use evaluations, may be necessary to gain insight and better define the problem areas before specific antibiotic stewardship strategies can be selected and implemented. Thus, we recommend that ASP annual plans include an outline for proposed evaluations for the coming year. This should include plans for monitoring the impact of ongoing ASP activities as well as new initiatives (see Chapter 7).

In addition to identifying needs, a careful assessment of key assets and resources available to the ASP should be well defined and utilized during strategic planning. For example, available personnel resources for daily antibiotic stewardship functions may determine if the implementation strategy takes on a centralized (e.g., specialized ASP pharmacist and physician using expertise and clinical judgment for patient-level interventions) or decentralized model (e.g., multiple clinical pharmacists making interventions by protocol or daily work routine). Similarly, other personnel that have expertise in infectious diseases (e.g., microbiology and infectious diseases physicians), established rapport with clinical staff (e.g., a hospitalist leader), and influence with hospital leadership can be recruited to serve key roles in ASP implementation. Data systems resources such as electronic medical records, computerized physician order entry (CPOE), surveillance software, and dedicated analyst time can be leveraged to improve the workflow and practical implementation of stewardship strategies (see Chapter 10). Educational avenues for clinical staff that are already well established can be used to deliver content specific to the aims of the ASP. A careful understanding of resources is essential for the ASP to develop realistic implementation plans for new initiatives and optimization of existing activities.

Prioritizing strategies that are both important for quality of care and achievable are key to ensure the program adopts reasonable goals and does not overcommit. Demonstration of cost savings may be necessary to gain support for the program, especially when seeking additional personnel resources for the ASP. Decisions on which strategies to pursue first should include careful estimates of the amount of effort and time necessary to achieve implementation. Strategic decisions and timelines should be based on urgency of institutional needs and available resources for implementation.

Once the ASP finds a strategy that works well, key characteristics and experience from prior successes should be utilized in implementation planning for new initiatives. The ASP team should be encouraged to appreciate and reflect on past successes. The satisfaction that comes from success can be used to highlight contributions from each team member, boost morale, and motivate the group to address the next challenge. These successes should be shared with frontline staff. Frontline staff should understand how they played a role in improving antibiotic use and potentially avoiding adverse events associated with unnecessary antibiotics use. Successful strategies can also be disseminated or adapted to other practice settings within the same institution or for health system or network-level ASP interventions.

After selection of antibiotic stewardship strategies, the ASP team must engage in implementation planning. Implementation is an iterative process that may result in many adjustments and changes as the team discovers how and where their efforts are successful. In 2012, the CDC partnered with the Institute for Healthcare Improvement to develop and define the drivers of change for reducing inappropriate antibiotic utilization.[13] In this exercise, a group of experts and pilot ASPs developed a "driver diagram and change package," which is a conceptual model that outlines several broad areas to explore and monitor stewardship efforts. The four primary drivers were as follows: 1) timely and appropriate initiation of antibiotics, 2) appropriate administration and de-escalation, 3) data monitoring, transparency, and stewardship infrastructure, and 4) availability of expertise at the point of care. Suggested areas to further pursue and define within each primary driver were included, which could then be used to develop detailed ASP implementation plans. Whichever implementation plan is pursued, the cycle of plan, do, study, act (PDSA) has been promoted to continue optimizing quality as an ongoing, evolving process.[14] The adaptive quality of antibiotic stewardship is a key advantage because the targets for improved antibiotic use, advances in medical knowledge, and new regulatory requirements dictate that ASPs keep pace with changing practice.

Successful Antibiotic Stewardship Strategies

One way to organize the different stewardship strategies into a conceptual framework is to place them into four categories based on two factors: 1) Do they occur before prescribing or after prescribing? and 2) Do they require an active or passive interaction with prescribers? [15] Active interventions require direct interaction with or action from a prescriber. Passive interventions provide indirect interactions in which the prescriber can seek out information in prescribing decisions if they chooses to do so. A mix of both active and passive approaches, before and after prescribing, is likely to have the greatest impact. Many passive interventions can be integrated with active interventions to maximize impact.

In this chapter, we will first discuss passive strategies that are most effective when integrated with active antibiotic stewardship interventions. Second, we discuss two active strategies that have a strong evidence basis: formulary restriction with preauthorization and prospective audit and feedback. Third, we discuss strategies that are targeted to specific clinical syndromes, clinical scenarios, practice settings, or antibiotics that have more limited evidence to support their use.

Passive Antibiotic Stewardship Strategies that Should Be Integrated with Active Interventions

Institution-specific treatment guidelines As a key resource for supporting ASP activities, institution-specific guidelines for the clinical management of infectious diseases should be a high priority for development. National guidelines, while a good starting point, may not provide the best options for local patient populations that carry their own specific clinical and epidemiologic risk factors. Institution-specific treatment guidelines for commonly encountered disease states should be tailored to local resistance data, local patient population characteristics, and the local formulary. Examples of common clinical syndromes to target for institution-specific treatment guidelines include skin and soft tissue infection, intra-abdominal infection, pneumonia (community- and hospital-acquired), urinary tract infection, and surgical prophylaxis (see Chapter 5). Implementation and adherence to these guidelines can help streamline and standardize antibiotic decision-making.

Convincing clinicians to use the guidelines, however, is the challenge and requires consideration of how the guidelines will be promoted and delivered to frontline providers.

The institution-specific guidelines can then be used as the standard reference when developing clinical pathways and order sets, performing one-on-one antibiotic stewardship interventions, and assessing adherence to local criteria for use of specific antibiotics. Guidelines can also be highlighted during formal educational sessions, posted on the hospital intranet, and integrated into clinical decision support systems. Guidelines must be reviewed regularly to incorporate changes in local data and updates in national guidelines to keep them relevant and useful for clinicians and the ASP.

Provider education Provider-focused educational initiatives aim to expand clinical providers' knowledge about antibiotics and infectious diseases. Educational strategies reinforce key principles of antibiotic stewardship, raise awareness of the need for the ASP, and can provide "face time" for ASP leaders to better establish their role as local experts in antibiotic stewardship. The importance of education for prescribers is highlighted in the IDSA/SHEA guidelines, the CDC Core Elements of Hospital and Outpatient Antibiotic Stewardship Programs, and The Joint Commission Antimicrobial Stewardship Standard.[1, 6–8] Traditional educational avenues such as lectures or didactic presentations to physician groups at grand rounds or continuing medical education presentations can reach many providers at one time. However, one-time or infrequent educational sessions without any ongoing active interventions do not reliably result in sustained change.[16, 17] Negative feedback, lack of participation, and/or lack of acceptance from some providers are nearly inevitable.

Innovation in delivery of educational content may help combat some of these barriers. Some examples include access to ASP resources and education at the point of care (e.g., through hospital intranet, mobile devices, or pocket cards), providing education at convenient times (e.g., through web-based modules or webinars), and maintaining interaction with providers in a convenient location (e.g., faculty lounges or physician work stations). In general, any major ASP initiative will require some education and informational communication with clinicians – especially if it may result in a change in workflow or is designed to impact prescriber decision-making.

An excellent demonstration of integrating educational interventions with an active intervention is available from the pediatric outpatient setting. A cluster-randomized study in outpatient pediatric clinics compared a one-hour educational intervention alone to education plus audit and feedback of prescriber-specific, aggregate, comparative antibiotic use data.[18] The audit and feedback intervention significantly reduced the use of broad-spectrum antibiotics for respiratory illness by approximately half and off-guideline use of antibiotics for pneumonia by approximately 75%, while education alone showed reductions of approximately 20% and 5%, respectively.[18] In another example, institutions using preauthorization incorporated educational counseling interviews with prescribers to improve their baseline knowledge rather than only providing directed feedback on the prescribed treatment.[19] As a result, antibiotic consumption was reduced by 26%, and appropriate antibiotic use was improved by 26%. Thus, education for providers has the most impact when integrated into ongoing, active interventions.

Recommended Active Interventions for Antibiotic Stewardship

Two evidence-based strategies, namely 1) preauthorization and 2) prospective audit and feedback, are the most commonly used interventions and have been recommended strategies for ASPs in multiple iterations of IDSA/SHEA guidelines.[20–22] These intervention strategies target prescribing decisions at different time points: before prescribing or after prescribing. Both strategies have proven effective in decreasing antibiotic use and costs while improving clinical outcomes.[3, 23] These strategies, however, are not without limitations and challenges (see **Table 2**).

Table 2 Antibiotic Stewardship Program Strategies

Strategy	Description	Benefits	Challenges
Preauthorization	Requirement for providers to seek ASP review and approval of antibiotic therapy prior to initiation	Improved antibiotic selection and clinical outcomes Decreased antibiotic consumption and expenditures "Mini-consult" with directed education for providers	Perceived loss of prescriber autonomy Time intensive Difficult to cover 24 hours, 7 days a week Unintended increases in non-restricted antibiotics Increased level of education and skill needed for ASP personnel
Prospective Audit and Feedback	ASP review of patients on select antibiotics after initiation of therapy with directed feedback to provider	Improved antibiotic selection and clinical outcomes Decreased antibiotic consumption and expenditures Directed education for provider	Recommendations are voluntary and may not be accepted Increased level of education and skill needed for ASP personnel Resource intensive Requires IT resources to accurately identify targeted patients for review
Institution-Specific Treatment Guidelines	Institutional guidelines that tailor recommendations from national guidelines to local resistance data, patient population, and formulary	Institution-specific recommendations increase relevance and utility compared to national guidelines Streamlined and standardized antibiotic decision-making Improved antibiotic selection and clinical outcomes	Clinician uptake and adherence Resources needed for assessment of adherence Need to maintain updates

Table 2 (cont.)

Strategy	Description	Benefits	Challenges
Education	Education provided in large-group format or through written ASP and hospital resources (e.g., policy) to expand clinical providers' knowledge about antibiotics and ID.	Large-group format may reach many providers at one time Reinforcement of key principles, raise awareness for ASP, and provide "face time" for ASP leaders	Does not result in sustained change without integration into an active strategy
Clinical Pathways and Order Sets	Syndrome-based guidance for antibiotic selection and diagnostics at the time of order entry	Integrates institutional guidelines into an implementation tool Encourages appropriate antibiotic selection and dosing for common infectious conditions Helps standardize antibiotic decisions	Limited uptake and use of the order sets Time consuming to design and maintain updates Requires IT resources to implement
Syndrome- or Culture-Based Audit and Feedback	ASP review of patients with specific clinical syndromes or positive microbiology culture results with directed feedback to providers	Improved antibiotic selection and clinical outcomes Corrects bug-drug mismatch events Encourages de-escalation based on microbiology result Messaging with frontline clinicians simplified by focus on syndrome-based decision-making	Requires notification system or process to identify eligible patients for review May require IT resources
Rapid Diagnostics	Diagnostic technologies which provide rapid identification and/or susceptibility information compared to traditional microbiology methods	Improves time to appropriate therapy compared to traditional microbiology methods. Encourages more rapid de-escalation decisions.	Clinician uptake and response to result For best effect, should integrate into active ASP activities (e.g., audit and feedback)
Allergy Initiatives	ASP-led initiatives to improve allergy assessments	Improve patient outcomes by increasing use of first-line therapies	Requires education at all levels (patient, nursing, pharmacy, providers)

Table 2 (cont.)

Strategy	Description	Benefits	Challenges
		Reduce use of non-beta-lactam alternative agents (e.g., vancomycin, clindamycin, aztreonam, fluoroquinolones)	May require IT support May require additional resources for skin-testing protocols
Dose-Optimization Protocols	Administration of an antibiotic dose based on patient-specific factors and antibiotic pharmacokinetic/ pharmacodynamic properties	More appropriate dosage regimen and better patient outcomes Improves safety by decreasing risk of adverse events Improvement in appropriate laboratory monitoring	Requires significant and ongoing educational efforts, routine re-assessments, and efforts to implement into pharmacy workflow.
Intravenous to Oral Conversion	Automatic conversion of intravenous to oral formulations for antibiotics with high oral bioavailability	"Low-hanging fruit" Significant cost savings without compromised effectiveness or safety Reduced incidence of catheter-related infections Decreased length of hospital stay Can be incorporated into routine pharmacy activities	Resources are necessary to enable real-time review Incorporating into pharmacy workflow when there are competing priorities
Automatic Infectious Diseases Consultation	"Automatic" ID consultation when required for eligible patients based on a hospital policy	Improved survival, reduced complications, and reduced readmissions Increased administration of appropriate therapy, improved standards for diagnostic testing, and appropriate durations of therapy	Cannot be applied where ID physicians are not available Acceptance of policy by non-ID physicians
ASP Rounds on High-Risk Units	Target high-priority practice areas by performing	Expanded ASP influence	Time intensive Labor intensive

Table 2 (cont.)

Strategy	Description	Benefits	Challenges
	multidisciplinary patient rounds on a routine basis	Direct provider education and influence on antibiotic therapy In-depth, patient-centered reviews	Difficulty engaging targeted prescriber groups
Antibiotic "Time-Outs"	Routine procedure for frontline providers to review and document agent choice, dose, duration, microbiology data, and indication	Potential for increased awareness of appropriate antibiotic therapy Viable option for ASPs with limited resources May be integrated into EMR processes	Paucity of data demonstrating impact on clinical outcomes and antibiotic consumption Prescribers may complete time-out documentation but not change their antibiotic decisions "Alert fatigue"
Automatic Stop Orders	Use of an antibiotic is permitted for a defined period of time and then requires approval for continuation	Decreased inappropriate use of antibiotics	Inadvertent and inappropriate discontinuation of antibiotics Resources required to maintain the procedures
Cascading or Tiered Antibiotic Susceptibility Reports	Collaborative effort with Microbiology to select specific susceptibility tests to include on clinical culture reports while censoring others	Improved antibiotic utilization Decreased resistance	Provider frustration Inaccurate assumption of susceptibility for agents not reported
Peer comparison data feedback to prescriber	Feedback of antibiotic use and/or appropriateness of prescribing data to the prescriber to allow comparison to other prescribers	Improved appropriateness of prescribing Identifies specific prescribers to target ASP educational effort and interventions Provides positive reinforcement to top performers as well as incentive to change behavior in poor performers	Requires a standardized EMR to collect and analyze data confidential for feedback Requires an adequate sample of prescribers or practices for valid comparison Requires development of an accepted definition of appropriate use

Preauthorization

Preauthorization has been utilized as early as the 1960s and is the longest standing ASP philosophy [24] An institutional formulary may be "open" without access limitations to a prescriber. Most institutions, however, have developed a system comprised of a selected list of approved medications to better control costs and manage supply. A "closed" formulary designates certain drugs as formulary versus non-formulary agents, which can limit availability by influencing decisions to stock them in the pharmacy. Designating high cost agents and infrequently used agents as non-formulary can be cost-saving as prescribers must choose among available lower cost alternatives or pursue a non-formulary process for obtaining the agent. Safety and efficacy of this approach is limited if drug-drug interaction software is not activated in the order entry of non-formulary antibiotics or prescribers are able to order through a request process that does not include review of appropriateness.[25] Non-formulary agents may be necessary and appropriate in certain clinical scenarios, so the non-formulary process must include reasonable expectations to obtain the agent when those scenarios are encountered.

Formulary system processes must be carefully considered and continually updated by a multidisciplinary group of pharmacists, physicians, and other experts to respond to changes in clinical practice and pharmaceutical markets. This designated group of practitioners commonly makes up what is known as the Pharmacy and Therapeutics (P&T) Committee. Generally, formulary decisions become hospital pharmacy policy after approval by the P&T Committee. Many ASPs influence formulary decisions by making recommendations to the P&T Committee through an Antibiotic Subcommittee or as voting members of P&T. Formulary management, including antibiotic restriction and streamlining the number of antibiotics available for use within the same class, is a crucial function of ASPs.

Formulary restriction is the act of limiting access of formulary medications to specific patients or clinical services based on areas of expertise (e.g., infectious diseases [ID] consultation), patient disease state, clinical scenario, or patient location. ASPs may use multiple sources of data to inform their rationales for antibiotic restriction including antibiograms, antibiotic use assessments, infection incidence, and costs. Restricting broad-spectrum agents, such as fluoroquinolones, have resulted in decreased incidence of *C. difficile* infections.[26, 27] ASPs have also restricted other broad-spectrum, expensive, or newly approved antibiotics, such as carbapenems, daptomycin, and ceftolozane-tazobactam. Formulary restrictions may be employed by requiring prescribers to enter either an infectious diagnosis or an appropriate indication for use based on established criteria at the time of prescribing either on paper order forms or electronically via CPOE.[28, 29] Criteria may be based on patient-specific factors, such as allergies, antibiotic history, concomitant medications, or presence of antibiotic-resistant pathogens. This method may be circumvented if prescribers falsely identify indications for use or are able to enter indications outside the predefined set of criteria.[30] In addition to an electronic medical record (EMR), monitoring and enforcing adherence with criteria for use may require substantial resources for personnel and real-time clinical decision support software to identify, review, and validate the appropriateness of the stated indications.

The most time-intensive method of directing use of restricted antibiotics requires the prescriber to obtain preauthorization from the ASP before the agent is dispensed from the pharmacy. The primary provider contacts the ASP by phone or pager and reviews antibiotic choices for specific patients. The goal of preauthorization is to provide appropriate therapy at the time of initiating antibiotics. This "mini-consult" serves to educate prescribers who are seeking advice concerning the appropriateness of an antibiotic, as well as those who are requesting authorization of a restricted agent. Providing coverage for preauthorization requests 24 hours a day, 7 days a week is not always feasible. Therefore, some institutions allow the first doses of the restricted agents to be used when review cannot be completed in a timely manner. The ASP then evaluates the appropriateness of the antibiotic choice at the next opportunity and determines whether the agent can be continued. Stewards involved in preauthorization processes are given authority to approve or deny requests for restricted antibiotics through hospital policies. Irrespective of the established approval policies, disputes may arise; therefore, it is important for institutions to establish an appeal process.

Restriction and preauthorization strategies have demonstrated significant benefits. These interventions decrease the consumption of targeted antibiotics and overall antibiotic expenditures.[22, 31–33] Reductions in inappropriate antibiotic use have also demonstrated short-term increases in susceptibilities as well as decreases in colonization and outbreaks with multidrug-resistant organisms and *C. difficile* infections.[23, 34, 35] However, the effects on drug resistance should be interpreted with caution since the follow-up times in studies have been short and other studies have not shown similar results.[36, 37] Additionally, there is concern that the restriction of one agent or restriction of an entire class may lead to a compensatory increase with another class or classes, otherwise known as "squeezing the balloon."[38, 39] Restriction of cephalosporins, for instance, have led to increases in imipenem-cilastatin use with subsequent increases in imipenem-cilastatin resistance among *P. aeruginosa* isolates.[39]

Limitations of the preauthorization strategy include perceived loss of prescriber autonomy, inappropriate recommendations stemming from inaccurate or misleading information from providers, and risk of delays in review and administration of appropriate antibiotics. Some surveys have shown that restriction policies have proven unpopular with prescribers.[40, 41] A survey conducted by Seemungal and colleagues found that of the 116 respondents, 50% expressed frustration and the perception that their time was wasted. Additionally, 41% felt that their autonomy was limited. Frustrated respondents were ten times more likely to report that they would intentionally provide inaccurate information, which has been significantly associated with inappropriate antibiotic recommendations.[10, 42, 43] In contrast to reported prescriber perceptions, studies have demonstrated that average response times for antibiotic requests were short (2.7 minutes), there was no delay in time to receipt of appropriate antibiotics, and length of stay decreased.[23, 31, 44] ASPs can overcome negative perceptions about autonomy by obtaining appropriate authority from institutional policy and committees, working to establish a positive, personal rapport with prescribers, and establishing a streamlined approval process that minimizes prescribers' time and effort. Further, ASPs must monitor patient outcomes and antibiotic use rates to identify if there are any unintended consequences from the restriction policies. For example, ASPs should identify instances of negative safety events resulting from unapproved requests and monitor any increases in other targeted antibiotics.

Prospective Audit and Feedback

Prospective audit and feedback is a strategy that promotes a team-based approach to patient care. ASP team members interact with prescribers to provide patient-specific therapy recommendations.[22, 45] They review targeted therapies after the initial prescribing and administration of antibiotics. Antibiotics targeted for audit may be identified based on their high potential for misuse (e.g., broad-spectrum antibiotics), cost, or high-risk of toxicity and safety concerns. Select patient populations, such as those with the highest antibiotic consumption, or those with specific syndromes, such as *Staphylococcus aureus* bacteremia, may also be prospectively monitored for audit and feedback interventions.

For prospective audit and feedback, the ASP physician or pharmacist performs the audit and provides direct feedback on rounds, via phone, or written communication.[46] The pharmacist who performs an audit may first review the case with the ASP physician prior to giving feedback.[47–49] The availability of trained personnel, culture of the institution, and the amount of time these team members are able to devote to antibiotic stewardship activities are primary drivers for the method of feedback chosen. Time is a precious resource that may not only influence the audit and feedback method but also how often it is performed. The size of the institution in relation to available ASP personnel time may dictate the frequency of audits, but some audit and feedback activity remains beneficial. For example, the provision of prospective audit and feedback three days a week in a smaller institution was able to demonstrate decreases in antibiotic use and expenditures to such a degree that it enabled them to support an ID physician part-time as well as a pharmacist.[50]

Prospective audit and feedback is significantly enhanced by the implementation of clinical decision support software (see Chapter 10). Clinical decision support software enables the real-time review of targeted antibiotics and patients with targeted clinical scenarios. Microbiology, laboratory, and pharmacy order, and/or administration data are integrated by this software and can be used to create specialized alerts for review. Specifically, these systems can be utilized to perform syndrome- or culture-based audit and feedback (see **Table 2**). Syndrome-based interventions such as the review of patients with *S. aureus* bacteremia, candidemia, or *C. difficile* infection are discussed elsewhere (see Chapter 5). ASPs can use this technology to identify bug-drug mismatches and opportunities for de-escalation based on pathogen susceptibilities. Bug-drug mismatches are events where patients are infected with pathogens identified on clinical culture that are non-susceptible to the prescribed antibiotics (e.g., patient treated with vancomycin with a culture positive for vancomycin-resistant Enterococci).

ASP interventions to correct inappropriate therapy can have a clear and meaningful impact on patient management and outcomes. De-escalation alerts also use microbiology and pharmacy information as a method to identify patients on broad-spectrum antibiotics with a cultured microorganism susceptible to agents with a narrower spectrum of activity. Other alerts can be crafted to identify unnecessary duplicative treatments (e.g., dual-anaerobic coverage). Interventions on these patients may result in avoided days of therapy or reduced days of broad-spectrum therapy, which may then reduce risks of unintended consequences such as *C. difficile* infections. For hospitals without clinical decision support software, de-escalation opportunities can be identified via a manual process of identifying patients on broad-spectrum agents or obtaining a list of positive microbiology cultures and performing many chart reviews.

When compared to programs lacking those resources, ASPs that used clinical decision support software for prospective audit and feedback provided greater sensitivity for identifying appropriate patients for review.[51] In fact, when targeting specific antibiotic combinations, the software decreased the number of patients requiring review by 84%.[52] Additionally, ASPs that have used clinical decision support software for audit have demonstrated decreased antibiotic use by up to 37%, decreased antibiotic expenditures by $400 per patient, and decreased lengths of stay when compared to standard of care.[53, 54] ASPs without clinical decision support software may work to build customized reports in which they capture patient identifiers, antibiotic dosages, and microbiology information to be reviewed and acted upon on a daily basis. This may be a reasonable alternative for smaller institutions who cannot afford expensive software and have a smaller number of reviewable patients per day.

When compared to supplemental antibiotic stewardship strategies, such as automatic stop orders and order forms, prospective audit and feedback was associated with significant cost savings, decreased median durations of therapy (two vs. five days), and decreased median lengths of stay (seven vs. eight days).[55, 56] Unlike the preauthorization strategy, prescribers do not perceive a loss of autonomy with prospective audit and feedback; therefore, there may be less opposition to the implementation of this method.[22, 45, 47] Additional advantages of this strategy are the opportunities to provide patient- or pathogen-specific education and therapy recommendations through feedback. In one institution's experience, therapies were generally not intervened on until 2.5 days after initiation, during which time more microbiology and patient data were available for review.[57]

Prospective audit and feedback is a labor-intensive strategy. The time and personnel necessary to carry out these functions are significant, particularly in larger institutions. Additionally, prescriber acceptance of ASP recommendations is voluntary and often dependent on the skill of the steward providing the intervention. The review and provision of feedback to prescribers requires a moderate degree of education and expertise for those performing the feedback interventions, which surpass that of standard schools of pharmacy coursework (see Chapter 2). A quasi-experimental study examined the implementation of audit and feedback in five academic medical centers, two of which had well-established ASPs and three of which had newly established ASPs. The intervention resulted in reduction of days of therapy per 1,000 patient days for targeted drugs in two of the five study hospitals; the two institutions with established ASPs.[58] In this study, the overall recommendation acceptance rate of 67% was lower than many ASPs can attain in practice. These results led the authors to conclude that audit and feedback can impact antibiotic use, but may be more effective in hospitals with well-established ASPs.

No rigorously designed studies directly compare preauthorization to prospective audit and feedback.[59] Although not a direct comparison, a large meta-analysis including 52 interrupted time-series analyses compared the relative effects of restrictive strategies versus "persuasive" strategies when compared to a standard of care without stewardship intervention.[3] Restrictive strategies had a 32% increase in appropriateness of antibiotic prescribing at one month compared to persuasive strategies, and had a 53% greater impact on the incidence of *C. difficile* infections and microbial resistance patterns within six months; however, there were no significant differences between the strategies at 12 or 24 months. The authors concluded that restrictive interventions may be more appropriate when the need is urgent, but that both persuasive and restrictive strategies are equally effective after approximately six months.

Another study in a single academic center described experience when preauthorization was subsequently replaced with audit and feedback for targeted agents. The use of targeted agents and all antibiotics significantly increased over a 24-month period, as did lengths of stay. However, study design without a comparator may have resulted in bias due to the changing complexity of patient populations or other unmeasured factors; thus definitive conclusions cannot be assumed.[59] Another single-center investigation used a 2-arm, quasi-experimental, crossover design to examine the effect of each strategy. Two general medicine teams in an academic medical center with a well-established ASP were randomized to each strategy for four months, and then switched to the other strategy for four months with a one-month washout in-between.[60] The time-series analysis of the main study outcome of days of therapy per 1,000 patient days, including both inpatient and post-discharge days, favored prospective audit and feedback over preauthorization with many of the saved days of therapy occurring in the post-discharge setting (median six vs. eight days of therapy per patient, $p = 0.03$). Inappropriate therapy on day 1 and 3 were also measured, with preauthorization exhibiting lower percent of inappropriate use on day 1 and prospective audit and feedback with lower percent on day 3. Patient outcomes, including *C. difficile* incidence, were not different between strategies. Thus, the choice of which strategy to implement must be tailored to the perceived need and goal for the targeted agents – namely, appropriate duration of therapy versus appropriate empiric choice. Both strategies are effective at changing antibiotic prescribing to improve adherence to prescribing guidelines and reduce durations when compared with no intervention.[61] We believe that a mix of both strategies is useful, with some consideration given to the type of agent targeted, availability of ASP personnel resources, goals (e.g., shorter duration versus appropriate empiric use), and likelihood of prescriber acceptance.

Targeted or Supplementary Strategies

Several additional strategies may be used to supplement the two strategies above (see **Table 2**). Many of these targeted strategies are effective in impacting antibiotic use and are discussed in detail in other chapters: use of clinical pathways and order sets (Chapter 5), implementation of rapid diagnostics (Chapter 9), antibiotic stewardship allergy initiatives (Chapter 11), and implementation of dose-optimization protocols or alternative dosing strategies (Chapter 8). Below, we will briefly discuss the other relevant targeted strategies.

Intravenous to oral conversion protocols As one of the simplest strategies for antibiotic management, intravenous to oral conversions are often considered "low-hanging fruit." By converting intravenous to oral formulations with high bioavailability, ASPs have demonstrated significant cost savings without compromising effectiveness of treatment or patient safety. Reductions in the incidence of catheter-related infections and decreases in length of hospital stay have been demonstrated.[62–66] This strategy is primarily pharmacy-driven and does not require expertise in ID. Pharmacists acting on an approved protocol containing defined criteria for conversion may either automatically change or contact the primary provider for approval to change the intravenous to oral formulation. However, agents for which there is not a direct intravenous to oral conversion (e.g., piperacillin-tazobactam) require more expertise and antibiotic stewardship input. In order to efficiently and accurately identify patients who meet the criteria for conversion, many institutions used CPOE systems to create real-time alerts for prescribers at the point of order entry or an electronically generated list of eligible patients for pharmacists to review.[64, 67] Implementation of an intravenous to oral policy involves consideration of how this activity will be incorporated into pharmacists' workflow, who may have other priorities and responsibilities.

Automatic infectious diseases consults An increasing number of institutions have implemented automatic ID consultations for certain serious infections that carry high risks of mortality, recurrence, and complications if not managed appropriately.[68, 69] ID consultations become "automatic" when a hospital policy strongly recommends ID consultation for eligible patients. The most evidence for the impact of automatic ID consultation is in *S. aureus* bacteremia but other clinical scenarios might also be targeted (e.g., Candidemia). There is mounting observational data that demonstrate the administration of appropriate therapy (e.g., nafcillin or cefazolin instead of vancomycin for methicillin-susceptible *S. aureus*), use of diagnostic testing (e.g., echocardiogram and repeat blood cultures), and appropriate durations of therapy are improved when ID consultants are involved in management of *S. aureus* bacteremia.[70–72] Also, comparative observational studies have demonstrated that ID consultation is associated with improved survival, reduced complications, and reduced readmissions.[68, 71, 73] The role of the ASP in implementing automatic ID consultations may include development of the formalized policy, championing its approval at relevant hospital committees, promoting its acceptance with physician groups, and serving as facilitator to rapidly identify eligible patients and notify providers to place formal ID consultations. The major limitation for this strategy is that it cannot be applied where ID physicians are not available. Telemedicine services have been suggested as a potential alternative, but comparative data suggests that "curbside" evaluations are not equivalent to bedside consults.[74, 75]

Antibiotic stewardship rounds on high-risk units ASPs that have a dedicated team can expand their influence and target high-priority practice areas by performing focused patient rounds on a routine basis. The best examples of this strategy include collaborations between stewards and critical care physicians to perform multidisciplinary rounds on intensive care unit (ICU) patients on active antibiotic treatment.[46, 76, 77] ICUs are a natural target population for ASP rounds due to patient complexity and high levels of antibiotic exposures; however, non-ICU wards or other specific units can also benefit.[78] Antibiotic stewardship rounds identify opportunities to optimize antibiotic therapies, which may include a variety of interventions such as de-escalation, dosing optimization, promoting shorter durations, avoiding certain agents (e.g., fluoroquinolones), and suggesting further diagnostic evaluations. Typically, the AS team will not see and examine patients as would be expected in formal consultations. Instead, the AS team meets with members of the primary team to review the patients on antibiotics verbally or by group chart review.

Although dedicated ASP rounds are time and personnel resource intensive, the advantages are multiple. This close interaction develops rapport with targeted prescriber groups. The multiple and repeated opportunities for one-to-one teaching and reinforcement of AS principles may lead to more sustained behavioral change. One strategy to offset this ongoing resource need is to implement frequent (e.g., daily) ASP rounds at the outset of the initiative and scale down (e.g., twice a week) once provider knowledge, outcomes, and practice improves. Process and outcome measures of interest for this intervention include the number of patient-level interventions, type of intervention made, antibiotic utilization (e.g., days of therapy per 1,000 patient days), and patient outcomes (e.g., ICU length of stay, *C. difficile* infections). Expected challenges include difficulty engaging the targeted prescriber groups and maintaining the rounding schedule when personnel time is limited.

Antibiotic "time-out" CDC promotes the antibiotic "time-out" procedure as an example of an "Action" to implement antibiotic stewardship in the Core Elements.[6] This intervention uses a design similar to the surgical "time-out" checklist that has been shown to reduce errors and promote teamwork in operating rooms. The time-out is an example of "self-stewardship" where the primary attending physician or treating team is prompted to routinely perform and document their review of each patient's antibiotic regimen to evaluate choice, dose, duration, microbiology data, and indication. The trigger for review may occur at a particular time point (e.g., 48 or 72 hours after initiation of antibiotics) and be integrated into the EMR (e.g., an EPIC "best practice alert").[79] It's an attractive alternative for ASPs that do not have robust personnel resources or a centralized ASP model to perform prospective audit and feedback. In addition, self-stewardship could reach a larger number of patients because it is not limited to targeted interventions by a centralized ASP. However, there is currently little evidence in the medical literature to demonstrate that the time-out strategy has an impact on either antibiotic utilization or patient outcomes.[80, 81] Strategies to promote antibiotic regimen review by frontline staff at the point of prescription may bear out as successful interventions in future studies, but at this point evidence is limited to pilot data.[82]

Automatic stop orders Automatic stop orders are another means by which ASPs have decreased the unnecessary use of antibiotics intended for both prophylaxis and treatment. In times of antibiotic shortages, this may also be a viable method for controlling use. With the institution of automatic stop orders, the use of an antibiotic is permitted for a defined period of time, after which the provider must obtain approval from the ASP for continuation. If approval is not sought, the antibiotic will automatically be discontinued. The purpose of automatic stop orders is to encourage reassessment of the antibiotic based on the patient's clinical condition, microbiology data, and other diagnostics and to promote safe and rational use. Prior to the implementation of this strategy, prescriber education is extremely important and warnings concerning the potential stop should be put into place. ASPs use different stop times, typically either 48–72 hours, but it could also be set to day 7 or 10 of treatment.

Automatic stop orders are enforced through CPOE systems or manually by ASP pharmacists who are empowered to do so. Without close monitoring, automatic stop orders may be circumvented if prescribers were to reenter the order at the time of discontinuation, which would allow for an additional 48–72 hours of the antibiotic. Automatic stop orders have been shown to significantly decrease the inappropriate use of antibiotics.[83, 84] Potential disadvantages of this strategy are the inadvertent and inappropriate discontinuation of antibiotics and the lack of resources to maintain the automatic stop procedures.

Cascading or selective reporting ASPs can collaborate with the microbiology laboratory to influence prescribing behavior by selecting specific antibiotic susceptibility tests to include on clinical culture reports while censoring others. In the United States, microbiology laboratories generally follow Clinical Laboratory Standards Institute (CLSI) guidelines to determine which drug susceptibilities are routinely tested and reported versus selectively reported.[85] (see Chapter 9). Collaborating with the Microbiology Lab. ASP input into the latter can prove beneficial to promote use of clinically appropriate, narrow-spectrum, cost-effective agents on formulary. The perceived withholding of information may frustrate clinicians, or they may inaccurately assume the organism is susceptible to drugs not included in the report. In general, susceptibilities not routinely reported due to cascade rules should be reported when there is resistance to avoid inaccurate assumptions and bug-drug mismatch. Carefully designed reporting protocols based on clinical scenarios must be developed to avoid situations where withholding information on specific drugs is detrimental. Objective data to demonstrate that cascaded susceptibility reporting improves antibiotic utilization and resistance is limited to single-center experiences.[86] and outpatient settings.[87, 88] However, to many, this practice is seen as a routine function of the microbiology laboratory.

Peer comparison data feedback to prescribers Changing prescriber behavior is a major challenge for ASPs when prescribers do not realize that their prescribing patterns differ from standard or optimal practice. Recent trials in the outpatient setting have used routine data feedback that analyzed prescribing data for an individual compared to other peer prescribers.[18, 89] These trials are based on the idea that being designated as an "outlier" or "not a top performer" will motivate prescribers to change. As described previously, Gerber et al. demonstrated that pediatric primary care providers responded to peer comparison feedback reports evaluating choice of antibiotic for upper respiratory infections. [18] However, when routine reporting stopped, prescribing rapidly returned to higher levels seen during the pre-intervention period, highlighting the challenge of sustained behavior change.[90] Meeker et al. performed a large, cluster-randomized trial in 47 primary care practices involving three different behavioral interventions implemented alone and in combination aiming to avoid antibiotics in patients diagnosed with nonbacterial upper respiratory conditions.[89] The three interventions included suggested alternatives to antibiotics presented at the time of order entry, accountable justification where clinicians were required to document free text rationales for prescribing antibiotics into the electronic medical record, and peer comparison reports sent by email to identify "top performers" with the lowest inappropriate prescribing rates. Both the accountable justification and peer comparison data feedback interventions led to significant reductions in inappropriate antibiotic prescribing compared to control practices.

Challenges in developing peer feedback reports are multiple. First, the intervention requires an EMR with retrievable data points for analysis as well as informatics resources to produce and deliver reports regularly and confidentially. Second, prior studies have targeted clinical scenarios that are relatively simple, straightforward conditions and patient populations in which electronic data points (e.g., billed diagnosis) are reliable enough to apply a reasonable definition of "inappropriate" use. More clinically complex populations, such as hospitalized patients, pose a distinct challenge in developing electronic definitions of "inappropriate" prescribing. Further, attributing decision-making to a single provider is challenging in team-based care models, particularly in academic institutions where multiple levels of clinicians and subspecialists may be involved in prescribing decisions. Finally, the reports must include a large enough number of prescribers to allow for meaningful comparisons that do not risk provider confidentiality and trust. Despite the challenges in applying this strategy to other practice settings, peer comparison data feedback in these studies was an effective tool in both gaining attention of prescribers and changing prescribing behavior and represents a promising area for future development.

Conclusions

Antibiotic stewardship strategic planning requires careful consideration of many factors: needs, resources, institutional culture, and anticipation of required resources for implementation. Although there are many potential interventions, the strategies of formulary restriction with preauthorization and prospective audit and feedback have the most evidence of effectiveness. Supplemental strategies, such as institution-specific guidelines and provider education, can be integrated into other strategies to provide the best mix for an individual institution. Regardless of which strategies are selected, we encourage tracking of outcomes, regular reflection on program successes and challenges, and an iterative process of intervention and reassessment. An adaptive and active ASP continually strives for an optimal fit for their institution, their prescribers, and, most importantly, the needs of the patients they serve.

References

1. Barlam, TF, SE Cosgrove, LM Abbo, et al. Implementing an Antibiotic Stewardship Program: Guidelines by the Infectious Diseases Society of America and the Society for Healthcare Epidemiology of America. *Clin Infect Dis* 2016; 62(10): e51–77.

2. Dellit, TH, RC Owens, JE McGowan, Jr., et al. Infectious Diseases Society of America and the Society for Healthcare Epidemiology of America guidelines for developing an institutional program to enhance antimicrobial stewardship. *Clin Infect Dis* 2007; 44(2): 159–77.

3. Davey, P, E Brown, E Charani, et al. Interventions to improve antibiotic prescribing practices for hospital inpatients. *Cochrane Database Syst Rev* 2013; 4: CD003543.

4. Centers for Medicare and Medicaid Programs; Hospital and Critical Access Hospital (CAH) Changes to Promote Innovation, Flexibility, and Imporvement in Patient Care: Proposed Rule. The Federal Register 2016 (Accessed August 26, 2016, at https://federalregister.gov/a/2016–13925.)

5. The Joint Commission. Antimicrobial Stewardship Standard. MM.09.01.01. (Accessed April 11, 2017 at www.jointcommission.org/new_antimicrobial_stewardship_standard/)

6. Pollack, LA and A Srinivasan. Core elements of hospital antibiotic stewardship programs from the Centers for Disease Control and Prevention. *Clin Infect Dis* 2014; 59 Suppl 3: S97–100.

7. Sanchez, GV, KE Fleming-Dutra, RM Roberts, and LA Hicks. Core Elements of Outpatient Antibiotic Stewardship. *MMWR Recomm Rep* 2016; 65(6): 1–12.

8. The Joint Commission Pre-Publication Standards for Antimicrobial Stewardship MM.09.01.01. (Accessed April 11, 2017 at ww.jointcommission.org/prepublication_standards_standards_revisions_for_critical_access_hospitals/.)

9. Centers for Disease Control and Prevention. National Healthcare Safety Network: Antimicrobial Use and Resistance (AUR) Options. (Accessed March 31, 2016 at www.cdc.gov/nhsn/acute-care-hospital/aur/index.html.)

10. Seemungal, IA and CJ Bruno. Attitudes of housestaff toward a prior-authorization-based antibiotic stewardship program. *Infect Control Hosp Epidemiol* 2012; 33(4): 429–31.

11. Centers for Disease Control and Prevention: The Core Elements of Hospital Antibiotic Stewardship Programs Checklist; Available from: www.cdc.gov/getsmart/healthcare/pdfs/checklist.pdf.

12. Centers for Disease Control and Prevention: Antimicrobial Management Program Gap Analysis Checklist.

13. Centers for Disease Control and Prevention and Institute for Healthcare Improvement. Antibiotic Stewardship Driver Diagram and Change Package: Centers for Disease Control and Prevention and Insitute for Healthcare Improvement 2012. (Accessed February 7, 2016 at www.cdc.gov/getsmart/healthcare/pdfs/antibiotic_stewardship_change_package.pdf.)

14. Langley, GL, R Moen, KM Nolan, et al. *The Improvement Guide: A Practical Approach to Enhancing Organizational Performance* 2nd ed. 2009, San Francisco, CA: Jossey-Bass Publishers.

15. Moehring, RW and DJ Anderson. Antimicrobial Stewardship as part of the infection prevention effort. *Curr Infect Dis Rep* 2012; 14(6): 592–600.

16. Ohl, CA and VP Luther. Antimicrobial stewardship for inpatient facilities. *J Hosp Med* 2011; 6 Suppl 1: S4–15.

17. Drew, RH, R White, C MacDougall, ED Hermsen, and RC Owens, Jr. Insights from the Society of Infectious Diseases Pharmacists on antimicrobial stewardship guidelines from the Infectious Diseases Society of America and the Society for Healthcare Epidemiology of America. *Pharmacotherapy* 2009; 29(5): 593–607.

18. Gerber, JS, PA Prasad, AG Fiks, et al. Effect of an outpatient antimicrobial stewardship intervention on broad-spectrum antibiotic

prescribing by primary care pediatricians: a randomized trial. *JAMA* 2013; 309(22): 2345–52.

19. Cisneros, JM, O Neth, MV Gil-Navarro, et al. Global impact of an educational antimicrobial stewardship programme on prescribing practice in a tertiary hospital centre. *Clin Microbiol Infect* 2014; 20(1): 82–8.

20. Drew, RH, R White, C MacDougall, et al. Insights from the Society of Infectious Diseases Pharmacists on antimicrobial stewardship guidelines from the Infectious Diseases Society of America and the Society for Healthcare Epidemiology of America. *Pharmacotherapy* 2009; 29(5): 593–607.

21. Owens, RC, Jr. Antimicrobial stewardship: concepts and strategies in the 21st century. *Diagn Microbiol Infect Dis* 2008; 61(1): 110–128.

22. Dellit, TH, RC Owens, JE McGowan, Jr., et al. Infectious Diseases Society of America and the Society for Healthcare Epidemiology of America guidelines for developing an institutional program to enhance antimicrobial stewardship. *Clin Infect Dis* 2007; 44(2): 159–177.

23. White, AC, Jr., RL Atmar, J Wilson, et al. Effects of requiring prior authorization for selected antimicrobials: expenditures, susceptibilities, and clinical outcomes. *Clin Infect Dis* 1997; 25(2): 230–239.

24. McGowan, JE, Jr. and M Finland. Usage of antibiotics in a general hospital: effect of requiring justification. *J Infect Dis* 1974; 130(2): 165–168.

25. MacDougall, C and RE Polk. Antimicrobial stewardship programs in health care systems. *Clin Microbiol Rev* 2005; 18(4): 638–656.

26. Kallen, AJ, A Thompson, P Ristaino, et al. Complete restriction of fluoroquinolone use to control an outbreak of *Clostridium difficile* infection at a community hospital. *Infect Control Hosp Epidemiol* 2009; 30(3): 264–272.

27. Dingle, KE, X Didelot, TP Quan, et al. Effects of control interventions on *Clostridium difficile* infection in England:

an observational study. *Lancet Infect Dis* 2017; 17(4): 411–421.

28. Standiford, HC, S Chan, M Tripoli, E Weekes, and GN Forrest. Antimicrobial stewardship at a large tertiary care academic medical center: cost analysis before, during, and after a 7-year program. *Infect Control Hosp Epidemiol* 2012; 33(4): 338–345.

29. Forrest, GN, TC Van Schooneveld, R Kullar, et al. Use of electronic health records and clinical decision support systems for antimicrobial stewardship. *Clin Infect Dis* 2014; 59 Suppl 3: S122–33.

30. Pope, SD, TH Dellit, RC Owens, et al. Results of survey on implementation of Infectious Diseases Society of America and Society for Healthcare Epidemiology of America guidelines for developing an institutional program to enhance antimicrobial stewardship. *Infect Control Hosp Epidemiol* 2009; 30(1): 97–98.

31. Reed, EE, KB Stevenson, JE West, KA Bauer, and DA Goff. Impact of formulary restriction with prior authorization by an antimicrobial stewardship program. *Virulence* 2013; 4(2): 158–162.

32. File, TM, Jr., A Srinivasan, and JG Bartlett. Antimicrobial stewardship: importance for patient and public health. *Clin Infect Dis* 2014; 59 Suppl 3: S93–96.

33. Ozkurt, Z, S Erol, A Kadanali, et al. Changes in antibiotic use, cost and consumption after an antibiotic restriction policy applied by infectious disease specialists. *Jpn J Infect Dis* 2005; 58(6): 338–343.

34. Quale, J, D Landman, G Saurina, et al. Manipulation of a hospital antimicrobial formulary to control an outbreak of vancomycin-resistant enterococci. *Clin Infect Dis* 1996; 23(5): 1020–1025.

35. Pear, SM, TH Williamson, KM Bettin, DN Gerding, and JN Galgiani. Decrease in nosocomial *Clostridium difficile*-associated diarrhea by restricting clindamycin use. *Ann Intern Med* 1994; 120(4): 272–277.

36. Toltzis, P, T Yamashita, L Vilt, et al. Antibiotic restriction does not alter endemic colonization with resistant gram-

negative rods in a pediatric intensive care unit. *Crit Care Med* 1998; 26(11): 1893–1899.

37. Stiefel, U, DL Paterson, NJ Pultz, et al. Effect of the increasing use of piperacillin/tazobactam on the incidence of vancomycin-resistant enterococci in four academic medical centers. *Infect Control Hosp Epidemiol* 2004; 25(5): 380–383.

38. Burke, JP. Antibiotic resistance–squeezing the balloon? *JAMA* 1998; 280(14): 1270–1271.

39. Rahal, JJ, C Urban, D Horn, et al. Class restriction of cephalosporin use to control total cephalosporin resistance in nosocomial Klebsiella. *JAMA* 1998; 280 (14): 1233–1237.

40. Dunagan, WC and G Medoff. Formulary control of antimicrobial usage: what price freedom? *Diagn Microbiol Infect Dis* 1993; 16(3): 265–274.

41. Bryan, CS. Strategies to improve antibiotic use. *Infect Dis Clin North Am* 1989; 3(4): 723–734.

42. Linkin, DR, S Paris, NO Fishman, JP Metlay, and E Lautenbach. Inaccurate communications in telephone calls to an antimicrobial stewardship program. *Infect Control Hosp Epidemiol* 2006; 27(7): 688–694.

43. Linkin, DR, NO Fishman, JR Landis, et al. Effect of communication errors during calls to an antimicrobial stewardship program. *Infect Control Hosp Epidemiol* 2007; 28(12): 1374–1381.

44. Mehta, JM, K Haynes, EP Wileyto, et al. Comparison of prior authorization and prospective audit with feedback for antimicrobial stewardship. *Infect Control Hosp Epidemiol* 2014; 35(9): 1092–1099.

45. Heineman, HS and VS Watt. All-inclusive concurrent antibiotic usage review: a way to reduce misuse without formal controls. *Infect Control* 1986; 7(3): 168–171.

46. DiazGranados, CA. Prospective audit for antimicrobial stewardship in intensive care: impact on resistance and clinical outcomes. *Am J Infect Control* 2012; 40(6): 526–529.

47. Seto, WH, TY Ching, M Kou, et al. Hospital antibiotic prescribing successfully modified by "immediate concurrent feedback". *Br J Clin Pharmacol* 1996; 41(3): 229–234.

48. Yeo, CL, DS Chan, A Earnest, et al. Prospective audit and feedback on antibiotic prescription in an adult hematology-oncology unit in Singapore. *Eur J Clin Microbiol Infect Dis* 2012; 31(4): 583–590.

49. Elligsen, M, SA Walker, R Pinto, et al. Audit and feedback to reduce broad-spectrum antibiotic use among intensive care unit patients: a controlled interrupted time series analysis. *Infect Control Hosp Epidemiol* 2012; 33(4): 354–361.

50. LaRocco, A, Jr. Concurrent antibiotic review programs–a role for infectious diseases specialists at small community hospitals. *Clin Infect Dis* 2003; 37(5): 742–743.

51. McGregor, JC, E Weekes, GN Forrest, et al. Impact of a computerized clinical decision support system on reducing inappropriate antimicrobial use: a randomized controlled trial. *J Am Med Inform Assoc* 2006; 13(4): 378–384.

52. Glowacki, RC, DN Schwartz, GS Itokazu, et al. Antibiotic combinations with redundant antimicrobial spectra: clinical epidemiology and pilot intervention of computer-assisted surveillance. *Clin Infect Dis* 2003; 37(1): 59–64.

53. Fraser, GL, P Stogsdill, JD Dickens, Jr., et al. Antibiotic optimization. An evaluation of patient safety and economic outcomes. *Arch Intern Med* 1997; 157(15): 1689–1694.

54. Solomon, DH, L Van Houten, RJ Glynn, et al. Academic detailing to improve use of broad-spectrum antibiotics at an academic medical center. *Arch Intern Med* 2001; 161 (15): 1897–1902.

55. Carling, PC, T Fung, and JS Coldiron. Parenteral antibiotic use in acute-care hospitals: a standardized analysis of fourteen institutions. *Clin Infect Dis* 1999; 29(5): 1189–1196.

56. Camins, BC, MD King, JB Wells, et al. Impact of an antimicrobial utilization program on antimicrobial use at a large teaching hospital: a randomized controlled trial. *Infect Control Hosp Epidemiol* 2009; 30(10): 931–938.

57. Owens, RC, Jr., AF Shorr, and AL Deschambeault. Antimicrobial stewardship: shepherding precious resources. *Am J Health Syst Pharm* 2009; 66 (12 Suppl 4): S15–22.

58. Cosgrove, SE, SK Seo, MK Bolon, et al. Evaluation of postprescription review and feedback as a method of promoting rational antimicrobial use: a multicenter intervention. *Infect Control Hosp Epidemiol* 2012; 33(4): 374–380.

59. Van Schooneveld, TC and ME Rupp. Antimicrobial stewardship strategies: preauthorization or postprescription audit and feedback? *Infect Control Hosp Epidemiol* 2014; 35(9): 1100–1102.

60. Tamma, PD, E Avdic, JF Keenan, et al. What is the more effective antibiotic stewardship intervention: preprescription authorization or postprescription review with feedback? *Clin Infect Dis* 2017; 64(5): 537–543.

61. Davey, P, CA Marwick, CL Scott, et al. Interventions to improve antibiotic prescribing practices for hospital inpatients. *Cochrane Database Syst Rev* 2017; 2: Cd003543.

62. Jones, M, B Huttner, K Madaras-Kelly, et al. Parenteral to oral conversion of fluoroquinolones: low-hanging fruit for antimicrobial stewardship programs? *Infect Control Hosp Epidemiol* 2012; 33(4): 362–367.

63. Kuti, JL, TN Le, CH Nightingale, DP Nicolau, and R Quintiliani. Pharmacoeconomics of a pharmacist-managed program for automatically converting levofloxacin route from i.v. to oral. *Am J Health Syst Pharm* 2002; 59(22): 2209–2215.

64. Lau, BD, BL Pinto, DR Thiemann, and CU Lehmann. Budget impact analysis of conversion from intravenous to oral medication when clinically eligible for oral intake. *Clin Ther* 2011; 33(11): 1792–1796.

65. Mertz, D, M Koller, P Haller, et al. Outcomes of early switching from intravenous to oral antibiotics on medical wards. *J Antimicrob Chemother* 2009; 64(1): 188–199.

66. Przybylski, KG, MJ Rybak, PR Martin, et al. A pharmacist-initiated program of intravenous to oral antibiotic conversion. *Pharmacotherapy* 1997; 17(2): 271–276.

67. Goff, DA, KA Bauer, EE Reed, et al. Is the "low-hanging fruit" worth picking for antimicrobial stewardship programs? *Clin Infect Dis* 2012; 55(4): 587–592.

68. Honda, H, MJ Krauss, JC Jones, MA Olsen, and DK Warren. The value of infectious diseases consultation in *Staphylococcus aureus* bacteremia. *Am J Med* 2010; 123(7): 631–637.

69. Jenkins, TC, CS Price, AL Sabel, PS Mehler, and WJ Burman. Impact of routine infectious diseases service consultation on the evaluation, management, and outcomes of *Staphylococcus aureus* bacteremia. *Clin Infect Dis* 2008; 46(7): 1000–1008.

70. Fowler, VG, Jr., LL Sanders, DJ Sexton, et al. Outcome of *Staphylococcus aureus* bacteremia according to compliance with recommendations of infectious diseases specialists: experience with 244 patients. *Clin Infect Dis* 1998; 27(3): 478–486.

71. Lahey, T, R Shah, J Gittzus, J Schwartzman, and K Kirkland. Infectious diseases consultation lowers mortality from *Staphylococcus aureus* bacteremia. *Medicine (Baltimore)* 2009; 88(5): 263–267.

72. Nagao, M, Y Iinuma, T Saito, et al. Close cooperation between infectious disease physicians and attending physicians can result in better management and outcome for patients with *Staphylococcus aureus* bacteraemia. *Clin Microbiol Infect* 2010; 16 (12): 1783–1788.

73. Vogel, M, RP Schmitz, S Hagel, et al. Infectious disease consultation for *Staphylococcus aureus* bacteremia – a systematic review and meta-analysis. *J Infect* 2016; 72(1): 19–28.

74. Forsblom, E, E Ruotsalainen, J Ollgren, and A Järvinen. Telephone consultation cannot replace bedside infectious disease consultation in the management of *Staphylococcus aureus* bacteremia. *Clinical Infectious Diseases* 2012; 56(4): 536–538.

75. Burden, M, E Sarcone, A Keniston, et al. Prospective comparison of curbside versus formal consultations. *J Hosp Med* 2013; 8 (1): 31–35.

76. Rimawi, RH, MA Mazer, DS Siraj, M Gooch, and PP Cook. Impact of regular collaboration between infectious diseases and critical care practitioners on antimicrobial utilization and patient outcome. *Crit Care Med* 2013; 41(9): 2099–2107.

77. Kollef, MH and ST Micek. Antimicrobial stewardship programs: mandatory for all ICUs. *Crit Care* 2012; 16(6): 179.

78. Boyles, TH, A Whitelaw, C Bamford, et al. Antibiotic stewardship ward rounds and a dedicated prescription chart reduce antibiotic consumption and pharmacy costs without affecting inpatient mortality or re-admission rates. *PLoS One* 2013; 8 (12): e79747.

79. Schulz, L, K Osterby, and B Fox. The use of best practice alerts with the development of an antimicrobial stewardship navigator to promote antibiotic de-escalation in the electronic medical record. *Infect Control Hosp Epidemiol* 2013; 34(12): 1259–1265.

80. Lee, TC, C Frenette, D Jayaraman, L Green, and L Pilote. Antibiotic self-stewardship: trainee-led structured antibiotic time-outs to improve antimicrobial use. *Ann Intern Med* 2014; 161(10 Suppl): S53–58.

81. Graber, CJ, MM Jones, PA Glassman, et al. Taking an antibiotic time-out: utilization and usability of a self-stewardship time-out program for renewal of vancomycin and piperacillin-tazobactam. *Hosp Pharm* 2015; 50(11): 1011–1024.

82. Hamilton, KW, JS Gerber, R Moehring, et al. Point-of-prescription interventions to improve antimicrobial stewardship. *Clin Infect Dis* 2015; 60(8): 1252–1258.

83. Guglielmo, BJ, V Dudas, I Maewal, et al. Impact of a series of interventions in vancomycin prescribing on use and prevalence of vancomycin-resistant enterococci. *Jt Comm J Qual Patient Saf* 2005; 31(8): 469–475.

84. Nickman, NA, HF Blissenbach, and JD Herrick. Medical committee enforcement of policy limiting postsurgical antibiotic use. *Am J Hosp Pharm* 1984; 41(10): 2053–2056.

85. Clinical and Laboratory Standards Institute. Performance standards for antimicrobial susceptibility testing; twenty-third informational supplement., in *CLSI document M100-S23*. Wayne, PA 2013.

86. Al-Tawfiq, JA, H Momattin, F Al-Habboubi, and SJ Dancer. Restrictive reporting of selected antimicrobial susceptibilities influences clinical prescribing. *J Infect Public Health* 2015; 8 (3): 234–241.

87. McNulty, CA, GM Lasseter, A Charlett, et al. Does laboratory antibiotic susceptibility reporting influence primary care prescribing in urinary tract infection and other infections? *J Antimicrob Chemother* 2011; 66(6): 1396–1404.

88. Arnold, SR and SE Straus. Interventions to improve antibiotic prescribing practices in ambulatory care. *Cochrane Database Syst Rev* 2005(4): CD003539.

89. Meeker, D, JA Linder, CR Fox, et al. Effect of behavioral interventions on inappropriate antibiotic prescribing among primary care practices: a randomized clinical trial. *JAMA* 2016; 315 (6): 562–570.

90. Gerber, JS, PA Prasad, AG Fiks, and et al. Durability of benefits of an outpatient antimicrobial stewardship intervention after discontinuation of audit and feedback. *JAMA* 2014; 312(23): 2569–2570.

Chapter 5

Syndrome-Based Antibiotic Stewardship

Trevor C. Van Schooneveld and Emily L. Heil

While decreasing antimicrobial resistance is an important goal, the primary focus of all antibiotic stewardship programs (ASPs) should be to improve patient outcomes and reduce avoidable harm caused by antibiotics.[1, 2] Such outcomes cannot be achieved through purely restrictive strategies (restriction or pre-authorization) nor can they be fully achieved through prospective audit and feedback. Providing the best care involves more than improving antibiotic selection; it involves improving all aspects of care for an infectious syndrome. This is the impetus for syndromic-based antibiotic stewardship.

Syndromic antibiotic stewardship promotes optimal, evidence-based care for a specific infectious syndrome such as community-acquired pneumonia (CAP), skin and soft tissue infections (SSTI), or *Clostridium difficile* infection (CDI). While misuse of antibiotics is often the stimulus for creating a syndrome-specific intervention, the interventions do not typically focus on restricting specific antibiotics (i.e., vancomycin or daptomycin) but rather on optimizing antibiotic use for common infectious syndromes. For example, SSTI antibiotic stewardship may include specific criteria to limit the use of certain anti-MRSA agents such as daptomycin. In a real world example, one facility targeted the overuse of broad-spectrum gram-negative agents for uncomplicated cellulitis and cutaneous abscess and instituted an SSTI treatment bundle that decreased the use of these agents with the additional benefits of more appropriate culture utilization and treatment duration.[3]

Syndromic antibiotic stewardship generally addresses multiple components of care including interventions to improve diagnosis, utilization and interpretation of various microbiologic and radiologic tests as well as selection of empiric therapy, de-escalation, treatment duration, and infection prevention. Syndromic antibiotic stewardship that addresses multiple areas of process improvement lends itself to the development of order sets, checklists, and bundles that consolidate evidence-based practices and improve outcomes. For example, introduction of a multifaceted care bundle for *Staphylococcus aureus* bacteremia (SAB) resulted in improvements in both evidence-based practice and mortality.[4] Similar improvements have been noted with interventions for CAP, sepsis, CDI, and candidemia.[5–8]

Syndromic stewardship efforts offer many advantages over other forms of stewardship. The inclusion of multidisciplinary input will improve both the quality and acceptability of the intervention. Syndromic stewardship approaches can improve diagnostic test utilization and help avoid diagnostic errors, which contribute significantly to inappropriate antibiotic use.[9] Syndromic antibiotic stewardship may offer the opportunity to improve efficiency of resource utilization including both laboratory and medications. For example, if an institution identified improper use of fluoroquinolones for acute exacerbations of chronic obstructive pulmonary disease (COPD), a syndromic intervention addressing diagnosis, testing, treatment choice, and duration could improve care much more holistically and efficiently than other stewardship methods. Syndromic approaches also allow for targeted messaging and education, which is often more effective and sustainable than simply focusing efforts on pre-prescription authorization or post-prescription review with feedback. Additionally, the syndromic focus may retrain the clinician's approach, allowing the clinician to improve the care they deliver for that syndrome in every health care setting. Finally, syndromic antibiotic stewardship interventions offer the opportunity to address prevention. A two-year study of the introduction of a 14-point ventilator-associated pneumonia (VAP) treatment and prevention bundle demonstrated non-significant improvements in antibiotic use, but significant declines in VAP rates likely due to major improvements in prevention practices.[10]

In general, a structured approach should be used for syndrome-specific stewardship (see Box 1). Identification of the syndrome needing intervention is step one. Focus should be placed on high frequency infections or those where antibiotic misuse is common. Once a syndrome is selected, key stakeholders should be identified and engaged for their input. These will vary depending on the syndrome targeted. For example, when creating a surgical prophylaxis guideline practice leaders in surgery and anesthesia should be recruited in contrast to a urinary tract infection (UTI) intervention where emergency department (ED) and inpatient clinicians should be included. Key stakeholders should provide input, feedback, and serve as clinical and educational liaisons to the groups they represent. The specific components of the intervention should include evidence-based practices, which are

Box 1 General Approach to Syndrome-Specific Stewardship	
Steps	**Examples/Comments**
1. Identify syndrome to target	• Choose high volume syndrome or syndrome with frequent antibiotic misuse • Examples: asymptomatic bacteriuria, community-acquired pneumonia, sepsis
2. Identify key stakeholders and collaborators	• Microbiology Laboratory Leadership • Infection Prevention • Hospitalists or Intensivists or Surgeons • Emergency Medicine • Information Technology
3. Develop facility-based guideline	• Engage stakeholders in development • Address diagnosis, treatment options and duration, prevention • Use multifaceted "bundle" approach
4. Implement guideline and educate on the new process	• Leverage EMR and clinical decision support systems in the implementation • Use stakeholders as educational liaisons • Educate key personnel prior to go-live with frequent educational reinforcement after go-live
5. Evaluate impact	• Evaluate impact on targeted interventions such as test utilization, antibiotic use, and patient related outcomes

customized, and facility specific. There are many strategies to promote implementation success, but targeted education of frontline personnel is essential to all efforts. For example, education regarding a surgical prophylaxis guideline must be provided to all parties involved in the process including pharmacists (provide agent), all surgeons (order agent), and anesthesiologists and nurses (administer agent). Frontline personnel such as residents and nurse practitioners must be included. Ideally, implementation should leverage the electronic medical record (EMR) or clinical decision support systems. Creation of a required standardized set of surgical prophylaxis options categorized by surgery type that is included in all pre-operative order sets would be an example. Measurement of the impact of an intervention should be planned with subsequent adjustments based on these data. A limited number of syndromic interventions should be introduced each year (suggest one to three interventions per year) to improve the ability of a program to focus resources on the effort and maximize its impact. Included below is a discussion of both potential and proven syndrome-based antibiotic stewardship interventions targeting common infectious syndromes including UTI and asymptomatic bacteriuria, pneumonia and lower-respiratory tract infection, SSTI, bacteremia and candidemia, and CDI.

Urinary Tract Infections

UTIs are among the most common bacterial infectious syndromes. However, UTIs are also frequently overdiagnosed and overtreated making them a natural target for antibiotic stewardship interventions. Antibiotic stewardship interventions related to UTIs lend themselves well to a bundled approach incorporating guidance for prevention, diagnosis, and treatment. All of the interventions discussed in this section – prevention strategies with urinary catheter use, optimization at the level of urinaylsis and subsequent culture orders, empiric treatment selection based on institutional, urine-specific antibiograms, and proper de-escalation and treatment durations – can be rolled out via a bundled management algorithm. The success of these interventions will require collaboration and engagement of multiple parties including ED physicians, urologists, nephrologists, hospitalists, nursing, and laboratory personnel. Education is central to the bundles that have demonstrated success in the literature and can be implemented via treatment algorithms included in electronic prescribing systems, pocket cards, presentations to house staff and other clinicians on management of catheter-associated UTI (CA-UTI) and asymptomatic bacteriuria, and audit and feedback of common antibiotics used for UTIs by ASP team members.[11, 12] Additionally, educating and engaging clinical pharmacists to provide treatment recommendations regarding asymptomatic bacteriuria management during patient care rounds can optimize treatment.[12]

Asymptomatic bacteriuria is a highly prevalent condition, particularly in the elderly, those with bladder dysfunction, or urinary catheter use.[13] With the exception of pregnant women and those about to undergo urologic procedures, treatment of asymptomatic bacteriuria has no clinical benefit and increases the risk of subsequent symptomatic UTIs, isolation of resistant organisms, and antibiotic-associated adverse effects.[13, 14] The treatment of patients with positive urine cultures despite low clinical suspicion for UTIs is widespread. In a survey, resident physicians showed major knowledge deficits regarding asymptomatic bacteriuria and admitted to prescribing antibiotics for this condition despite knowing they were not indicated.[15]

Overdiagnosis will lead to inappropriate antibiotic use making appropriate urinalysis and urine culture practice an important target for stewardship intervention. Urinalysis and/ or urine culture should only be performed in the context of symptoms suggestive of UTIs. However, it has been shown that more than half of urinaylses and urine cultures obtained at admission lack clear indications.[16, 17] Unfortunately, positive test results drive antibiotic utilization, often more than symptoms.[16–18] Interventions at the time of urine test ordering can decrease the frequency of inappropriate testing. For example, a mandatory field can be placed into an electronic order for a urinanalysis or urine culture requiring documentation of signs or symptoms of a UTI. The presence of pyuria (white blood cells in the urine) is not diagnostic of a UTI, but lack of pyuria is highly valuable in the exclusion of infection.[19, 20] Changing urine culture ordering practices to only allow urine cultures when a urinalysis (UA) indicates pyuria can significantly reduce the number of urine cultures performed (a significant cost avoidance) and the subsequent detection of bacteriuria in patients.[21, 22] However, implementation of urine "reflex" testing alone is not sufficient to prevent unnecessary urine cultures and antibiotic use as there is still a high prevalence of pyuria in patients with asymptomatic bacteriuria.[23] An alternative method that has successfully reduced treatment in these patients is a selective reporting strategy where the laboratory only provides positive urine culture results for these patients upon request.[24] Other options include reporting culture results only when the colony-forming units per milliliter (CFU/mL) exceeds 100,000 or providing education along with results that urine culture with <100,000 CFUs/mL may not be clinically relevant as colony counts of >100,000 CFUs/mL are more likely to be associated with clinically significant UTIs. [25] Processes that lead to the ordering of a urine culture can be evaluated and revised. A single center decreased the urine cultures in their ED by 24% using a quality improvement mechanism that revised nursing and ED test ordering processes.[26]

Catheter-associated bacteriuria is very common, and CA-UTI is one of the most common healthcare-associated infections.[27] These conditions are of particular interest to ASPs as not only do they drive antibiotic use, but CA-UTI is also publicly reported and associated with non-payment of claims or financial penalties. Prevention is the most effective strategy for the reduction of catheter-associated bacteriuria and CA-UTI. ASPs often work with infection control programs to promote evidence-based prevention strategies as part of syndrome-based antibiotic stewardship. First, urinary catheters should only be placed for appropriate indications and should not be used for the management of incontinence. Second, urinary catheters must be inserted with appropriate aseptic technique and maintained properly. Finally, prompt removal of urinary catheters when they are no longer indicated is essential. Nursing-driven protocols and electronic physician-reminder systems can reduce inappropriate catheterization days and may reduce CA-UTI as well.[28–31] A checklist outlining appropriate indications, insertion and maintenance, and indications for removal can be incorporated into an EMR and/or made available in areas frequented by staff (e.g., break rooms). Numerous resources for healthcare-associated infection prevention including CA-UTI are available from the CDC (http://www.cdc.gov/hai/prevent/tap/resources.html).

For symptomatic UTIs, ASPs should consider collaborating with microbiology laboratories to create urine-specific antibiograms to guide treatment as hospital-wide antibiograms may lead to unnecessarily broad-spectrum antibiotic coverage. This is especially important in the ED where uncomplicated UTIs in otherwise healthy community patients are frequently encountered. Hospital and even ED-specific antibiograms may be skewed toward patients with multiple comorbidities and higher rates of antibiotic resistance as otherwise healthy patients frequently receive empiric treatment and may not have cultures performed or represent a minority of patients presenting to EDs with UTIs.[32] Education on local resistance patterns in the ED can increase use of narrow-spectrum agents such as cephalexin or urine-specific agents like nitrofurantoin, and minimize use of broad-spectrum agents such as fluoroquinolones.[33] As national rates of fluoroquinolone resistance have neared 20%, it is important to use local resistance data to customize treatment recommendations for conditions such as pyelonephritis.[34] Finally, previous urine culture results can assist in current therapy choice. A study of >4,000 patients with multiple paired urine cultures found 57% and 83% concordance in the identity and susceptibility pattern respectively of urine pathogens when a culture was performed four to eight weeks later in the same patient.[35]

Selection of therapy for uncomplicated cystitis should cover the predominant organisms (namely *Escherichia coli*) with a narrow-spectrum agent based on local susceptibility patterns. For complicated UTI, factors such as the presence of urinary catheters, recent or prolonged hospitalization, and antibiotic exposure must be accounted for in addition to local susceptibility patterns. Pharmacokinetic properties of the antibiotic are important to assure adequate concentration of the drug at the site of infection. For example, agents such as nitrofurantoin and fosfomycin, while excellent choices for cystitis, do not achieve adequate renal concentrations to treat upper tract infections. Literature regarding optimal duration of treatment for simple cystitis suggests that shorter courses are adequate and regimens ranging from a single dose to five days, depending on the agent used, are recommended.[36] Treatment duration for complicated UTIs, including pyelonephritis and CA-UTI, should be driven by the agent used and patient characteristics.[29, 36] A detailed review of duration of therapy can be found in Chapter 6.

Pneumonia and Lower-Respiratory Tract Infections

Pneumonia is the most common infectious syndrome requiring hospitalization with an estimated 1.1 million discharges with a primary diagnosis of pneumonia in 2010 [37]. In a review of antibiotic use at 183 hospitals, treatment of lower-respiratory tract infection (LRTI) accounted for 38% of all use and was the most common indication for prescribing antibiotics.[38] Unfortunately, much of this use is both broad spectrum and inappropriate. At one center, only 48% of pneumonia diagnoses by the treating team were corroborated upon expert case review.[9] Similarly, only 42% of 231 suspected VAP cases were confirmed upon review, resulting in 1,183 excess antibiotic days.[39]

There are numerous opportunities for ASPs to improve clinical care for patients with all forms of pneumonia using a syndromic antibiotic stewardship approach. These efforts include diagnostic issues such as optimizing microbiologic testing or implementing bio-marker testing; selecting empiric therapy including when to cover for resistant pathogens; optimizing therapy once culture data are known and the clinical picture becomes clearer; and preventing pneumonia with pneumococcal vaccines and VAP prevention bundles. Included below is a discussion of these approaches with, where applicable, specific recommendations for the various pneumonia syndromes including CAP, hospital-acquired pneumonia (HAP), and VAP.

The diagnosis of pneumonia can be difficult and empiric antibiotics are often started where respiratory issues are later found to be noninfectious in nature; thus, ASP facilitation of diagnosis and test utilization is important. In addition, viral LRTI may present similarly to bacterial infection and differentiation can be difficult. ASPs may choose to implement algorithms that incorporate biomarkers such as procalcitonin (PCT) to assist in pneumonia diagnosis. PCT has been shown to be useful in differentiating bacterial from nonbacterial causes of LRTIs including bronchitis, exacerbations of COPD, CAP, HAP, and VAP. PCT is ubiquitously produced in situations of systemic infection such as pneumonia and sepsis; rises rapidly (typically within six to twelve hours); is not generally impaired by immuno-suppression; correlates with severity of illness; and declines when an infection is appropriately treated. Numerous randomized trials have shown PCT-guided therapy can safely decrease antibiotic use in a variety of LRTIs (VAP, CAP, exacerbations of chronic bronchitis, and acute LRTI) and in a variety of settings (ambulatory, ED, inpatient, and ICU). [40–43] The largest study of PCT use was a randomized, multicenter, non-inferiority trial comparing PCT-guided therapy to usual care which enrolled 1381 patients presenting to the ED with LRTI.[43] PCT levels were used to assist clinician decision-making about antibiotic initiation and to prompt discontinuation when it normalized. PCT-based management was associated with a 12.2% absolute decrease in antibiotic initiation (87.7% vs. 75.4%), three fewer days of antibiotic exposure (5.7 vs. 8.7 days), and an 8.2% absolute decrease in antibiotic adverse events (28.1% vs. 19.8%). There was no difference in mortality, ICU admission, recurrence, and disease-specific complications between the groups. A meta-analysis found PCT-guided therapy in LRTI was associated with lower antibiotic exposures across all settings and diagnoses, without any increase in mortality.[44] These data suggest that integrating PCT into pneumonia and LRTI management can result in significant improvements in antibiotic use if suggested protocols are followed. Unfortunately, little US data exists, and it is unclear if PCT outside of the research setting results in such robust changes in antibiotic use.[45] If procalcitonin is implemented, ASP driven educational efforts are essential to successful implementation of PCT and should be targeted toward clinicians who will be interpreting the data including intensivists, hospitalists, and ED clinicians. Treating clinicians must recognize when to order a PCT, what conditions can cause noninfectious elevations in PCT, when to repeat, and how to interpret the results as different levels imply different likelihoods of bacterial infection. Audit and feedback of patients with negative PCT values who are on antibiotics may be a useful activity for ASP teams. The combination of various diagnostic tools such as biomarkers, clinical predictions scores, and/or rapid viral testing may also be useful to ASPs in promoting appropriate antibiotic use.[46, 47]

ASPs should be engaged in guiding the use of antibiotics in pneumonia, in particular they should focus on determining when to use combination therapy and broad-spectrum agents targeting multidrug-resistant organisms (MDRO) such as MRSA and *Pseudomonas aeruginosa*. Targeting typical respiratory-tract pathogens (*Streptococcus pneumoniae, Haemophilus influenzae, Legionella pneumophila*, etc.) with combination therapy is recommended for all patients with severe CAP or CAP treated in the ICU. Interventions that assist clinicians in identifying these patients such as the creation of order sets with the definition of severe CAP included or clinical decision support systems which suggest appropriate regimens based on the level of care can be considered.

Current American Thoracic Society and Infectious Diseases Society of America (IDSA) guidelines recommend that decisions on when to provide therapy active against MDRO organisms be based on the presence of risk factors for these pathogens.[48, 49] A significant proportion of pneumonia cases may be considered high risk for MDRO pathogens including late-onset (>5 days in hospital) HAP, VAP, and potentially healthcare-associated pneumonia (HCAP). While HCAP is no longer included in the HAP/VAP guidelines it is an ingrained driver of antibiotic use and facilities should consider how to guide antibiotic use in these cases. HCAP is typically defined as the presence of any of the following risk factors: recent hospital stay or antibiotic use, residence in a long-term care facility, receipt of hemodialysis, participation in home IV or wound therapy, or previous colonization with MDRO pathogens.[50] While there are clear data supporting MDRO risk in VAP, much less data are available for non-ventilated HAP or HCAP. Although retrospective studies including culture-positive HCAP patients have found high MDRO rates, prospective studies and studies including culture-negative patients have not corroborated this.[51–53] For example, a single center study of community-onset pneumonia in the US ($N = 521$, 49.5% HCAP) found MDROs to be uncommon (3.8% overall) with slightly higher rates in HCAP vs. CAP (5.9% vs. 1.9% respectively).[52] In this study, the HCAP definition was not associated with MDRO isolation, but specific risk factors for MDRO isolation included long-term care facility (LTCF) residence, previous isolation of *Pseudomonas aeruginosa*, antibiotic exposure in the last 90 days, and duration of hospitalization in the last 90 days. Similarly, a meta-analysis of 24 studies judged the overall quality of evidence available to be poor and found the HCAP definition poorly discriminatory for MDRO isolation.[54] Unfortunately, the HCAP definition has driven expanded use of broad-spectrum antibiotic use with the percent of pneumonia patients at Veterans Affairs hospitals treated with vancomycin and piperacillin/tazobactam rising from 16% to 31% and 16% to 27% respectively.[55] MDRO incidence rates vary by region and facility, and ASPs should use local data to better identify those patients needing broad-spectrum antibiotics. The current HAP/VAP guidelines recommend creation of a respiratory tract specific antibiogram as one method to better target MDRO therapy.[48] ASPs should work to identify local risk factors for MDRO infection and put processes in place to ensure broad-spectrum antibiotics are restricted to only those at increased risk.

Syndromic interventions should provide guidance on when and what microbiologic data should be obtained along with information on how to interpret these data. Not all patients with CAP require extensive microbiologic evaluation. The utility of blood cultures in hospitalized CAP patients has been debated due to low yield and false-positive results. For example, 84% of 209 CAP patients had blood cultures but nearly half of the positive results were for contaminants.[56] Sputum cultures, while only able to be obtained in 40–50% of patients and not indicated in all patients, can be useful. Gram-stain and culture can diagnose up to 80% of pneumococcal pneumonias if obtained early in the course of evaluation (< 12 hours after antibiotics). [57] In addition, negative sputum cultures can be used for de-escalation as noted in the IDSA CAP guidelines: "Failure to detect S. *aureus* or gram-negative bacilli in good-quality specimens is strong evidence against the presence of these pathogens."[49] Thus, negative respiratory-tract cultures should prompt ASPs to recommend de-escalation, particularly if therapy targeting MRSA or *Pseudomonas* has been initiated. Urine antigens for pneumococcus and *Legionella pneumophila* should be reserved for those at high risk for these pathogens but offer the advantages of reasonable diagnostic performance and a readily available specimen. In a study of 474 CAP episodes (36% caused by pneumococci), 75 cases were diagnosed by urine antigen only with 41 clinicians adjusting therapy based on this data alone.[58] Finally, centers that perform nasal swabs to evaluate for MRSA colonization may find this data useful in deciding when to use vancomycin. For example, a negative MRSA nasal polymerase chain reaction (PCR) in a single center study had a negative predictive value for MRSA pneumonia of 99%.[59] Conversely, Sarikonda et al. found that MRSA colonization detected by PCR was poorly predictive of MRSA pneumonia in the ICU with a negative predictive value of 84% and a positive predictive value of 18%.[60] ASP programs should develop processes such as order sets which facilitate evidence-based use of diagnostic studies in CAP.

For patients who are at risk of MDRO (HCAP/HAP/VAP), ASPs should institute processes to guide when and how to obtain respiratory-tract specimens in addition to assisting clinicians to use these data to adjust therapy. Detection of colonization is common, particularly in patients who have chronic lung disease or are ventilated, and ASP should develop clinical criteria guiding when and how to obtain respiratory-tract specimens. Interestingly, the lack of an adequate respiratory-tract specimen in patients diagnosed with VAP has been associated with failure to de-escalate antibiotics and increased mortality.[61, 62] The type of sample should be individualized as a randomized trial comparing outcomes of various respiratory-tract sampling (directed bronchoalveolar lavage/brushing [BAL] vs. endotracheal aspiration [ETA]) for VAP diagnosis found no difference in antibiotic use and mortality between the diagnostic modalities.[62]

Based on these data, current guidelines recommend using noninvasive sampling to obtain a semi-quantitative respiratory-tract culture in all patients with suspected HAP or VAP.[48] ASPs should target patients with VAP and negative cultures for potential antibiotic discontinuation. In support of this recommendation, Raman et al. found antibiotic discontinuation in patients with suspected VAP and negative BALs did not increase mortality compared to continuation of therapy.[63] In fact, therapy discontinuation was associated with a decrease in the number of subsequent superinfections, respiratory superinfections, and multidrug-resistant superinfections.[63] Some facilities use routine respiratory-tract surveillance cultures to direct empiric therapy in VAP.[64–66] If this practice is employed, programs must enact processes to avoid overtreatment of colonized patients and ensure the data are used to guide therapy.

With the frequent use of empiric broad-spectrum antibiotics in pneumonia, de-escalation and appropriate duration of therapy should be included in any pneumonia ASP effort. De-escalation in pneumonia and sepsis has been associated with decreased mortality, and both positive and negative respiratory-tract cultures can assist in de-escalation.[67, 68] Duration of therapy in pneumonia is often longer than necessary and further information on appropriate antibiotic durations can be found in Chapter 6. In the ICU where the majority of antibiotic use is for respiratory-tract infections, collaboration between ICU teams and Infectious Diseases (ID) physicians and/or ASP experts can improve antibiotic use.[69] Additionally, clinical decision support systems can improve both empiric and culture-directed antibiotic therapy and may improve clinical outcomes.[70, 71]

Implementing these interventions using a "bundle" approach has improved both antibiotic use and patient outcomes in pneumonia. Receipt of guideline concordant therapy is associated with improved clinical outcomes in CAP and should be a component of any CAP bundle recommended by the ASP.[72, 73] The ED is a natural setting for CAP bundle implementation. A CAP-treatment algorithm including education, printed forms, and automated pharmacy technology improved appropriate antibiotic selection from 55% to 93%.[74] CAP bundle implementation at another center resulted in earlier initiation of antibiotics, improved mortality (11% vs. 14%), and shortened length of hospital stay (8 vs. 9 days) [8]. Finally, a multicenter study randomized hospitals to usual care or implementation of a CAP bundle that included the following: a clinical prediction rule for admission; standardized antibiotic selection and duration recommendations; and guidelines for the timing of intravenous (IV) to oral (PO) switch and hospital discharge.[75] Bundle use decreased admission rates, bed usage, and length of stay for CAP without any increase in adverse outcomes. Duration of IV antimicrobial antibiotic therapy also decreased by 1.7 days. Similar improvements have been documented when clinical guidelines have been introduced in pediatric CAP patients.[76, 77]

As mentioned previously, ASP efforts can be coupled with prevention strategies. While VAP prevention efforts have been successful at decreasing VAP rates, improvements in antibiotic use have been less common. [78] The multicenter implementation of a VAP clinical practice guideline addressing prevention, diagnosis, and treatment through education and implementation team engagement, improved VAP prevention practices and decreased VAP rates but not antibiotic appropriateness.[10] ASP should work with infection control and critical care to implement strategies proven to decrease both time on the ventilator and VAP. Finally, pneumococcal vaccination has been associated with decreased incidence of CAP and improved outcomes when pneumonia does develop.[79] Improvement in pneumococcal and influenza vaccination rates of inpatients and/or outpatients is a worthy target for stewardship efforts and can be integrated into the syndromic approach.

Skin and Soft Tissue Infections

ED visits and hospital admissions related to SSTIs have been increasing, potentially attributable to the emergence of community-associated MRSA.[80] SSTI is an important target for antibiotic stewardship intervention as management of these infections has been associated with unnecessary diagnostic studies, overly broad-spectrum antibiotic therapy, and prolonged treatment duration. A study of 322 SSTIs at a single center found >70% of cases were treated with both broad-spectrum gram-negative and anti-anaerobic therapy; furthermore, 46% of cases were treated with three or more antibiotics.[81]

The first step to appropriate management of SSTIs is correct diagnosis of the specific type of SSTI (abscess vs. cellulitis vs. surgical wound infection, etc.) as this will allow clinicians to target the anticipated pathogens. Education regarding how to differentiate SSTI from other common conditions is useful and should be considered. An understanding of the microbial epidemiology of common SSTIs is essential to appropriate antibiotic use. Beta-hemolytic streptococci cause the vast majority of non-suppurative cellulitis and targeting these pathogens alone using a beta-lactam antibiotic is appropriate.[82, 83] *Staphylococcus aureus* is frequently associated with skin abscesses, infections with significant purulence, open wounds, penetrating trauma, and sites of intravenous drug use. Greater than half of *S. aureus* causing these types of SSTI are methicillin-resistant and therapy recommendations must take this into account.[84] Gram-negative and anaerobic pathogens are typically only causative of SSTI in the setting of animal bites, water associated injuries, neutropenia and other severe states of immunosuppression, and very severe infections such as necrotizing fasciitis, severe diabetic foot infections, and gas gangrene. [85] Severe SSTI in diabetic patients may be appropriate for use of agents active against gram-negative and anaerobic pathogens, but superficial infections (cellulitis, etc.) and mild to moderate diabetic foot ulcers are usually monomicrobial and caused by Staphylococci or Streptococcal spp. [91]. Therefore, empiric therapy for almost all SSTI should be limited to gram-positive coverage only. If parenteral therapy is initiated, prompt de-escalation to oral therapy is recommended once clinical improvement is observed. Oral agents for the treatment of SSTI, specifically agents that cover MRSA, should be selected based on local antibiograms as susceptibility to oral agents, particularly clindamycin, may vary. Many patients with cutaneous abscesses can be managed with incision and drainage alone and guidance on when to use antibiotics can be useful. The optimal duration of treatment of cellulitis or cutaneous abscesses in the hospital setting is not well established, but in general, treatment durations of 5–7 days are adequate, although longer courses may be appropriate in severe or poorly responding infections.[85]

Another important aspect of antibiotic stewardship in SSTI is guiding the utilization of laboratory tests or imaging. Antibiotic stewardship protocols should discourage the routine use of radiographs, blood cultures, and labs such as C-reactive protein and erythrocyte sedimentation rate. Blood cultures are low yield (positive in <5%of cases) and not cost-effective to perform for all patients but should be obtained in those with severe signs of systemic illness, neutropenia, malignancy or other immunodeficiency, or predisposing factors like animal bites or immersion injury.[85, 86] Tissue cultures or skin biopsies in cellulitis are exceedingly low yield and not recommended. When an abscess is drained, cultures should be obtained, particularly if an antibiotic is being utilized.[85] Imaging in SSTI is common but of low diagnostic yield, as described by Jenkins et al. who found 83% of patients with SSTIs underwent imaging with diagnostic yields of <2%.[81] Use of computed tomographic (CT) and magnetic resonance imaging (MRI) should be discouraged except in cases of suspected pyomyositis, severe infection including necrotizing fasciitis, lack of response to therapy, and potentially neutropenic cancer patients.[85, 87]

Clinical practice guidelines generated by ASPs encompassing both diagnosis and treatment can optimize the management of SSTI. Denver Health implemented a guideline for cellulitis and cutaneous abscess that was disseminated broadly and incorporated into an electronic admission order set. [3] The guideline recommended selective use of plain film radiographs and blood cultures and discouraged CT, MRI, and superficial wound cultures. Therapeutic guidance included empiric therapy recommendations, use of nonsteroidal anti-inflammatory agents, oral transition options based on culture results, and standardized durations of therapy. Post-implementation of the guideline, use of microbiologic cultures decreased from 80% to 66% and median duration of antibiotic therapy decreased (13 vs. 10 days), both of which were significant. Additionally, fewer patients received broad-spectrum gram-negative antibiotics or anti-anaerobic therapy with no change in clinical failure rates.[3]

Antibiotic stewardship interventions for SSTI are especially important for patients in the ED where the potential for subsequent admission is high if managed inappropriately. Interventions targeting the inappropriate use of intravenous agents such as vancomycin for patients who will be discharged from the ED may be useful as vancomycin overuse is common.[88] The utility of real-time determination of S. aureus and methicillin-susceptibility in the ED has been associated with more targeted antibiotic selection. In one study, the use of rapid identification of S. aureus and differentiation of methicillin-resistant strains in the ED was associated with improvements in antibiotic appropriateness, although absolute changes in antibiotic use were small.[89] The role of rapid diagnostics is explored further in Chapter 9.

Another novel intervention to optimize SSTI therapy and minimize readmissions is the use of "to-go" medications in the ED (i.e., when the remainder of the antibiotic course is given to the patient at the time of ED discharge to continue in the outpatient setting rather than a prescription). A comparison of patients with cellulitis who received their full course of medications "to-go" compared to those who received a prescription found a reduction in return visits (2% vs. 7%) at a cost of only $1,123 to the institution.[90] "To-go" medications can be applied to other common infections seen in the ED such as UTIs or dental infections through ASP and ED collaboration.[90] Developing strategies to improve compliance with post-discharge medications, such as a "to-go" program could facilitate treatment success as noncompliance with post-discharge oral therapy increases the risk for poor clinical outcomes.[91]

Bacteremia and Candidemia

Bacteremia

Bacteremia and candidemia are common targets for ASP efforts and a wealth of emerging rapid diagnostic technologies can be easily coupled to antibiotic stewardship interventions to optimize therapy (Chapter 9). Even in the absence of such rapid diagnostic tests, there is much potential for antibiotic stewardship involvement in the management of bacteremia. *Staphylococcus aureus* bacteremia has a 30-day mortality of roughly 25% and is associated with metastatic infection and excess morbidity and mortality.[92] Quality performance measures for the management of SAB can be found in IDSA clinical practice guidelines for the treatment of MRSA and can generally be extrapolated to methicillin-sensitive *Staphylococcus aureus* MSSA management [93] Infectious diseases expert consultation for patients with SAB has been shown to improve outcomes including reduced infection relapse or recurrence, hospital readmission, and mortality.[94–96] ASP teams can help coordinate evidence-based care for patients with SAB and also facilitate timely ID consultation. Similar to other infectious syndromes discussed in this chapter, antibiotic stewardship interventions related to SAB are best implemented as a multifaceted bundle. The University of Michigan Hospitals and Health System implemented a SAB care bundle that improved adherence with the SAB performance measures and decreased readmissions for SAB.[97] A pharmacy member of their ASP team received real-time alerts every time *S. aureus* was identified in the blood. Using guidance from the SAB care bundle, the ASP pharmacist made recommendations to the primary care team or the ID consult service and followed the patients for the duration of their hospitalization. SAB bundle elements included initiation of effective antibiotics within 24 hours of Gram-stain, achievement of therapeutic vancomycin concentrations, recommendations for IV beta-lactam therapy for MSSA, blood cultures every 48 hours until clearance, elimination of the foci of infection if feasible, an echocardiogram for complicated bacteremia, and ID consultation.[97] While ASP interventions have not been directly compared to bedside ID consultation, there are data suggesting that bedside consultation is superior to telephone consultation.[98]

Antibiotic stewardship interventions in SAB should focus on rapid transition to optimal therapy and appropriate dosing. Vancomycin remains the mainstay of treatment for MRSA bacteremia, and beta-lactams such as oxacillin/nafcillin or cefazolin are preferred for MSSA. As MSSA bacteremia outcomes are significantly worse if treated with non-beta-lactam agents, early transition to beta-lactams is a potential target for ASP intervention. ASPs can also create protocols to promote optimal vancomycin dosing as achievement of target troughs of 15–20 mg/L early in therapy is associated with improved clinical outcomes.[99]

ASP interventions can also influence the management of gram-negative bacteremia where time to appropriate therapy is an important modifiable risk factor for mortality.[100] The ASP for a three-hospital system implemented a program where pharmacists received automated pages during business hours when gram-negative bacilli were found in blood cultures and when results were updated. After-hours and weekend results were emailed for review the following workday. The ASP pharmacist reviewed the patient record and contacted the team with recommendations. Time to appropriate therapy was significantly lower, 8 vs. 14 hours, in the intervention group as was attributable length of stay, that decreased by 2.2 days. Most important, in patients not on appropriate therapy at the time of culture positivity, ASP intervention resulted in significant reductions in length of stay and infection-related mortality.[101] Microbiologists from the ASP team can also have a positive impact on bacteremia management. A four-year pre/post-intervention evaluating clinical microbiologist participation on rounds in a cardiothoracic ICU found that appropriate empirical therapy, compliance with guidelines, therapy de-escalations, and time to optimization of therapy were all significantly improved.[102] While at most institutions it is unlikely that ASPs have the resources to round with all ICU teams, data suggest that having an ASP team member provide recommendations early in bacteremia management is beneficial.

Another important aspect of care that ASPs can impact through their recommendations is de-escalation of antibiotics in the setting of negative blood cultures. Some centers do not report a preliminary negative blood culture result for three to five days, despite data suggesting that 98% of aerobic gram-positive and gram-negative bloodstream infections are detected within 48 hours.[103] This promotes antibiotic continuation until cultures are finalized. An evaluation of 416 monomicrobial bloodstream infections and 210 contamination episodes demonstrated a 99.8% negative predictive value of negative culture results at 48 hours, potentially facilitating earlier de-escalation or discontinuation of empiric antibiotic therapy.[103]

Cost effectiveness data focusing on bacteremia management can be utilized to support the development of ASPs or continued support. A study using a decision analysis model compared costs and outcomes of patients with bacteremia when managed with or without antibiotic stewardship intervention. [104] The authors found that ASP bacteremia review cost $39,737 compared to standard treatment (no stewardship) costing $39,563. The probabilistic sensitivity analysis demonstrated there was more than a 90% likelihood that antibiotic stewardship would be cost-effective at a level of $10,000 per quality-adjusted life year (QALY), and the cost of operating an ASP per QALY gained was estimated to be $2367.[104]

Candidemia and Antifungal Stewardship

Multiple studies have investigated the role of stewardship in improving the quality of management of candidemia. Similar to bacteremia, successful programs have utilized a bundled approach with multiple interventions to optimize treatment with real-time intervention by stewardship team members. Implementation of a comprehensive care bundle based on elements from the IDSA Candidiasis Guidelines [105] at a single center improved compliance with evidence-based practices, but did not improve length of stay, time to candidemia clearance, or incidence of recurrence.[106] The bundle focused on selection of appropriate antifungal therapy, removal of intravascular catheters, obtainment of blood cultures at least every 48 hours until clearance of candidemia, appropriate duration of antifungal treatment, and coordination of ophthalmologic exams to assess for *Candida* endophthalmitis. A similar study using a comprehensive candidemia guideline and ASP notification for all Candida-positive blood cultures found time to effective therapy decreased in the post-intervention period from a median of 13.5 hours to 1.3 hours. Effective therapy was administered more frequently in the post-intervention period [88% vs. 99%). There were no differences demonstrated for in-hospital mortality, infection-related length-of-stay, or hospital costs.[107]

While antibiotic stewardship has traditionally focused on antibiotics, the health and economic burden of invasive fungal infections are substantial. Additionally, antifungal agents are associated with high drug costs and potential toxicities making antifungal stewardship an important area for intervention. An antifungal stewardship program that focused on cost-effective management of invasive Aspergillus infections and candidemia decreased total antifungal prescriptions and expenditures during the six-year program. Specific recommendations for invasive aspergillosis included galactomannin antigen testing, CT scans, voriconazole therapeutic drug monitoring, and minimal use of combination therapy. The recommendations for candidemia included optimal timing and duration of antifungal therapy and removal of central venous catheters.[108]

Clostridium difficile Infections

CDI has become the most common healthcare-associated infection with an estimated 250,000–500,000 infections and 14,000–29,000 deaths per year in the United States.[109, 110] CDI recurrence is also common, occurring in 20–30% of cases. The initiating factor in CDI pathogenesis is the disruption of normal intestinal flora, usually due to antibiotic exposure, although other agents (chemotherapy, proton pump inhibitors [PPI]) likely contribute as well. Use of any antibiotic for even short durations can precipitate CDI, but certain classes are associated with greater CDI risk including clindamycin, broad-spectrum cephalosporins (3rd and 4th generation), carbapenems, and fluoroquinolones.[111, 112] Thus antibiotic use, particularly inappropriate use, is a driver for CDI with one center finding 26% of patients diagnosed with CDI had been unnecessarily treated with antibiotics. [113] There is a large body of evidence associating changes in antibiotic use with decreased CDI occurrence. Valiquette et al. described a severe CDI outbreak that was not controlled with infection control practices alone, but when an ASP intervention reduced high-risk antibiotic use by 50%, the outbreak was halted.[114] Data from the UK and Scotland demonstrate how changes in antibiotic use can influence national CDI rates.[115, 116] CDI risk increases with the number of antibiotics, duration of therapy, and total antibiotic dose, which suggests antibiotic stewardship interventions that improve any of these factors are likely to be beneficial.[117]

Other medications, such as PPIs, that increase the risk of CDI or recurrence, can also be targeted by ASPs. There is accumulating data that PPI use, even without antibiotics, can result in CDI.[118–120] Unfortunately, PPIs are widely prescribed (often for non-evidence-based indications) and infrequently discontinued, even when CDI has occurred. One study found 61% of CDI cases were on a PPI with less than half prescribed for an evidence-based indication. PPI use was discontinued in only three of 458 patients.[119]

Other antibiotics in use at the time of CDI diagnosis should be discontinued, if possible, as continued use has been associated with slower resolution of symptoms, lower cure rates, and increased likelihood of relapse.[121] A large multicenter retrospective analysis of CDI found continuation of non-CDI treatment antibiotics after diagnosis associated with a 63% increase in length of stay and an increased odds of mortality and readmission.[122]

C. difficile test ordering and interpretation is another potential target for antibiotic stewardship intervention. CDI testing should only be performed when patients are clearly symptomatic as asymptomatic carriage is not uncommon. In addition, other reasons for diarrhea should be evaluated before ordering a CDI test including use of laxatives or recent receipt of oral contrast. At one center, only 96 of 150 patients tested for CDI had clinically significant diarrhea and at another center 44% of persons tested for CDI had received a laxative within the last 48 hours.[123, 124] Ordering *C. difficile* tests can be highly variable. Under-testing can miss CDI cases and over-testing can result in unnecessary treatment of asymptomatic individuals.[125] Testing of infants (<1 year of age), testing for cure, and repeat testing should be strongly discouraged. Education on appropriate testing can improve both diagnostic performance and appropriateness of therapy.[124] Many tests are available to diagnose CDI with varying performance characteristics and turnaround times, and ASP recommendations for interpretation must be customized to the characteristics of the method used and population tested. Of note, recent data have suggested that PCR-based testing may be "over-sensitive" and detect very low levels of *C. difficile* not associated with adverse outcomes.[126, 127] Whatever testing method is used, ASPs should provide specific guidance on when to test for CDI while working with clinicians and the microbiology laboratory to ensure appropriate test use and interpretation.

C. difficile treatment should be based upon disease severity which is classified into mild-moderate, severe, and severe-complicated disease. ASPs should develop systems to promote severity-based treatment. Oral vancomycin has been shown to be superior to metronidazole for CDI treatment, especially for moderate to severe CDI.[128, 129] Despite the superiority of vancomycin for CDI, a number of studies show low vancomycin utilization.[124, 130, 131] A single center review of CDI found only 52% compliance with national treatment guidelines. Noncompliance was most common in severe *C. difficile* disease and was associated with increased mortality and recurrence.[130, 132] Jardin and colleagues implemented ASP directed automatic substitution of vancomycin for metronidazole in severe CDI cases and increased vancomycin use from 14% to 91%.[133] ASP guided and enforced institutional standards of when and how to use combination therapy can be developed. In addition, identifying severely ill patients and promoting involvement of experts such as infectious disease and surgery is critical.

CDI bundles have become common and these generally focus on improving test use/interpretation, providing appropriate treatment based on severity of disease, and reducing the use of other medications that promote CDI such as PPIs and concomitant antibiotics. They also may be coupled with processes that target reduction of antibiotics in patients at high risk for developing CDI and improved infection control practices. In one example, education of nurses and house officers improved the appropriateness of test ordering and the treatment of severe CDI with vancomycin, which increased guideline compliance from 57% to 93%.[124] The education also included teaching on how CDI is transmitted and the prevention practices that should be used (i.e., contact precautions, hand washing with soap and water, cleaning of equipment and the environment with bleach, and avoiding unnecessary antibiotics). Jury et al. implemented a series of steps including education of clinicians, EMR-based clinical decision support, timely notification of *C. difficile* positive results, and audit and feedback of CDI therapy.[134] These interventions were associated with significant improvements in CDI treatment in response to testing, time to starting CDI therapy, and appropriate use of vancomycin for severe CDI. Finally, Brumley et al. implemented CDI education, ASP review of CDI cases, and an electronic care bundle which prompted discontinuation of concomitant antibiotics and acid suppressive medications, severity-based antibiotic selection, appropriate duration of therapy decisions, and consultation with experts. [7] Compliance with the overall bundle increased from 45% to 81% with significant improvements in discontinuation of acid suppression (18% vs. 90%) and increased administration of appropriate therapy (64% vs. 82%).

Infection control practices are essential to preventing the spread of CDI and control of antibiotic use without effective infection control will likely be unsuccessful at controlling CDI spread. ASPs should work with local infection control experts to implement recommended practices including rapid CDI identification with implementation of contact isolation, dedicated equipment for CDI positive patients, hand hygiene upon room exit, and disinfection of contaminated equipment and the environment with sporicidal agents. [123] Other strategies are available if these primary strategies are unsuccessful at controlling CDI, and readers are referred to the SHEA Compendium of Strategies to Prevent *Clostridium difficile* Infections in Acute Care Hospitals for further information.[123]

Conclusion

One of the most common tools used for syndromic antibiotic stewardship is the development of a clinical guideline or treatment algorithm often in conjunction with an order set. Figure 1 illustrates how clinical and laboratory data can be used to develop an algorithm for diagnosis and management of UTI, which can be paired with treatment recommendations based upon the type of UTI diagnosed (simple vs. complicated). As mentioned, syndromic antibiotic stewardship can be bundled with prevention practices. Figure 2 is an example of a therapeutic and prevention component of a syndromic antibiotic stewardship intervention focusing on CDI management. To promote uptake, an order set could be created that automatically presents severity-based treatment recommendations to clinicians when a patient tests positive for CDI. This illustrates how clinical decision support systems (CDSS) can be integrated into syndromic antibiotic stewardship. CDSS can provide patient-specific information filtered or presented at opportune times with a goal of enhancing care. Guidance in the EMR may utilize alerts, templates, reference information, order sets, or other tools which can also be implemented using paper forms. Further information on EMR and CDSS is in Chapter 10. Education that targets end users should always be a part of syndromic antibiotic stewardship and is essential to its success. Education can take the form of handouts, academic detailing, lectures, case presentations, electronic modules, and point of care statements.

The key ingredients for successful syndromic antibiotic stewardship are not defined, but the following are suggested as essential to success: leadership, accountability, expert input, integration into usual care, ease of use, implementation in appropriate populations, education which includes framing the reasons for change, process evaluation, and feedback. Leadership commitment to antibiotic stewardship and an accountable leader are essential. The creation of syndrome-based efforts requires multidisciplinary input; experts from relevant disciplines affected should be included. For example, development of an ED CAP protocol should involve ED physicians, hospitalists, along with ID and critical care experts. ED nurses and pharmacists are important for process implementation and should also be consulted. Clinical leaders should be engaged to provide onsite support and validation of any efforts. For example, if a surgical antibiotic prophylaxis effort is being developed,

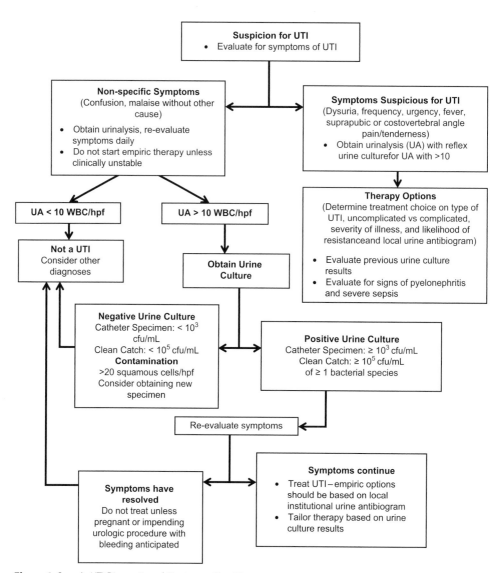

Figure 1 Sample UTI Diagnosis and Treatment Algorithm

leaders from each surgical area, anesthesia, and pharmacy should all be involved so they can then promote best practices among their peers. Finally, changing antibiotic use requires changing clinician behavior and the reasons for adjusting practice should be framed appropriately. When approaching clinicians, the discussion should focus on clinical value and improved patient care. It is easier to obtain "buy-in" from clinicians if the focus is improving care around a specific condition rather than restricting antibiotic use. Furthermore, interventions viewed as collaborative, educational, and promoting optimized care rather than restricting clinician choice are likely to be better accepted and may lead to sustained behavior change. Local practice data can be exceedingly useful in this situation to highlight areas for improvement.

Mild-Moderate *C. difficile* Infection (CDI): Diarrhea not meeting criteria for severe or complicated
- Vancomycin 125 mg PO q6h x 10 days
- Alternative: Metronidazole 500 mg PO q8h x 10 days
  - Avoid IV metronidazole as data suggests inferior to PO.

Severe CDI: CDI associated with development of any of the following: WBC > 20,000, serum creatinine ≥ 1.5 X baseline, albumin <3.0 g/dl, severe abdominal tenderness, or requires ICU care for CDI
- Vancomycin 125 mg PO q6h x 10 days (DO NOT treat with IV vancomycin)

Severe, Complicated CDI: (i.e., hypotension or shock, ileus, toxic megacolon, fulminant colitis):
- Consult Infectious Diseases Service
- Consult Gastroenterology and General Surgery for evaluation for possible colectomy
- Vancomycin 500 mg PO q6h + metronidazole 500 mg IV q8h +/- vancomycin enema 500 mg in 100 mL of 0.9% NaCl; instill via Foley catheter q6h and retain for 1h

Recurrent CDI:
- Vancomycin 125 mg PO q6h x 10 days followed by,
- Vancomycin 125 mg PO q12h x 7 days, 125 mg PO q24h x 7 days, then 125 mg PO every 3 days x 14 days
- Consider referral for fecal microbiota transplant if recurrence after taper

Discontinue acid suppressive medications and other antibiotics if possible: The use of acid suppressive medications (ASM), especially proton pump inhib itors, has been associated with an increased risk of CDI. Patients with CDI continued on ASM have a higher recurrence rate of CDI. The use of concomitant antibiotics is associated with prolonged time to resolution and recurrence. Discontinue other antibiotics if medically possible.

Isolation/Infection Control

- All patient care units will use the same procedures for testing, treatment, and isolation
- Only patients with a positive *C. difficile* antigen (CDAg) and toxin OR positive CDAg, negative toxin, and positive PCR test should be placed on enteric isolation
- Enteric isolation procedures include:
  - Universal glove use for all contact with patient or environment
  - Gown use for any substantial patient or environmental contact
  - Soap and water hand hygiene after patient or environment contact
- Patients remain in isolation for 1 week after treatment is completed and they are asymptomatic (no diarrhea), whichever is longer
- Environmental Services will perform routine bleach cleaning of all CDI patient rooms weekly and at discharge
- UV irradiation will be included in terminal clean after CDI patient discharge

Figure 2 Sample *Clostridium difficile* Treatment and Isolation Guidelines
*Note, treatment recommendations represent examples, adjust based on institutional formulary, current guidelines, and literature.

The "how" of implementing syndrome-based antibiotic stewardship efforts is also important, and ASPs should try to consolidate efforts into an integrated approach. Rather than generating multiple guidance documents on CDI diagnosis, treatment, and isolation, consolidation into a one-stop shop is ideal. As described, this bundled approach is more likely to improve multiple aspects of care and result in direct patient outcome improvement. Development of syndromic efforts should take into account the current processes of care and attempt to work within these. Making resources available for clinicians is essential, and they can be distributed via forms, posters, websites, order sets, electronic alerts, or apps. These products should be concise, easy to locate, and easy to interpret. If CDSS or alerts are used, they should be directed toward the clinicians most likely to make use of them and be directly actionable. For example, when an alert fires for a positive CDI test, it should include the ability to order therapy as well. Finally, when any sort of improvement process is begun, a system for monitoring and providing performance feedback is essential. ASPs should develop ways to measure their success and identify areas for further improvement.

As described in this chapter, syndromic antibiotic stewardship is a frequently used tool and can address many issues of antibiotic misuse encountered by ASPs. It can be integrated with other strategies such as pre-authorization, IV to PO switch, education, de-escalation, and dose optimization. Syndrome-focused ASP efforts provide a clinically relevant method for driving improvements in antibiotic use and patient care.

References

1. Dellit TH, Owens RC, McGowan JE, Jr, et al. Infectious Diseases Society of America and the Society for Healthcare Epidemiology of America guidelines for developing an institutional program to enhance antimicrobial stewardship. *Clin Infect Dis* 2007; 44(2):159–177.

2. Barlam TF, Cosgrove SE, Abbo LM, et al. Executive summary: Implementing an antibiotic stewardship program: Guidelines by the Infectious Diseases Society of America and the Society for Healthcare Epidemiology of America. *Clin Infect Dis* 2016; 62(10):1197–1202.

3. Jenkins TC, Knepper BC, Sabel AL, et al. Decreased antibiotic utilization after implementation of a guideline for inpatient cellulitis and cutaneous abscess. *Arch Intern Med* 2011; 171(12):1072–1079.

4. Lopez-Cortes LE, Del Toro MD, Galvez-Acebal J, et al. Impact of an evidence-based bundle intervention in the quality-of-care management and outcome of *Staphylococcus aureus* bacteremia. *Clin Infect Dis* 2013; 57(9):1225–1233.

5. Takesue Y, Ueda T, Mikamo H, et al. Management bundles for candidaemia: The impact of compliance on clinical outcomes. *J Antimicrob Chemother* 2015; 70(2):587–593.

6. Miller RR, III, Dong L, Nelson NC, et al. Multicenter implementation of a severe sepsis and septic shock treatment bundle. *Am J Respir Crit Care Med* 2013; 188 (1):77–82.

7. Brumley PE, Malani AN, Kabara JJ, Pisani J, Collins CD. Effect of an antimicrobial stewardship bundle for patients with *Clostridium difficile* infection. *J Antimicrob Chemother* 2016; 71(3):836–840.

8. Hortmann M, Heppner HJ, Popp S, Lad T, Christ M. Reduction of mortality in community-acquired pneumonia after implementing standardized care bundles in the emergency department. *Eur J Emerg Med* 2014; 21(6):429–435.

9. Filice GA, Drekonja DM, Thurn JR, Hamann GM, Masoud BT, Johnson JR. Diagnostic errors that lead to inappropriate antimicrobial use. *Infect Control Hosp Epidemiol* 2015; 36(8):949–956.

10. Sinuff T, Muscedere J, Cook DJ, et al. Implementation of clinical practice guidelines for ventilator-associated pneumonia: A multicenter prospective study. *Crit Care Med* 2013; 41(1):15–23.

11. Trautner BW, Grigoryan L, Petersen NJ, et al. Effectiveness of an antimicrobial stewardship approach for urinary catheter-associated asymptomatic bacteriuria. *JAMA Intern Med* 2015; 175(7) 1120–1127.

12. Kelley D, Aaronson P, Poon E, McCarter YS, Bato B, Jankowski CA. Evaluation of an antimicrobial stewardship approach to minimize overuse of antibiotics in patients with asymptomatic bacteriuria. *Infect*

Control Hosp Epidemiol 2014; 35 (2):193–195.

13. Nicolle LE, Bradley S, Colgan R, et al. Infectious Diseases Society of America guidelines for the diagnosis and treatment of asymptomatic bacteriuria in adults. *Clin Infect Dis* 2005; 40(5):643–654.

14. Cai T, Nesi G, Mazzoli S, et al. Asymptomatic bacteriuria treatment is associated with a higher prevalence of antibiotic resistant strains in women with urinary tract infections. *Clin Infect Dis* 2015; 61(11):1655–1661.

15. Lee MJ, Kim M, Kim NH, et al. Why is asymptomatic bacteriuria overtreated?: A tertiary care institutional survey of resident physicians. *BMC Infect Dis* 2015; 15:289.

16. Yin P, Kiss A, Leis JA. Urinalysis orders among patients admitted to the general medicine service. *JAMA Intern Med* 2015; 175(10):1711–1713.

17. Hartley S, Valley S, Kuhn L, et al. Inappropriate testing for urinary tract infection in hospitalized patients: An opportunity for improvement. *Infect Control Hosp Epidemiol* 2013; 34 (11):1204–1207.

18. Cope M, Cevallos ME, Cadle RM, Darouiche RO, Musher DM, Trautner BW. Inappropriate treatment of catheter-associated asymptomatic bacteriuria in a tertiary care hospital. *Clin Infect Dis*, 2009; 48(9):1182–1188.

19. Tambyah PA, Maki DG. The relationship between pyuria and infection in patients with indwelling urinary catheters: A prospective study of 761 patients. *Arch Intern Med*, 2000; 160(5):673–677.

20. Stovall RT, Haenal JB, Jenkins TC, et al. A negative urinalysis rules out catheter-associated urinary tract infection in trauma patients in the intensive care unit. *J Am Coll Surg* 2013; 217 (1):162–166.

21. Jones CW, Culbreath KD, Mehrotra A, Gilligan PH. Reflect urine culture cancellation in the emergency department. *J Emerg Med* 2014; 46(1):71–76.

22. Sarg M, Waldrop G, Beier M, et al. Impact of changes in urine culture ordering practices on antimicrobial utilization in intensive care units at an academic medical center. *Infect Cont Hosp Epidemiol* 2016; 37 (4):448–454.

23. Humphries RM, Dien Bard J. Point-counterpoint: Reflex cultures reduce laboratory workload and improve antimicrobial stewardship in patients suspected of having urinary tract infections. *J Clin Microbiol* 2016; 54 (2):254–258.

24. Leis JA, Rebick GW, Daneman N, et al. Reducing antimicrobial therapy for asymptomatic bacteriuria among noncatheterized inpatients: A proof-of-concept study. *Clin Infect Dis* 2014; 58 (7):980–983.

25. Kwon JH, Fausone MK, Du H, Robicsek A, Peterson LR. Impact of laboratory-reported urine culture colony counts on the diagnosis and treatment of urinary tract infection for hospitalized patients. *Am J Clin Pathol* 2012; 137(5):778–784.

26. Chironda B, Clancy S, Powis JE. Optimizing urine culture collection in the emergency department using frontline ownership interventions. *Clin Infect Dis* 2014; 59(7):1038–1039.

27. National Nosocomial Infections Surveillance System. National nosocomial infections surveillance (NNIS) system report, data summary from January 1992 through June 2004, issued October 2004. *Am J Infect Control* 2004; 32 (8):470–485.

28. Cornia PB, Amory JK, Fraser S, Saint S, Lipsky BA. Computer-based order entry decreases duration of indwelling urinary catheterization in hospitalized patients. *Am J Med* 2003; 114(5):404–407.

29. Hooton TM, Bradley SF, Cardenas DD, et al. Diagnosis, prevention, and treatment of catheter-associated urinary tract infection in adults: 2009 international clinical practice guidelines from the Infectious Diseases Society of America. *Clin Infect Dis* 2010; 50 (5):625–663.

30. Loeb M, Hunt D, O'Halloran K, Carusone SC, Dafoe N, Walter SD. Stop orders to reduce inappropriate urinary catheterization in hospitalized patients: A randomized controlled trial. *J Gen Intern Med* 2008; 23(6):816–820.

31. Topal J, Conklin S, Camp K, Morris V, Balcezak T, Herbert P. Prevention of nosocomial catheter-associated urinary tract infections through computerized feedback to physicians and a nurse-directed protocol. *Am J Med Qual* 2005; 20 (3):121–126.

32. Hines MC, Al-Salamah T, Heil EL, et al. Resistance patterns of *Escherichia coli* in women with uncomplicated urinary tract infection do not correlate with emergency department antibiogram. *J Emerg Med* 2015; 49(6):998–1003.

33. Hudepohl NJ, Cunha CB, Mermel LA. Antibiotic prescribing for urinary tract infections in the emergency department based on local antibiotic resistance patterns: Implications for antimicrobial stewardship. *Infect Control Hosp Epidemiol* 2015:1–2.

34. Sanchez GV, Master RN, Karlowsky JA, Bordon JM. In vitro antimicrobial resistance of urinary *Escherichia coli* isolates among U.S. outpatients from 2000 to 2010. *Antimicrob Agents Chemother* 2012; 56(4):2181–2183.

35. MacFadden DR, Ridgway JP, Robicsek A, Elligsen M, Daneman N. Predictive utility of prior positive urine cultures. *Clin Infect Dis* 2014; 59(9):1265–1271.

36. Gupta K, Hooton TM, Naber KG, et al. International clinical practice guidelines for the treatment of acute uncomplicated cystitis and pyelonephritis in women: A 2010 update by the Infectious Diseases Society of America and the European Society for Microbiology and Infectious Diseases. *Clin Infect Dis* 2011; 52(5): e103–120.

37. CDC. National hospital discharge survey. (Accessed August 2016, at www.cdc.gov/nchs/nhds/nhds_tables.htm#number.)

38. Fridkin S, Baggs J, Fagan R, et al. Vital signs: Improving antibiotic use among hospitalized patients. *MMWR Morb Mortal Wkly Rep* 2014; 63(9):194–200.

39. Nussenblatt V, Avdic E, Berenholtz S, et al. Ventilator-associated pneumonia: Overdiagnosis and treatment are common in medical and surgical intensive care units. *Infect Control Hosp Epidemiol* 2014; 35 (3):278–284.

40. Briel M, Schuetz P, Mueller B, et al. Procalcitonin-guided antibiotic use vs a standard approach for acute respiratory tract infections in primary care. *Arch Intern Med* 2008; 168(18):2000–2007.

41. Stolz D, Christ-Crain M, Bingisser R, et al. Antibiotic treatment of exacerbations of COPD: A randomized, controlled trial comparing procalcitonin-guidance with standard therapy. *Chest* 2007; 131(1):9–19.

42. Stolz D, Smyrnios N, Eggimann P, et al. Procalcitonin for reduced antibiotic exposure in ventilator-associated pneumonia: A randomised study. *Eur Respir J* 2009; 34(6):1364–1375.

43. Schuetz P, Christ-Crain M, Thomann R, et al. Effect of procalcitonin-based guidelines vs standard guidelines on antibiotic use in lower respiratory tract infections: The ProHOSP randomized controlled trial. *JAMA* 2009; 302 (10):1059–1066.

44. Schuetz P, Briel M, Christ-Crain M, et al. Procalcitonin to guide initiation and duration of antibiotic treatment in acute respiratory infections: An individual patient data meta-analysis. *Clin Infect Dis* 2012; 55(5):651–662.

45. Albrich WC, Dusemund F, Bucher B, et al. Effectiveness and safety of procalcitonin-guided antibiotic therapy in lower respiratory tract infections in "real life": An international, multicenter poststudy survey (ProREAL). *Arch Intern Med* 2012; 172 (9):715–722.

46. Zagli G, Cozzolino M, Terreni A, Biagioli T, Caldini AL, Peris A. Diagnosis of ventilator-associated pneumonia: A pilot, exploratory analysis of a new score based on procalcitonin and chest echography. *Chest* 2014; 146(6):1578–1585.

47. Branche AR, Walsh EE, Vargas R, et al. Serum procalcitonin measurement and viral testing to guide antibiotic use for respiratory infections in hospitalized adults: A randomized controlled trial. *J Infect Dis* 2015; 212(11):1692–1700.

48. Kalil AC, Metersky ML, Klompas M, et al. Management of adults with hospital-acquired and ventilator-associated pneumonia: 2016 clinical practice guidelines by the Infectious Diseases Society of America and the American Thoracic Society. *Clin Infect Dis* 2016; 63 (5):e61–e111.

49. Mandell LA, Wunderink RG, Anzueto A, et al. Infectious Diseases Society of America and the American Thoracic Society Consensus Guidelines on the management of community-acquired pneumonia in adults. *Clin Infect Dis* 2007; 44 Suppl 2:S27–72.

50. American Thoracic Society, Infectious Diseases Society of America. Guidelines for the management of adults with hospital-acquired, ventilator-associated, and healthcare-associated pneumonia. *Am J Respir Crit Care Med* 2005; 171 (4):388–416.

51. Kollef MH, Shorr A, Tabak YP, Gupta V, Liu LZ, Johannes RS. Epidemiology and outcomes of health-care-associated pneumonia: Results from a large US database of culture-positive pneumonia. *Chest* 2005; 128(6):3854–3862.

52. Gross AE, Van Schooneveld TC, Olsen KM, et al. Epidemiology and predictors of multidrug-resistant community-acquired and health care-associated pneumonia. *Antimicrob Agents Chemother* 2014; 58 (9):5262–5268.

53. Chalmers JD, Taylor JK, Singanayagam A, et al. Epidemiology, antibiotic therapy, and clinical outcomes in health care-associated pneumonia: A UK cohort study. *Clin Infect Dis* 2011; 53(2):107–113.

54. Chalmers JD, Rother C, Salih W, Ewig S. Healthcare-associated pneumonia does not accurately identify potentially resistant pathogens: A systematic review and meta-analysis. *Clin Infect Dis* 2014; 58 (3):330–339.

55. Jones BE, Jones MM, Huttner B, et al. Trends in antibiotic use and nosocomial pathogens in hospitalized veterans with pneumonia at 128 medical centers, 2006–2010. *Clin Infect Dis* 2015; 61 (9):1403–1410.

56. Jenkins TC, Stella SA, Cervantes L, et al. Targets for antibiotic and healthcare resource stewardship in inpatient community-acquired pneumonia: A comparison of management practices with national guideline recommendations. *Infection* 2013; 41(1):135–144.

57. Musher DM, Montoya R, Wanahita A. Diagnostic value of microscopic examination of gram-stained sputum and sputum cultures in patients with bacteremic pneumococcal pneumonia. *Clin Infect Dis* 2004; 39(2):165–169.

58. Sorde R, Falco V, Lowak M, et al. Current and potential usefulness of pneumococcal urinary antigen detection in hospitalized patients with community-acquired pneumonia to guide antimicrobial therapy. *Arch Intern Med* 2011; 171 (2):166–172.

59. Dangerfield B, Chung A, Webb B, Seville MT. Predictive value of methicillin-resistant *Staphylococcus aureus* (MRSA) nasal swab PCR assay for MRSA pneumonia. *Antimicrob Agents Chemother* 2014; 58(2):859–864.

60. Sarikonda KV, Micek ST, Doherty JA, Reichley RM, Warren D, Kollef MH. Methicillin-resistant Staphylococcus aureus nasal colonization is a poor predictor of intensive care unit-acquired methicillin-resistant *Staphylococcus aureus* infections requiring antibiotic treatment. *Crit Care Med* 2010; 38 (10):1991–1995.

61. Rello J, Vidaur L, Sandiumenge A, et al. De-escalation therapy in ventilator-associated pneumonia. *Crit Care Med* 2004; 32(11):2183–2190.

62. Canadian Critical Care Trials Group. A randomized trial of diagnostic techniques for ventilator-associated pneumonia. *N Engl J Med* 2006; 355 (25):2619–2630.

63. Raman K, Nailor MD, Nicolau DP, Aslanzadeh J, Nadeau M, Kuti JL. Early antibiotic discontinuation in patients with clinically suspected ventilator-associated pneumonia and negative quantitative bronchoscopy cultures. *Crit Care Med* 2013; 41(7):1656–1663.

64. De Bus L, Saerens L, Gadeyne B, et al. Development of antibiotic treatment algorithms based on local ecology and respiratory surveillance cultures to restrict the use of broad-spectrum antimicrobial drugs in the treatment of hospital-acquired pneumonia in the intensive care unit: A retrospective analysis. *Crit Care* 2014; 18 (4):R152.

65. Brusselaers N, Labeau S, Vogelaers D, Blot S. Value of lower respiratory tract surveillance cultures to predict bacterial pathogens in ventilator-associated pneumonia: Systematic review and diagnostic test accuracy meta-analysis. *Intensive Care Med* 2013; 39 (3):365–375.

66. Luna CM, Sarquis S, Niederman MS, et al. Is a strategy based on routine endotracheal cultures the best way to prescribe antibiotics in ventilator-associated pneumonia? *Chest* 2013; 144(1):63–71.

67. Cremers AJ, Sprong T, Schouten JA, et al. Effect of antibiotic streamlining on patient outcome in pneumococcal bacteraemia. *J Antimicrob Chemother* 2014; 69(8): 2258–2264.

68. Garnacho-Montero J, Gutierrez-Pizarraya A, Escoresca-Ortega A, et al. De-escalation of empirical therapy is associated with lower mortality in patients with severe sepsis and septic shock. *Intensive Care Med* 2014; 40(1):32–40.

69. Rimawi RH, Mazer MA, Siraj DS, Gooch M, Cook PP. Impact of regular collaboration between infectious diseases and critical care practitioners on antimicrobial utilization and patient outcome. *Crit Care Med* 2013; 41 (9):2099–2107.

70. Evans RS, Pestotnik SL, Classen DC, et al. A computer-assisted management program for antibiotics and other antiinfective agents. *N Engl J Med* 1998; 338(4):232–238.

71. Paul M, Andreassen S, Tacconelli E, et al. Improving empirical antibiotic treatment using TREAT, a computerized decision support system: Cluster randomized trial. *J Antimicrob Chemother* 2006; 58 (6):1238–1245.

72. McCabe C, Kirchner C, Zhang H, Daley J, Fisman DN. Guideline-concordant therapy and reduced mortality and length of stay in adults with community-acquired pneumonia: Playing by the rules. *Arch Intern Med* 2009; 169 (16):1525–1531.

73. Grenier C, Pepin J, Nault V, et al. Impact of guideline-consistent therapy on outcome of patients with healthcare-associated and community-acquired pneumonia. *J Antimicrob Chemother* 2011; 66 (7):1617–1624.

74. Ostrowsky B, Sharma S, DeFino M, et al. Antimicrobial stewardship and automated pharmacy technology improve antibiotic appropriateness for community-acquired pneumonia. *Infect Control Hosp Epidemiol* 2013; 34(6):566–572.

75. Marrie TJ, Lau CY, Wheeler SL, Wong CJ, Vandervoort MK, Feagan BG. A controlled trial of a critical pathway for treatment of community-acquired pneumonia. CAPITAL study investigators: Community-acquired pneumonia intervention trial assessing levofloxacin. *JAMA* 2000; 283 (6):749–755.

76. Newman RE, Hedican EB, Herigon JC, Williams DD, Williams AR, Newland JG. Impact of a guideline on management of children hospitalized with community-acquired pneumonia. *Pediatrics* 2012; 129 (3):e597–604.

77. Smith MJ, Kong M, Cambon A, Woods CR. Effectiveness of antimicrobial guidelines for community-acquired pneumonia in children. *Pediatrics* 2012; 129(5):e1326–1333.

78. Weireter LJ, Jr, Collins JN, Britt RC, Reed SF, Novosel TJ, Britt LD. Impact of a monitored program of care on incidence of ventilator-associated pneumonia: Results of a longterm performance-improvement project. *J Am Coll Surg* 2009; 208 (5):700–704.

79. Fisman DN, Abrutyn E, Spaude KA, Kim A, Kirchner C, Daley J. Prior pneumococcal vaccination is associated with reduced death, complications, and length of stay among hospitalized adults with community-acquired pneumonia. *Clin Infect Dis* 2006; 42 (8):1093–1001.

80. Edelsberg J, Taneja C, Zervos M, et al. Trends in US hospital admissions for skin and soft tissue infections. *Emerg Infect Dis* 2009; 15(9):1516–1518.

81. Jenkins TC, Sabel AL, Sarcone EE, Price CS, Mehler PS, Burman WJ. Skin and soft-tissue infections requiring hospitalization at an academic medical center: Opportunities for antimicrobial stewardship. *Clin Infect Dis* 2010; 51 (8):895–903.

82. Bruun T, Oppegaard O, Kittang BR, Mylvaganam H, Langeland N, Skrede S. Etiology of cellulitis and clinical prediction of streptococcal disease: A prospective study. *Open Forum Infect Dis* 2015; 3(1): ofv181.

83. Jeng A, Beheshti M, Li J, Nathan R. The role of beta-hemolytic streptococci in causing diffuse, nonculturable cellulitis: A prospective investigation. *Medicine (Baltimore)* 2010; 89(4):217–226.

84. Moran GJ, Krishnadasan A, Gorwitz RJ, et al. Methicillin-resistant *S. aureus* infections among patients in the emergency department. *N Engl J Med* 2006; 355 (7):666–674.

85. Stevens DL, Bisno AL, Chambers HF, et al. Practice guidelines for the diagnosis and management of skin and soft tissue infections: 2014 update by the Infectious Diseases Society of America. *Clin Infect Dis* 2014; 59(2):e10–52.

86. Perl B, Gottehrer NP, Raveh D, Schlesinger Y, Rudensky B, Yinnon AM. Cost-effectiveness of blood cultures for adult patients with cellulitis. *Clin Infect Dis* 1999; 29(6):1483–1488.

87. Blankenship RB, Baker T. Imaging modalities in wounds and superficial skin infections. *Emerg Med Clin North Am* 2007; 25(1):223–234.

88. Mueller K, McCammon C, Skrupky L, Fuller BM. Vancomycin use in patients discharged from the emergency department: A retrospective observational cohort study. *J Emerg Med* 2015; 49 (1):50–57.

89. May LS, Rothman RE, Miller LG, et al. A randomized clinical trial comparing use of rapid molecular testing for *Staphylococcus aureus* for patients with cutaneous abscesses in the emergency department with standard of care. *Infect Control Hosp Epidemiol* 2015; 36 (12):1423–1430.

90. Hayes BD, Zaharna L, Winters ME, Feemster AA, Browne BJ, Hirshon JM. To-go medications for decreasing ED return visits. *Am J Emerg Med* 2012; 30 (9):2011–2014.

91. Eells SJ, Nguyen M, Jung J, Macias-Gil R, May L, Miller LG. Relationship between adherence to oral antibiotics and postdischarge clinical outcomes among patients hospitalized with *Staphylococcus aureus* skin infections. *Antimicrob Agents Chemother* 2016; 60(5):2941–2948.

92. Kalil AC, Van Schooneveld TC, Fey PD, Rupp ME. Association between vancomycin minimum inhibitory concentration and mortality among patients with *Staphylococcus aureus* bloodstream infections: A systematic review and meta-analysis. *JAMA* 2014; 312 (15):1552–1564.

93. Liu C, Bayer A, Cosgrove SE, et al. Clinical practice guidelines by the Infectious Diseases Society of America for the treatment of methicillin-resistant *Staphylococcus aureus* infections in adults and children. *Clin Infect Dis* 2011; 52(3): e18–55.

94. Bai AD, Showler A, Burry L, et al. Impact of infectious disease consultation on quality of care, mortality, and length of stay in *Staphylococcus aureus* bacteremia: Results from a large multicenter cohort study. *Clin Infect Dis* 2015; 60(10):1451–61.

95. Jenkins TC, Price CS, Sabel AL, Mehler PS, Burman WJ. Impact of routine infectious diseases service consultation on the

evaluation, management, and outcomes of *Staphylococcus aureus* bacteremia. *Clin Infect Dis* 2008; 46(7):1000–1008.

96. Robinson JO, Pozzi-Langhi S, Phillips M, et al. Formal infectious diseases consultation is associated with decreased mortality in *Staphylococcus aureus* bacteraemia. *Eur J Clin Microbiol Infect Dis*, 2012; 31(9):2421–2428.

97. Nguyen CT, Gandhi T, Chenoweth C, et al. Impact of an antimicrobial stewardship-led intervention for *Staphylococcus aureus* bacteraemia: A quasi-experimental study. *J Antimicrob Chemother* 2015; 70 (12):3390–3396.

98. Forsblom E, Ruotsalainen E, Ollgren J, Jarvinen A. Telephone consultation cannot replace bedside infectious disease consultation in the management of *Staphylococcus aureus* bacteremia. *Clin Infect Dis* 2013; 56(4):527–535.

99. Kullar R, Davis SL, Kaye KS, Levine DP, Pogue JM, Rybak MJ. Implementation of an antimicrobial stewardship pathway with daptomycin for optimal treatment of methicillin-resistant *Staphylococcus aureus* bacteremia. *Pharmacotherapy* 2013; 33 (1):3–10.

100. Micek ST, Welch EC, Khan J, et al. Resistance to empiric antimicrobial treatment predicts outcome in severe sepsis associated with gram-negative bacteremia. *J Hosp Med* 2011; 6(7):405–410.

101. Pogue JM, Mynatt RP, Marchaim D, et al. Automated alerts coupled with antimicrobial stewardship intervention lead to decreases in length of stay in patients with gram-negative bacteremia. *Infect Control Hosp Epidemiol* 2014; 35 (2):132–138.

102. Arena F, Scolletta S, Marchetti L, et al. Impact of a clinical microbiology-intensive care consulting program in a cardiothoracic intensive care unit. *Am J Infect Control* 2015; 43(9):1018–1021.

103. Pardo J, Klinker KP, Borgert SJ, Trikha G, Rand KH, Ramphal R. Time to positivity of blood cultures supports antibiotic de-escalation at 48 hours. *Ann Pharmacother* 2014; 48(1):33–40.

104. Scheetz MH, Bolon MK, Postelnick M, Noskin GA, Lee TA. Cost-effectiveness analysis of an antimicrobial stewardship team on bloodstream infections: A probabilistic analysis. *J Antimicrob Chemother* 2009; 63(4):816–825.

105. Pappas PG, Kauffman CA, Andes D, et al. Clinical practice guidelines for the management of candidiasis: 2009 update by the Infectious Diseases Society of America. *Clin Infect Dis* 2009; 48(5):503–535.

106. Antworth A, Collins CD, Kunapuli A, et al. Impact of an antimicrobial stewardship program comprehensive care bundle on management of candidemia. *Pharmacotherapy* 2013; 33(2):137–143.

107. Reed EE, West JE, Keating EA, et al. Improving the management of candidemia through antimicrobial stewardship interventions. *Diagn Microbiol Infect Dis* 2014; 78(2):157–161.

108. Mondain V, Lieutier F, Dumas S, et al. An antibiotic stewardship program in a french teaching hospital. *Med Mal Infect* 2013; 43 (1):17–21.

109. Lessa FC, Mu Y, Bamberg WM, et al. Burden of *Clostridium difficile* infection in the United States. *N Engl J Med* 2015; 372 (9):825–834.

110. CDC. Antibiotic resistance threats in the United States, 2013. (Accessed August 2016, at www.cdc.gov/drugresistance/ threat-report-2013/.)

111. Slimings C, Riley TV. Antibiotics and hospital-acquired *Clostridium difficile* infection: Update of systematic review and meta-analysis. *J Antimicrob Chemother* 2014; 69(4):881–891.

112. Deshpande A, Pasupuleti V, Thota P, et al. Community-associated *Clostridium difficile* infection and antibiotics: A meta-analysis. *J Antimicrob Chemother* 2013; 68 (9):1951–1961.

113. Shaughnessy MK, Amundson WH, Kuskowski MA, DeCarolis DD, Johnson JR, Drekonja DM. Unnecessary antimicrobial use in patients with current or recent *Clostridium difficile* infection. *Infect Control Hosp Epidemiol* 2013; 34 (2):109–116.

114. Valiquette L, Cossette B, Garant MP, Diab H, Pepin J. Impact of a reduction in the use of high-risk antibiotics on the course of an epidemic of *Clostridium difficile*-associated disease caused by the hypervirulent NAP1/ 027 strain. *Clin Infect Dis* 2007; 45 Suppl 2: S112–121.

115. Hernandez-Santiago V, Marwick CA, Patton A, Davey PG, Donnan PT, Guthrie B. Time series analysis of the impact of an intervention in Tayside, Scotland to reduce primary care broad-spectrum antimicrobial use. *J Antimicrob Chemother* 2015; 70(8): 2397–2404.

116. Quarterly surveillance report on the surveillance of *Clostridium difficile* infection (CDI) in Scotland. (Accessed October 2017, at www.hps.scot.nhs.uk/ haiic/sshaip/publicationsdetail.aspx?id= 50174.)

117. Stevens V, Dumyati G, Fine LS, Fisher SG, van Wijngaarden E. Cumulative antibiotic exposures over time and the risk of *Clostridium difficile* infection. *Clin Infect Dis* 2011; 53(1):42–48.

118. Chitnis AS, Holzbauer SM, Belflower RM, et al. Epidemiology of community-associated *Clostridium difficile* infection, 2009 through 2011. *JAMA Intern Med* 2013; 173(14):1359–1367.

119. McDonald EG, Milligan J, Frenette C, Lee TC. Continuous proton pump inhibitor therapy and the associated risk of recurrent *Clostridium difficile* infection. *JAMA Intern Med* 2015; 175(5):784–791.

120. Kwok CS, Arthur AK, Anibueze CI, Singh S, Cavallazzi R, Loke YK. Risk of *Clostridium difficile* infection with acid suppressing drugs and antibiotics: Meta-analysis. *Am J Gastroenterol* 2012; 107 (7):1011–1019.

121. Mullane KM, Miller MA, Weiss K, et al. Efficacy of fidaxomicin versus vancomycin as therapy for *Clostridium difficile* infection in individuals taking concomitant antibiotics for other concurrent infections. *Clin Infect Dis* 2011; 53(5):440–447.

122. Harpe SE, Inocencio TJ, Pakyz AL, Oinonen MJ, Polk RE. Characterization of continued antibacterial therapy after diagnosis of hospital-onset *Clostridium difficile* infection: Implications for antimicrobial stewardship. *Pharmacotherapy* 2012; 32(8):744–754.

123. Dubberke ER, Han Z, Bobo L, et al. Impact of clinical symptoms on interpretation of diagnostic assays for *Clostridium difficile* infections. *J Clin Microbiol* 2011; 49 (8):2887–2893.

124. Buckel WR, Avdic E, Carroll KC, Gunaseelan V, Hadhazy E, Cosgrove SE. Gut check: *Clostridium difficile* testing and treatment in the molecular testing era. *Infect Control Hosp Epidemiol* 2015; 36 (2):217–221.

125. Davies KA, Longshaw CM, Davis GL, et al. Underdiagnosis of *Clostridium difficile* across Europe: The European, multicentre, prospective, biannual, point-prevalence study of *Clostridium difficile* infection in hospitalised patients with diarrhoea (EUCLID). *Lancet Infect Dis* 2014; 14(12): 1208–1219.

126. Planche TD, Davies KA, Coen PG, et al. Differences in outcome according to *Clostridium difficile* testing method: A prospective multicentre diagnostic validation study of *C. difficile* infection. *Lancet Infect Dis* 2013; 13 (11):936–945.

127. Dionne LL, Raymond F, Corbeil J, Longtin J, Gervais P, Longtin Y. Correlation between *Clostridium difficile* bacterial load, commercial real-time PCR cycle thresholds, and results of diagnostic tests based on enzyme immunoassay and cell culture cytotoxicity assay. *J Clin Microbiol* 2013; 51 (11):3624–3630.

128. Zar FA, Bakkanagari SR, Moorthi KM, Davis MB. A comparison of vancomycin and metronidazole for the treatment of *Clostridium difficile*-associated diarrhea, stratified by disease severity. *Clin Infect Dis* 2007; 45(3):302–307.

129. Drekonja DM, Butler M, MacDonald R, et al. Comparative effectiveness of *Clostridium difficile* treatments: A systematic review. *Ann Intern Med* 2011; 155(12):839–847.

130. Brown AT, Seifert CF. Effect of treatment variation on outcomes in patients with *Clostridium difficile. Am J Med* 2014; 127 (9):865–870.

131. Curtin BF, Zarbalian Y, Flasar MH, von Rosenvinge E. *Clostridium difficile*-associated disease: Adherence with current guidelines at a tertiary medical center. *World J Gastroenterol* 2013; 19 (46):8647–8651.

132. American Society of Microbiology. A practical guidance document for the laboratory detection of toxigenic *Clostridium difficile*. 2010. (Accessed August 2016, at www.asm.org/images/pdf/Clinical/clostridiumdifficile9–21.pdf.)

133. Jardin CG, Palmer HR, Shah DN, et al. Assessment of treatment patterns and patient outcomes before vs after implementation of a severity-based *Clostridium difficile* infection treatment policy. *J Hosp Infect* 2013; 85(1):28–32.

134. Jury LA, Tomas M, Kundrapu S, Sitzlar B, Donskey CJ. A *Clostridium difficile* infection (CDI) stewardship initiative improves adherence to practice guidelines for management of CDI. *Infect Control Hosp Epidemiol* 2013; 34(11):1222–1224.

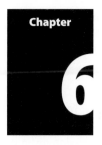

Chapter

6

Duration of Therapy
Our Role as Stewards

George E. Nelson and Annie Wong-Beringer

Introduction

The development of antibiotic resistance is a natural phenomenon in microorganisms, but the risk of developing resistance is increased when antibiotics are used for unnecessarily prolonged durations.[1–3] Historically, longer antibiotic treatment courses were pursued for myriad reasons: antibiotics seemed plentiful, resistance was a less pressing concern, and long durations were used by default in clinical trials. The prevailing attitude among clinicians was that antibiotics were at worst risk neutral, but with the increased recognition of the emergence of resistance, *Clostridium difficile* infections, and organ specific toxicities, this attitude has become an antiquated belief. In the past, published data comparing durations of therapy were modest [4] with minimal incentives for pharmaceutical companies to investigate limiting antibiotic durations and a paucity of funding resources available for academic investigation of this subject. As such, there are limited recommendations or conclusive guidelines on durations of therapy.[4] In recent years, evidence is mounting that shorter durations of therapy can be prescribed without a negative impact on patient outcomes.

A cornerstone of antibiotic stewardship is optimizing the duration of therapy but duration is not often targeted in programmatic interventions. Limiting duration optimizes patient safety by reducing adverse drug events such as *Clostridium difficile*; facilitates earlier removal of invasive devices; and improves drug compliance. Limiting duration of therapy can also reduce the development of resistance – the shortest duration needed for cure reduces the selection for resistant organisms.

In this chapter, we will focus on infectious syndromes that are commonly encountered in the inpatient and outpatient settings and provide guidance on durations of therapy. Special populations, such as pediatrics and immunosuppressed populations, will be included in the discussions where high-quality evidence supports recommended treatment durations. Clinical syndromes are discussed in order of most to least studied with respect to treatment duration. In addition, we will discuss how ASPs can assist with reducing treatment durations.

Pneumonia

Pneumonia is a common cause of infection-related morbidity and mortality worldwide. Much progress has been made on withholding antibiotics for upper respiratory infections, especially in the outpatient setting.[5] But once the diagnosis of pneumonia has been made and the clinical decision to initiate antibiotic treatment has been determined, a number of variables impact proper duration of therapy. In this section, we will discuss the historical approach to antibiotic treatment durations for pneumonia and evidence that informs current guidelines for duration of therapy for community-acquired pneumonia (CAP), hospital-acquired pneumonia (HAP), and ventilator-associated pneumonia (VAP).

Community-Acquired Pneumonia

The American Thoracic Society (ATS) 2001 Guidelines recommended a 7- to 10-day course of antibiotics for *Streptococcus pneumoniae* pneumonia and a 10- to 14-day course for "atypical" pathogens, based on low-grade evidence.[6] There was some concession given to shorter courses (i.e., 5 to 7 days) when antibiotics with extended half-lives, such as azithromycin, were used. Multiple randomized studies and two meta-analyses support shorter treatment duration (3 to 7 days).[7–9] Details on three key studies are provided below.

Leophonte et al. conducted a multicenter, randomized, double-blind trial in 244 hospitalized adults receiving ceftriaxone for the treatment of CAP comparing a standard 10-day vs. 5-day course. Study patients had at least one of the following risk factors: age $\geq$ 65 years, tobacco use ($\geq$10 packs per year), chronic alcohol use, obesity, nutritional deficiency, or at least one underlying medical condition [7]; the most common isolated pathogen (either by blood culture or bronchial culture) was *S. pneumoniae* followed by *Haemophilus influenzae*. Identification of atypical pathogens was considered an exclusion criterion. The 5-day course was noninferior to the 10-day course for clinical cure evaluated at days 10, 30, and 45.

Dunbar et al. demonstrated in a multicenter, randomized, double-blind trial that a 5-day regimen of high-dose levofloxacin was noninferior to standard dose levofloxacin given for 10 days for the treatment of mild to severe CAP.[8] The investigators note that increasing the dose of levofloxacin exploits pharmacokinetic parameters allowing for a shorter course of treatment without diminishing the therapeutic benefit. In the clinically evaluable population, the clinical success rates were 92% (183/198) for the high-dose group and 91% (175/192) for the standard-dose, extended-duration group. Resolution of fever was faster in the group receiving high-dose, short-course therapy (49.1% vs. 38.5%; $P = 0.03$), and microbiologic eradication rates were similar between groups.

El Moussaoui et al. then performed a prospective, blinded, randomized trial for CAP, ranging from mild to severe disease. All patients received intravenous amoxicillin for 3 days and (if clinical improvement was noted) transitioned to either oral amoxicillin ($n = 63$) or placebo ($n = 56$) for an additional 5-day course.[9] Clinical cure was similar between the groups while length of stay, mild adverse drug reactions and allergic reactions trended higher in the 8-day treatment group.

In trials of antibiotic therapy for CAP, azithromycin has been used for 3–5 days as oral therapy for outpatients with infections caused by both classic bacterial as well as atypical pathogens.[10–12] Duration of therapies comparing different antibiotic classes can be difficult to define in a uniform fashion, because some antibiotics (such as azithromycin) are administered for a short time yet have a long half-life at respiratory sites of infection. Results with azithromycin should not be extrapolated to other drugs with significantly shorter half-lives.

Several meta-analyses evaluating duration of therapy for CAP have been performed. A 2007 meta-analysis included 15 randomized controlled trials (RCTs) with 2,796 patients.[13] A variety of antibiotic regimens were included (azithromycin [$n = 10$]; beta-lactams [$n = 2$], fluoroquinolones [$n = 2$], and ketolides [$n = 1$]). Short-course therapy varied between 3 and 7 days while extended-course therapy ranged from 10 to 14 days. There was no difference in the risk of clinical failure between the short-course and extended-course regimens, nor were any differences noted in mortality or bacteriologic eradication. In subgroup analyses, there was a trend toward favorable clinical efficacy for the short-course regimens in all antibiotic classes. The authors concluded that adults with mild to moderate CAP could be treated with regimens of 7 days or fewer without compromising clinical outcomes.

A second meta-analysis included seven double-blind RCTs evaluating either adults or children (5 studies of adults; two studies of children between 2 and 59 months) with mild to moderately severe CAP.[14] Durations varied (short course [adults 3–7 days; children 3 days]; extended course [adults 7–10 days; children 5 days]). No differences were found between short- and extended-courses in clinical success at the end of therapy, clinical success at late follow-up, microbiological success, relapses, mortality, or adverse events. A Cochrane review that appeared the same year focusing specifically on children aged 2–59 months included four trials [15–18], two of which [15, 18] were in the preceding meta-analysis. These four studies included a total of 6,177 children and compared the same antibiotic given for either 3 or 5 days for non-severe CAP. No differences in clinical cure, treatment failure, or relapses were found.

Results from the above studies have led to the recommendation for a shortened duration of treatment for CAP in the 2007 Infectious Diseases Society of America (IDSA) Guidelines: "Patients with CAP should be treated for a minimum of 5 days, should be afebrile for 48–72 hours, and should have no more than 1 CAP-associated sign of clinical instability before discontinuation of therapy."[19] The British Thoracic Society (BTS) guidelines released in 2009 recommended a 7-day course of antibiotic therapy for adult patients hospitalized with mild to moderately severe CAP.[20]

For mild to moderately severe CAP, 5 days of therapy is likely to be sufficient if clinical response has been promptly noted. Durations longer than 7 days are infrequently necessary; notable exceptions include patients with CAP who also have bacteremia or meningitis or are infected with more difficult to treat pathogens (endemic fungi, *Pseudomonas* spp., etc). It should be noted that nearly all studies that have evaluated shorter courses have not found deleterious effects in CAP in either inpatients or outpatients.[19]

Hospital-Acquired Pneumonia and Ventilator-Associated Pneumonia

Most of the data presented are derived from studies evaluating VAP. While the data are frequently extrapolated to HAP, duration of treatment remains to be studied in the latter populations since they constitute a heterogeneous patient group with differences in under-lying comorbid conditions, severity at presentation, and causative pathogens.[21] Micro-biologic sampling and diagnostic evaluation may be easier to complete in intubated patients, but the importance of early, directed therapy and impact of drug-resistant patho-gens remains important.

Dennesen and colleagues demonstrated rapid eradication of *H. influenzae* and *S. pneumoniae* from tracheal aspirates in VAP patients though Enterobacteriaceae, *S. aureus*, and *P. aeruginosa* persisted despite *in vitro* susceptibility to the antibiotics administered.[22] In this study, significant clinical improvements were noted within the first 6 days of antibiotic treatment, and extended therapy ≥ 14 days created additional colonization of gram-negative pathogens, notably *P. aeruginosa* and Enterobacteriaceae. The early clinical improvement and emergent resistance noted in Dennesen's study informed future studies examining duration of therapy in VAP patients.

Consistent with results from the above study, Luna et al. found that patients who survived VAP after receiving adequate therapy tended to demonstrate clinical improvement by days 3–5 in contrast to nonresponding patients who did not demonstrate improvement during days 3–5.[23] These data supported the premise that most patients with VAP who receive appropriate antibiotic therapy have a favorable clinical response within the first 6 days. Prolonged therapy simply leads to colonization with antibiotic-resistant bacteria, which may precede a recurrent episode of VAP.

Reducing the duration of therapy in patients with VAP without compromising outcomes has been demonstrated in several studies using different approaches. Ibrahim et al. evaluated an ICU-specific antibiotic protocol focusing on pathogen-directed treatment, de-escalation and a 7-day course of appropriate antibiotics.[24] In a prospective before-and-after study design, the primary outcome was initial administration of antibiotic treatment based on respiratory tract cultures; secondary outcomes included duration of antibiotic therapy, in-hospital mortality, ICU length of stay (LOS), and VAP recurrence. Fifty patients with VAP in the group prior to protocol implementation were compared with 52 patients after protocol implementation. The guideline, based on antibiotic resistance patterns at their institution, provided empiric antibiotic recommendations for a planned 7-day course; patients with lack of improvement in clinical and laboratory parameters could receive extended-course therapy or therapy based on the treating physicians' clinical judgment. *Pseudomonas* was the most common bacterial pathogen isolated followed by staphylococci (MRSA/MSSA). Use of the guideline was associated with a significant reduction in the total duration of antibiotic treatment to 8 ± 5 days from 15 ± 8 days ($p < 0.001$) without differences in outcome. Mortality was similar (21/50 [42%] vs. 27/52 [52%]) as was ICU LOS (23 vs. 22 days); recurrence of VAP was lower in the de-escalation group (4/52 [8%] vs. 12/50 [24%]; $p = 0.03$).

Using a modified clinical pulmonary infection score (CPIS), Singh and colleagues identified low-risk patients with suspected VAP and conducted a randomized trial to evaluate duration of therapy. Patients with a CPIS score ≤ 6 were treated either with conventional therapy (10–21 days, 42 subjects) or were randomized to antibiotics for 3 days (39 subjects). CPIS score was recalculated after 3 days and if still ≤ 6, it was recommended that antibiotics be discontinued. The study was terminated early as it became apparent that physicians began treating patients in the control group with 3 days of therapy instead of the extended-course duration. As expected, patients in the short-course arm received fewer days of therapy, and importantly, they had shorter lengths of ICU stay (9 vs. 15 days) and less emergence of antibiotic-resistant organisms or superinfection (14% vs. 38%).[25] While some proposed that many of these patients may not have had VAP, the study did demonstrate that for patients where the likelihood of infection at the start of antibiotic therapy is not always clear, use of the CPIS can assist with reassessing and guiding duration of therapy.

Micek et al. performed an RCT for an antibiotic discontinuation policy in patients with clinically suspected VAP.[26] The discontinuation policy recommended cessation of antibiotics if any of the following criteria were met: non-infectious etiology of infiltrate was identified (e.g. edema, atelectasis), signs and symptoms of active infection had resolved (temperature $\leq 38.3°C$, circulating leukocyte count $<10,000/\mu L$ [$10 \times 10^9/L$] or decreased by $>25\%$ from the peak value, improvement or lack of progression on the chest radiograph, absence of purulent sputum, and a Pao_2/Fio_2 ratio >250). Severity of illness and CPIS were similar between discontinuation and conventional treatment groups. Compared to patients receiving conventional management, those in the discontinuation group had shorter duration of antibiotic treatment for VAP (6.0 ± 4.9 days vs. 8.0 ± 5.6 days) while hospital mortality (32% vs. 37%), ICU LOS (6.8 ± 6.1 days vs. 7.0 ± 7.3 days), and occurrence of a recurrent episode of VAP (17.3% vs. 19.3%) were similar. It should be noted that the percent of VAP caused by *Pseudomonas* and MRSA/MSSA were also similar between groups.

A multicenter RCT conducted by Chastre et al. demonstrated that patients receiving appropriate, initial empiric therapy of VAP for 8 days compared to 15 days had no excess mortality (19% vs. 17%) or recurrent infections (29% vs. 26%) and similar ventilation-free days, organ failure-free days, ICU LOS, and had more antibiotic-free days (13.1 vs. 8.7 days $p < 0.001$).[27] Subgroup analysis demonstrated a trend toward higher rates of relapse for *P. aeruginosa* or an *Acinetobacter* species (41% vs. 25%) though among those who had recurrent infections multidrug-resistant pathogens were noted less frequently in the 8-day treatment group (42% vs. 62% of pulmonary recurrences, $p = 0.04$).

Following Chastre's study, Hendrick and colleagues retrospectively evaluated their institutional experience treating VAP in surgical and trauma ICUs over a nearly 8-year period to determine if non-glucose fermenting gram-negative bacteria required longer treatment courses as suggested by Chastre and colleagues.[28] They identified 154 (154/452; 34%) episodes of VAP caused by non-fermenters. Twenty-seven (27/154; 18%) patients received between 3 and 8 days (mean 6.4) of antibiotics, and 127 (127/154; 82%) received ≥ 9 days (mean 17.1) of therapy. The differences were non-significant between short and extended durations for recurrence (22% vs. 34%) or mortality (22% vs. 14%). These data suggest that not all patients with VAP due to non-fermenting gram-negative bacteria required prolonged treatment based on 27 patients treated for 8 days or less; however, the findings will need confirmation with a larger sample size in a prospective comparative study.

Two systematic reviews of RCTs evaluating duration of therapy for VAP have been published [29, 30] which have informed the recently released IDSA/ATS guidelines for management of HAP and VAP.[31] The first review included 4 RCTs comparing short course (7–8 days) with extended duration (10–15 days) for treatment of VAP and found no differences in mortality or relapses, though increase in antibiotic-free days was noted in short-course treatment as expected (mean difference 3.4 days; 95% CI, 1.43–5.37).[29] The most recent review included 6 RCTs (including the 4 RCTs in prior review) with 1088 participants with pneumonia (92% with VAP).[30] Short-course therapy (7–8 days) compared with extended duration (10–15 days) demonstrated significantly higher 28-day antibiotic-free days (mean difference 4.02 days; 95% CI, 2.26–5.78) without any significant increase in mortality, duration of ventilation, or length of stay. This also held true regardless of pathogen isolated, though VAP due to non-fermenters treated with short-course therapy was associated with higher rates of recurrence (OR 2.18; 95% CI, 1.14–4.16). The IDSA/ATS guidelines conducted their own meta-analyses, including the above systematic reviews, and confirmed the lack of difference in mortality, clinical cure, and recurrence with the additional finding that when limited to the subpopulation of non-fermenting gram-negative bacilli also yielded no observed differences in recurrence (OR 0.94; 95% CI, 0.56–1.59).[31] These data informed the recommendations to treat VAP, regardless of pathogen, for 7 days. While the panel acknowledged this recommendation was based on moderate confidence, they recognized that short-course therapy decreases antibiotic exposure and antibiotic resistance without impacting mortality or recurrence and surely reduces costs and side effects in the setting of the very uncommon scenario of recurrent VAP for individual patients. The panel distinguished between HAP and VAP, but offered the same recommendations for HAP given there were no useful studies evaluating duration of therapy specifically for HAP and therefore based their recommendations on extrapolations from the above studies evaluating VAP.

Based on the studies above, treatment duration for uncomplicated VAP should be limited to 7 days of therapy if patients have received appropriate initial therapy and have demonstrated an appropriate clinical response. Short-course therapy may be associated with a higher rate of recurrent disease when infection is caused by non-fermenting gram-negative bacilli, but this is likely a very uncommon event based on recently published data. However, vigilance for signs and symptoms consistent with recurrence is warranted. Patients without microbiologic confirmation of causative organism may be managed with shorter courses. Extrapolation to HAP should be performed with caution; large studies have not specifically evaluated patients who may have different responses than patients with VAP. More studies are needed to address those patient populations as well as those with additional risk factors, including immunosuppression, who were frequently excluded from the above studies.

Successful Stewardship Interventions to Optimize Duration of Therapy: Pneumonia

A variety of antibiotic stewardship (AS) methodologies have been investigated to optimize management and reduce the duration of therapy for patients presenting with CAP which include education, algorithm development, and direct feedback. Avdic and colleagues [32] performed a single-center, prospective study evaluating a 3-part intervention: a baseline knowledge and practice survey, educational offerings to providers, and a post-prescription review and feedback (PPRF) by the AS team for CAP patients in addition to pre-prescription authorization (PPA) for certain antibiotics. The pre- and post-intervention periods (approximately 3 months each period) included 62 and 65 patients respectively. In the intervention period, 48 stewardship recommendations were made in 34 patients with an acceptance rate of 69%. The duration of therapy decreased from a median of 10 to 7 days ($p = 0.001$) and duplicate therapy avoided (90% vs. 55%) while length of stay remained similar. To evaluate whether this short-term intervention conferred sustained results, a follow-up study was conducted in the same institution 3 years after the initial intervention [33] and showed that these results were sustained.

Haas et al. conducted a study evaluating syndrome-specific interventions aimed at CAP to improve resource utilization (imaging and diagnostic cultures) as well as to shorten duration of antibiotic therapy.[34] After performing a baseline survey of CAP management, a multidisciplinary team was convened to create a local clinical practice guideline for management of non-ICU patients based on national guidelines. The guideline was disseminated to providers via email with periodic reminders, discussions at house staff conferences, grand rounds, staff meetings, postings on the AS website and in work areas. After implementation of the guidelines, a pre-post-intervention study was performed. There were 166 cases in pre-intervention period (April 15, 2008–May 31, 2009) and 84 cases in the intervention period (July 1, 2011–July 31, 2012). The median duration of therapy decreased from 10 to 7 days ($p<0.0001$) while frequency of clinical failure was similar between the two periods.

Urinary Tract Infection

Infections of the urinary tract are generally classified as lower tract disease (i.e., cystitis) and upper tract disease (i.e., pyelonephritis) and are a frequent reason for antibiotic use in the inpatient and outpatient settings. Asymptomatic bacteriuria is defined as the presence of bacteria in urine specimens without symptoms. In general, treatment is not recommended for asymptomatic bacteriuria with the exception of pregnant women or prophylaxis prior to transurethral prostate resection or urologic procedures with anticipated mucosal bleeding.[35]

Antibiotic treatment of urinary tract infections (UTIs) account for 8% of the antibiotics prescribed during >100 million ambulatory care visits in the US annually.[36] Numerous studies and meta-analyses have addressed antibiotic treatment duration for cystitis. Most published studies have evaluated the following agents as single-dose, 3-day or 7-day treatment course: trimethoprim/sulfamethoxazole (TMP/SMX), fluoroquinolones, oral beta-lactam agents, nitrofurantoin, or fosfomycin.

Two studies [37, 38] compared 3 days of TMP/SMX with longer durations and demonstrated that bacterial eradication was similar, though there were more frequent recurrences in shorter-course therapy groups (19% vs. 12%; $P = 0.05$). The authors concluded that the trend toward higher recurrence rate was counterbalanced by trends toward fewer adverse effects (18% vs. 30%; $P = 0.06$).[39] Single-dose therapy was noted to be generally less effective based on a meta-analysis of seven trials [37, 40–45] comparing single-dose TMP/SMX with longer durations of therapy; single-dose therapy had less bacterial eradication (87% vs. 94%; $P = 0.014$), though recurrence rates were similar.[39]

Fluoroquinolones have also been studied extensively; however, many of the studies included agents no longer in use. Six studies compared single-dose therapy with longer durations; four studies [46–49] showed lower bacterial eradication rates with single-dose therapy. Two studies showed high rates of eradication but those studies were small, with fewer than 50 patients each.[50, 51] Three studies compared a fluoroquinolone for 3 days vs. a longer duration.[49, 52, 53] A double-blind multi-clinic study randomized 373 patients to either 3 or 7 days of therapy with norfloxacin and found both regimens had equivalent short-term efficacy, defined as elimination of significant bacteriuria at 3–13 days posttreatment.[52] One publication analyzed three multicenter, prospective, randomized, double-blind trials that included a total of 970 women with acute, symptomatic, uncomplicated cystitis to determine the minimum effective dose.[48] Patients received oral ciprofloxacin (200 to 500 mg in one or two divided doses for 1, 3, 5, or 7 days) or norfloxacin (400 mg twice daily for 7 days). Both 3- and 5-day therapy with ciprofloxacin was equivalent to 7-day therapy with either ciprofloxacin or norfloxacin; all groups had bacteriologic and clinical response >90% 4–9 days posttreatment. The authors concluded that 3 days of ciprofloxacin was the minimum effective duration.

Six studies evaluated a single dose of a beta-lactam antibiotic compared with longer durations of therapy.[54–59] Fang et al. demonstrated that a single dose of amoxicillin offered equivalent clinical cure rates compared with conventional (i.e., 10 days) treatment (22/22 vs. 21/21) [54], but a follow-up study comparing single-dose amoxicillin with 14 days of therapy found a trend toward reduced bacterial eradication with the single-dose regimen (43/71, 61% vs. 67/91, 74%; $p = 0.07$).[56] Rubin et al. randomized patients with uncomplicated cystitis to single doses of amoxicillin or conventional ten-day courses of TMP/SMX or ampicillin and found comparable rates of eradication with the three regimens (90%, 100%, and 96%, respectively).[57] In a randomized double-blind placebo-controlled trial, Raz et al. compared single-dose amoxicillin-clavulanate with a 3-day course in 109 patients with uncomplicated cystitis and found similar clinical cure rates at 7 and 28 days posttreatment: 78% vs. 87% and 67% vs. 78%, respectively.[55] One study compared 3 days vs. 7 days and found equivalent bacterial eradication rates but higher rates of recurrence.[60] Most studies demonstrate that beta-lactams are inferior in cure rates compared with fluoroquinolones [61] when given for the same duration, possibly because of persistence of the vaginal bacterial reservoir. Another study evaluated a 3-day regimen of TMP/SMX ($n = 70$) compared with cefpodoxime proxetil ($n = 63$) and demonstrated equivalence in clinical outcomes, recurrence, and microbiologic outcomes.[62] The small sample size and overall cure rates (70/70 early clinical cure in TMP/SMX arm and 62/63 in cefpodoxime arm) limited the ability of the study to find differences between the two drugs.

Nitrofurantoin for 5 days has been shown to have equivalent clinical and microbiological cure rates as a 3-day regimen of TMP/SMX.[63] Four RCTs [63–66] demonstrate that a 7-day nitrofurantoin therapy has similar clinical cure rates as ciprofloxacin for 3 days, TMP/SMX for 7 days, and 3-g single-dose of fosfomycin. Taken together, the above studies demonstrate a clinical cure rate with nitrofurantoin of 88% to 93% and a bacterial cure rate of 81% to 92%. A meta-analysis of nitrofurantoin for cystitis was recently conducted and included 27 controlled trials with over 4,800 patients; most patients were female and were over 20 years old.[67] The more robust studies included in the analysis indicated overall equivalence between 3 and 7 days of nitrofurantoin when compared with TMP/SMX (3–7 days), ciprofloxacin (3 days) and amoxicillin (3 days). Similar clinical cure rates were seen for nitrofurantoin given for 5–7 days vs. one of eight comparator antibiotics, but microbiologic efficacy was slightly higher in comparator antibiotics (RR 0.93, 95% CI 0.89–0.97). When nitrofurantoin was given for only 3 days, clinical cure was reduced (range, 60–70%) compared to studies with longer duration.

Data suggest that TMP/SMX for 3 days is an appropriate treatment course for cystitis if local resistance does not exceed 20% or the pathogen is not known to be resistant. Nitrofurantoin for 5 days is an alternative regimen with minimal resistance and good tolerability. Fosfomycin single-dose therapy given its prolonged half-life is another alternative. The fluoroquinolones have shown high cure rates among susceptible infections with 3-day regimens, but given the side-effect profile and rising resistance patterns these agents are not recommended when other oral options exist. Beta-lactam agents may be appropriate for 3–7 days in patients for whom other recommended agents cannot be used, but have reduced efficacy and comparably higher side-effect profile.

Pyelonephritis

The 1999 IDSA guidelines recommended 14 days of therapy for pyelonephritis in most situations. More recent RCTs demonstrated that ≤ 7 days of ciprofloxacin achieved greater bacteriologic and clinical cure rates than trimethoprim-sulfamethoxazole given for 14 days [68] and that high-dose levofloxacin given for 5 days was equivalent to 10 days of ciprofloxacin.[69, 70]

Other investigators compared 1 week versus 3 weeks of treatment with pivampicillin plus pivmecillinam for pyelonephritis.[71] Clinical success was achieved in 29/32 (91%) and in 28/29 (97%) patients treated for one vs. three weeks, respectively; bacterial eradication was much lower in the 1-week group (28% vs. 69%) with a large number of those patients experiencing recurrences of cystitis secondary to emergence of drug-resistant strains. Thus, the authors concluded that 1 week of treatment was an insufficient duration of therapy for those agents.

With the advent of antibiotics with improved urinary penetration, and more importantly tissue penetration in cases of pyelonephritis, a randomized trial in the Netherlands evaluated sequential IV and oral fleroxacin therapy for total duration of 7 or 14 days for treatment of UTI.[72] It should be noted that this group included patients with pyelonephritis, but also those with complicated cystitis. No significant difference in bacteriologic cure was found between the two groups (7 days: 78%; 14 days: 75%).

Talan compared short-course fluoroquinolone treatment (7 day) with longer course (14 day) TMP/SMX therapy.[68] This randomized double-blind comparative trial studied 255 women with pyelonephritis and a causative bacterial organism on urinary culture. Bacteriologic cure rates were 99% (112/113) vs. 89% (90/101) ($p = 0.004$) with clinical cure rates of 96% (109/113) and 83% (92/111) ($p = 0.002$) for ciprofloxacin and TMP/SMX, respectively. The authors noted that *E. coli*, which caused more than 90% of infections, was more frequently resistant to TMP/SMX (18%) than to ciprofloxacin (0%; $p < 0.001$). This accounted for the greater bacteriologic and clinical failure rates with TMP/SMX despite a longer treatment course than ciprofloxacin. It is important to note that the study was conducted in an era of minimal fluoroquinolone resistance, and demonstrated that short-course therapy is sufficient with an active antibiotic with adequate urinary penetration.

Two subsequent studies evaluated whether high-dose therapy over a shorter duration improved outcomes. Klausner performed a double-blind, non-inferiority trial comparing 5 days of levofloxacin with 10 days of ciprofloxacin in acute pyelonephritis in both males and females.[69] There were no differences in microbiological eradication or clinical success. It should be noted that fluoroquinolone resistance was low (2%) in this study. Another report using data from the same study confirmed equivalence of the above regimens when complicated urinary tract infections were combined with pyelonephritis.[70]

A meta-analysis evaluated short- and long-course therapy for the treatment of pyelonephritis including 4 RCTs where the same antibiotic was used in each arm.[73] Short course therapy ranged from 7 to 14 days and long-course therapy ranged from 14 to 42 days. While this meta-analysis showed no differences in terms of clinical success (OR, 1.27; 95% CI, 0.59–2.70), bacteriologic efficacy (OR, 0.80; 95% CI, 0.13–4.95), or relapse (OR, 0.65; 95% CI, 0.08–5.39), results from this analysis had low applicability in that the duration of therapy defined as "short course" was in essence extended-course therapy and the antibiotics evaluated were largely not first-line agents. However, for each of the studies included, no difference was observed with treatment duration given beyond 2 weeks. The added risks of adverse effects and emergence of resistant pathogens were not addressed in patients receiving prolonged treatment.

Pyelonephritis requires longer durations of antibiotic treatment than cystitis. Understanding local resistance patterns and selecting an agent that can achieve high and reliable tissue penetration are key factors in recommending short-course therapy (5–7 days). Patients with complicated pyelonephritis, perinephric abscess, or associated bacteremia may require longer durations and were not included in the above studies. Ciprofloxacin given for 7 days is an appropriate regimen if local resistance is <10% or the isolate is known to be sensitive. High-dose levofloxacin (750 mg) given once daily for 5 days is another acceptable regimen given the above conditions are met. TMP/SMX for 14 days is an alternative for susceptible isolates. Beta-lactams are generally less effective and are considered second-line therapy; insufficient evidence exists to confirm an optimal duration though 10–14 days has been recommended in the past.

Successful Stewardship Interventions to Optimize Duration of Therapy: UTI

Many of the stewardship interventions related to UTI management have focused on reducing treatment for asymptomatic bacteriuria and selection of appropriate empiric antibiotics. Two studies evaluated AS interventions aimed at reducing prolonged durations of therapy for UTI in different settings. Hecker and colleagues assessed guideline adherence and antibiotic use in the emergency department (ED) before and after an AS intervention that consisted of implementing an electronic order set followed by audit and feedback.[74] Patients were identified by using ICD-9 codes for cystitis. They conducted the analysis of 200 patients randomly selected in each of three time periods: baseline, electronic order set intervention (period 1), and audit and feedback intervention (period 2) over a 2-year period. Adherence to guidelines increased from 44% (baseline) to 68% (period 1) to 82% (period 2) ($p \leq 0.015$ for each). Unnecessary antibiotic days decreased from 250 to 119 to 52 days ($p < 0.001$ for each period). Another study evaluated an AS care bundle to shorten duration of therapy for UTI in hospitalized adults.[75] They created institutional guidelines based on national guidelines for UTI treatment and distributed as pocket cards along with posting on the institutional website accompanied by an educational campaign. The bundle was pharmacist-driven and included a real-time alert targeting patients with abnormalities on urinalysis who were receiving an antibiotic. The ASP care bundle included five elements: 1) confirmation of UTI based on ASP review with case definitions, 2) initiation of empiric therapy based on institutional guidelines, 3) changing to optimal agent based on culture results within 48 hours, 4) conversion of IV to oral (PO) therapy within 72 hours, and 5) continuing treatment for a total duration (inpatient plus outpatient) per institutional recommendations. They compared patients managed under the bundle to historical controls and found compliance with all bundle elements was increased after the intervention period (75% vs. 38%, $p<0.001$) and that more patients treated for appropriate durations following bundle implementation (89 vs. 64%, $p = 0.001$) with average duration shortened by 2 days in the bundle group (2.3 vs. 4.9 days, $p = 0.001$).

Intra-Abdominal Infections

Intra-abdominal infections (IAIs) are a heterogenous collection of diagnoses with a variety of empiric antibiotic choices for which risk factors, knowledge of local resistance patterns, and source control are essential to achieving clinical cure. Guidelines on duration of therapy for IAIs first appeared in 2002 [76] and 2003.[77] At that time, treatment of fewer than 7 days was thought adequate unless source control could not be achieved. Since that time several studies have emerged to help inform some of the knowledge gaps. Recent literature has provided high-quality evidence for durations of therapy for complicated intra-abdominal infections (cIAIs).[78]

The initial multidisciplinary guidelines featured consensus of the IDSA, the Surgical Infection Society, the American Society for Microbiology, and the Society of Infectious Disease Pharmacists. The section on duration of therapy was brief and included only a single reference that by that time was already more than 20 years old. The guidelines stated the following: "Antimicrobial therapy for established infections should be continued until resolution of clinical signs of infection occurs, including normalization of temperature and white blood cell count and return of gastrointestinal function."[79] This was relatively vague, but was based on the dated evidence that risk of treatment failure appeared to be low when the above clinical parameters had been met.[79] The minimal risk of subsequent treatment failure for those that had no evidence of infection at time of antibiotic cessation has since been confirmed.[80] For patients who did not meet those clinical parameters by day 5, 6, or 7, additional diagnostic evaluation was suggested. The 2009 update [81] of the guidelines contains more specific guidance for duration of therapy based on accrual of evidence. Source control greatly influences treatment duration for these infections. The guidelines suggest that antibiotic therapy should be limited to 4 to 7 days, unless source control is inadequate as longer durations have not been associated with improved outcomes.

Even shorter durations are thought to be effective for prophylaxis of intra-abdominal conditions at high risk for infection. Twenty-four hours of prophylactic anti-infective therapy is thought adequate for traumatic or iatrogenic bowel injuries operated on within 12 hours, upper gastrointestinal perforations operated on within 24 hours, non-perforated appendicitis, cholecystitis, bowel obstruction, and bowel infarction, in which the focus of infection is completely eliminated by a surgical procedure and there is no extension of infection.[81]

Despite the aforementioned studies, the appropriate duration of antibiotic therapy for cIAIs remained unclear. Sawyer et al. performed a randomized, prospective trial to evaluate the duration of therapy for cIAI.[78] Confirming that source control was an important part of cure, they randomly assigned 518 patients with cIAI and adequate source control to receive antibiotics until 2 days after the resolution of fever, leukocytosis, and ileus, with a maximum of 10 days of therapy (control) or to receive a fixed course of antibiotics (short course) for 4 ± 1 calendar days. There was no difference in the composite outcome of surgical-site infection, recurrent IAI, or death within 30 days between the short course and control group (56/257 [21.8%] vs. 58/260 [22.3%]; $p = 0.92$) though median duration of antibiotic therapy was significantly lower in the short-course group (4.0 vs. 8.0 days; $p < 0.001$). The authors concluded that among patients with IAIs who had undergone adequate source control procedures, no additional benefit was conferred by extending antibiotics beyond 4 days.

Duration of antibiotics for cIAIs depends heavily on adequate source control. Recent guidelines have suggested that 4 to 7 days of antibiotics is sufficient, provided source control is achieved and longer durations do not improve outcomes. Newer data suggest there is no benefit of prolonging durations beyond 4 days after adequate source control. There is insufficient evidence to suggest an optimal treatment duration when source control is inadequate or unable to be achieved, though treatment should typically be continued until resolution of fever, normalization of leukocytosis, and clinical stability is reached.

Successful Stewardship Interventions to Optimize Duration of Therapy: IAI

Translating evidence into clinical practice requires multifaceted interventions and behavioral change. Popovski and colleagues implemented a multimodal intervention including educational sessions, guideline pocket cards, and posters emphasizing new data focusing on risk stratification, IV to PO conversion, empiric therapy, and duration of therapy for IAI.[82] They performed a pre- and post-implementation study in a surgical unit at a single institution. There was no statistical difference in the percentage of patients who had a surgical procedure to achieve source control between periods [97/152 (64%) vs. 105/145 (72%); $p = 0.11$]; completeness of source control was not described. There were 152 patients with IAI in the pre-intervention period (April–November 2010) and 145 in the post-intervention period (April–November 2011). One of the primary endpoints was to reduce ciprofloxacin use based on data from their local antibiogram, and they found a reduction in patients receiving this agent [74% to 34% (OR 0.18, 95% CI 0.11–0.31] with an associated decrease in DOT/1000 PD from 221 to 74 (OR 0.3, 95% CI 0.2–0.3). They also found a decrease in DOT/1000 PD for piperacillin/tazobactam (116 to 67; OR 0.6, 95% CI 0.5–0.7) which was offset by increase in patients receiving ceftriaxone (1.3% to 53% [OR 85, 95% CI 20–515]) with corresponding increases in DOT/1000 PD from 6 to 92 (OR 17, 95% CI 10–25). They did not find a statistically significant reduction in overall duration which was thought to be related to their inability to capture outpatient duration of therapy. They found that the mean duration of in-hospital antibiotic was reduced by one day, though the result was not statistically significant (6 vs. 5 days; mean difference 1.0, 95% CI −0.82–2.82). The ability for their multidisciplinary approach to drive down DOT/1000 PD for targeted antibiotics holds promise though they were unable to demonstrate an overall benefit for total duration of therapy. The relatively recent trial by Sawyer [78] demonstrated that shorter courses have similar outcomes for a variety of IAI and this will be a target for AS interventions in the future.

Skin and Soft Tissue Infections

Skin and soft tissue infections (SSTIs) are a common infectious syndrome present in both inpatient and outpatient settings. SSTIs encompass a heterogeneous collection of diagnoses. Cases of cellulitis with or without abscess offer the greatest opportunities for stewardship intervention. The diagnosis of SSTIs are typically made on clinical grounds rather than direct microbiologic or imaging confirmation.

Uncomplicated Cellulitis

A retrospective analysis demonstrated that prolonged durations of antibiotics are frequently prescribed for the treatment of SSTIs in hospitalized patients and provides an antibiotic stewardship opportunity.[83] This study reported that the median duration of therapy was 13–14 days for cellulitis, cutaneous abscess, and SSTI with additional complicating factors. Hepburn et al. performed a randomized, double-blind, placebo-controlled trial evaluating levofloxacin for 5 days followed by five days of either placebo or levofloxacin to complete a 10-day course.[84] Patients met inclusion criteria if they had clinical improvement by 5 days and no persistent focus of infection or abscess formation. The majority of patients included in the analysis were treated as outpatients (75/87; 86%). Clinical success was similar for the 10-day and 5-day regimens at both 14 and 28 days (42/43 [98%] vs. 43/44 [98%] respectively). Thus, 5-day treatment appears to be sufficient for uncomplicated cellulitis in those with prompt improvement.

Newer agents provide additional opportunities for short-course therapy for SSTIs. Prokcocimer et al. evaluated the efficacy and safety of a 6-day oral tedizolid regimen in acute bacterial SSTIs vs. 10-day oral linezolid therapy (ESTABLISH-1) in a phase 3, randomized, double-blind, noninferiority multicenter trial.[85] The analysis included 332 patients who received tedizolid for 6 days vs. 335 patients who received linezolid for 10 days. Tedizolid was noninferior to linezolid in early clinical response (at 48 to 72 hours), end of therapy (day 11), and post-therapy evaluation 1–2 weeks after completion of treatment. This study again demonstrated that when comparing antibiotics within the same class, shorter durations were equally effective. It is important to note that tedizolid had a broad-range of gram-positive activity and narrower spectrum agents are often equally effective, less costly, and less likely to induce resistance.

Cellulitis with Abscess Formation

While many prescribers will treat cutaneous abscesses with antibiotics, the addition of systemic antibiotics after incision and drainage of cutaneous abscesses has not been shown to improve cure rates [86–90], though the development of new lesions may be reduced in the short term.[86, 90] Nonetheless, current guidelines do not recommend systemic antibiotics if drainage is achieved, but should be administered for patients with systemic infections or compromised immune systems.[91]

Two important studies have been published since the release of the 2014 IDSA SSTI guidelines. The first study evaluated whether a 3 or 10-day course of antibiotics after surgical drainage of skin abscesses in children (age 3 months-17 years) had equivalent treatment failure and recurrence rates.[92] Of the 249 patients studied, 87% of wound cultures grew staphylococci (64% MRSA; 36% MSSA). Overall failure rate was low (13/249, 5% total) which precluded any observable differences between groups, if they existed. In a subgroup analysis, patients with *S. aureus* were more likely to experience treatment failure in the 3-day group compared with the 10- day group (7.2%, 9/125 vs. 1.6%, 2/124; $p = 0.03$). Recurrent infection within 1 month was higher in the short-course therapy group (18.2%, 21/115 vs. 7.6%, 9/118; $p = 0.02$) and in patients with MRSA (13% [8/60] vs. 3% [2/67]; $p = 0.0546$). These differences were noted at 3 months (39% in 3 day group vs. 25% in 10 day group, $p = 0.03$); but not by 6 months (43% in 3 day group vs. 40% in 10 day group). Current guidelines include a recommendation that recurrent abscesses should be treated with a 5- to 10-day course of antibiotics active against the isolated pathogen. The increasing prevalence of MRSA in cutaneous abscesses has challenged whether oral antibiotics in conjunction with incision and drainage has benefit.

The second study published in 2016 by Talan et al. [93] was a large randomized placebo-controlled trial at five emergency departments that evaluated treatment outcomes after incision and drainage of cutaneous abscesses with the addition of either twice daily TMP/SMX or placebo for 7 days.[93] The clinical cure of abscesses was higher in the TMP/SMX than placebo groups (80.5%, 507/603 vs. 73.6%, 454/617; $p = 0.0005$). This study reflects a population with a high prevalence of MRSA infections (at 45%). The strength of this newer study is that it was powered to detect a smaller difference than other studies described above.

Uncomplicated cellulitis can be managed with as few as 5 days of therapy if prompt clinical improvement is seen. Cellulitis with cutaneous abscess formation currently holds no recommendations to give adjunctive antibiotics in addition to incision and drainage, though recent data may demonstrate slight improvement with 7 days of TMP/SMX and should be balanced with consideration of antibiotic-related adverse effects or selection of bacterial resistance. Immunocompromised hosts are recommended to receive systemic antibiotics for cutaneous abscesses and have similar recommendations for other SSTI presentations.

Successful Stewardship Interventions to Optimize Duration of Therapy: SSTI

SSTI management has provided an AS opportunity to reduce therapy duration. Jenkins et al. performed a baseline descriptive analysis of a cohort of consecutive patients ($n = 322$) with SSTI at a single institution and found that median duration of therapy for cellulitis, cutaneous abscess, and SSTI with complicating factors was 13, 13, and 14 days respectively. [83] A follow-up study used evidence-based guidelines regarding empiric therapy and duration that were circulated via email and posted on the institutional intranet and in work areas, creation of an order set, educational campaigns with peer champions, followed by an audit and feedback program.[94] The median duration of therapy was reduced from 13 to 10 days post-intervention ($p < 0.001$) without differences in clinical failure, LOS, or rehospitalization. Agents prescribed with broad gram-negative coverage also decreased from 66% to 36% in the post-intervention period.

Conclusion

Antibiotic stewardship has become ever more important with the increasing threat of antibiotic resistance. Our role as stewards demands that we utilize evidence to provide guidance on appropriate duration to achieve optimal treatment outcomes while reducing the collateral damage of antibiotic resistance and medication adverse effects. Selecting the appropriate duration of therapy has been proposed as the most promising stewardship intervention to reduce antibiotic resistance.[95] While there remains a strong need for well-designed research to answer complex clinical questions about the optimal duration of therapy, evidence continues to mount demonstrating that shorter durations reduce overall antibiotic exposure, cost, and adverse effects without worsening length of stay, mortality, recurrence, or clinical cure.

Multiple, well-designed studies have been conducted evaluating CAP and VAP with subsequent meta-analyses demonstrating that CAP can safely be treated with 5 days of therapy and HAP/VAP with 7 days duration. Urinary tract infections also have been studied extensively with as few as 3 days sufficient for most scenarios of cystitis; pyelonephritis requires longer durations than cystitis, but even 5–7 days achieves cure. Complicated intra-abdominal infections with adequate source control show no benefit with treatment durations extended beyond 4 days, though no consensus exists for cases when source control is incomplete. Skin and soft tissue infections can be managed with as few as 5 days of therapy provided prompt clinical improvement is seen. The above conditions are frequently encountered in both the inpatient and outpatient settings and have evidence to support the treatment duration recommendations, but consideration for the individual patient complexities must be taken into account. It remains important for clinicians to understand that shorter durations should be the norm with extenuating circumstances for longer durations considered on a case-by-case basis. ASPs have utilized a variety of strategies to effectively reduce treatment duration for various infectious syndromes through educational campaigns, development of local guidelines, implementation of electronic order set, and prospective audit with feedback; these AS activities should be given a high institutional priority.

References

1. Martin SJ, Micek ST, Wood GC. Antimicrobial resistance: consideration as an adverse drug event. *Crit Care Med* 2010; 38(Suppl 6):S155–S1561.

2. File TM, Jr. Clinical efficacy of newer agents in short-duration therapy for community-acquired pneumonia. *Clin Infect Dis* 2004; 39 (Suppl 3):S159–164.

3. File TM, Jr. Duration and cessation of antimicrobial treatment. *J Hosp Med* 2012; 7 (Suppl 1):S22–33.

4. Hayashi Y, Paterson DL. Strategies for reduction in duration of antibiotic use in

hospitalized patients. *Clin Infect Dis* 2011; 52(10):1232–1240.

5. Centers for Disease Control and Prevention. Delayed Prescribing Practices. 2015. (Accessed March 23, 2016, at www.cdc.gov/getsmart/community/improving-prescribing/interventions/delayed-prescribing-practices.html.)

6. Niederman, MS, Mandell LA, Anzueto A, et al. Guidelines for the management of adults with community-acquired pneumonia: diagnosis, assessment of severity, antimicrobial therapy, and prevention. *Am J Respir Crit Care Med* 2001; 163(7):1730–1754.

7. Leophonte PC, Choutet P, Gaillat J, et al. Efficacy of a ten day course of ceftriaxone compared to a shortened five day course in the treatment of community-acquired pneumonia in hospitalized adults with risk factors. *Medecine et Maladies Infectieuses* 2002; 32(7):369–381.

8. Dunbar LM, Wunderink RG, Habib MP, et al. High-dose, short-course levofloxacin for community-acquired pneumonia: a new treatment paradigm. *Clin Infect Dis* 2003; 37(6):752–60.

9. el Moussaoui R, de Borgie CA, van den Broek P, et al. Effectiveness of discontinuing antibiotic treatment after three days versus eight days in mild to moderate-severe community acquired pneumonia: randomised, double blind study. *BMJ* 2006; 332(7554):1355.

10. Rizzato G, Montemurro L, Fraioli P, et al. Efficacy of a three day course of azithromycin in moderately severe community-acquired pneumonia. *Eur Respir J* 1995; 8(3):398–402.

11. Schonwald S, Skerk V, Petricevic I, et al. Comparison of three-day and five-day courses of azithromycin in the treatment of atypical pneumonia. *Eur J Clin Microbiol Infect Dis* 1991; 10(10):877–880.

12. Yanagihara K, Izumikawa K, Higa F, et al. Efficacy of azithromycin in the treatment of community-acquired pneumonia, including patients with macrolide-resistant *Streptococcus pneumoniae* infection. *Intern Med* 2009; 48(7):527–535.

13. Li JZ, Winston LG, Moore DH, Bent S. Efficacy of short-course antibiotic regimens for community-acquired pneumonia: a meta-analysis. *Am J Med* 2007; 120 (9):783–790.

14. Dimopoulos G, Matthaiou DK, Karageorgopoulos DE, et al. Short- versus long-course antibacterial therapy for community-acquired pneumonia: a meta-analysis. *Drugs* 2008; 68(13):1841–1854.

15. Agarwal G, Awasthi S, Walter SD, et al. Three day versus five day treatment with amoxicillin for non-severe pneumonia in young children: a multicentre randomised controlled trial. *BMJ* 2004; 328(7443):791.

16. Kartasasmita C, Saha S., Short Course Cotrimoxazole Study Group. *Three days versus five days oral cotrimoxazole for non-severe pneumonia: Consultative meeting to review evidence and research priorities in the management of acute respiratory infections (ARI).* Geneva: World Health Organization 2003.

17. Lupison SP, Medalla MF, Miguel CA, Nisperos E, Sunico ES. A randomised, placebo controlled trial of short course cotrimoxazole for the treatment of pneumonia in Filipino children. *Philippine Journal of Microbiology and Infectious Diseases* 1999; 28(1):15–20.

18. Pakistan Multicentre Amoxycillin Short Course Therapy (MASCOT) Pneumonia Study Group. Clinical efficacy of 3 days versus 5 days of oral amoxicillin for treatment of childhood pneumonia: a multicentre double-blind trial. *Lancet* 2002; 360(9336):835–841.

19. Mandell LA, Wunderink RG, Anzueto A, et al. Infectious Diseases Society of America/American Thoracic Society consensus guidelines on the management of community-acquired pneumonia in adults. *Clin Infect Dis* 2007; 44(Suppl 2): S27–72.

20. Lim WS, Baudouin SV, George RC, et al. BTS guidelines for the management of community acquired pneumonia in adults: update 2009. *Thorax* 2009; 64(Suppl 3):iii–55.

21. American Thoracic Society and Society of American Infectious Diseases. Guidelines for the management of adults with hospital-acquired, ventilator-associated, and healthcare-associated pneumonia. *Am J Respir Crit Care Med* 2005; 171 (4):388–416.

22. Dennesen PJ, van der Ven AJ, Kessels AG, Ramsay G, Bonten MJ. Resolution of infectious parameters after antimicrobial therapy in patients with ventilator-associated pneumonia. *Am J Respir Crit Care Med* 2001; 163(6):1371–1375.

23. Luna CM, Blanzaco D, Niederman MS, et al. Resolution of ventilator-associated pneumonia: prospective evaluation of the clinical pulmonary infection score as an early clinical predictor of outcome. *Crit Care Med* 2003; 31(3):676–682.

24. Ibrahim EH, Ward S, Sherman G, et al. Experience with a clinical guideline for the treatment of ventilator-associated pneumonia. *Crit Care Med* 2001; 29 (6):1109–1115.

25. Singh N, Rogers P, Atwood CW, Wagener MM, Yu VL. Short-course empiric antibiotic therapy for patients with pulmonary infiltrates in the intensive care unit: a proposed solution for indiscriminate antibiotic prescription. *Am J Respir Crit Care Med* 2000; 162(2 Pt 1):505–511.

26. Micek ST, Ward S, Fraser VJ, Kollef MH. A randomized controlled trial of an antibiotic discontinuation policy for clinically suspected ventilator-associated pneumonia. *Chest* 2004; 125(5):1791–1799.

27. Chastre J, Wolff M, Fagon JY, et al. Comparison of 8 vs. 15 days of antibiotic therapy for ventilator-associated pneumonia in adults: a randomized trial. *JAMA* 2003; 290(19):2588–2598.

28. Hedrick TL, McElearney ST, Smith RL, et al. Duration of antibiotic therapy for ventilator-associated pneumonia caused by non-fermentative gram-negative bacilli. *Surg Infect (Larchmt)* 2007; 8(6):589–597.

29. Dimopoulos G, Poulakou G, Pneumatikos IA, et al. Short- vs. long-duration antibiotic regimens for ventilator-associated pneumonia: a systematic review and meta-analysis. *Chest* 2013; 144(6):1759–1767.

30. Pugh R, Grant C, Cooke RP, Dempsey G. Short-course versus prolonged-course antibiotic therapy for hospital-acquired pneumonia in critically ill adults. *Cochrane Database Syst Rev* 2015; 8:CD007577.

31. Kalil AC, Metersky ML, Klompas M, et al. Management of adults with hospital-acquired and ventilator-associated pneumonia: 2016 clinical practice guidelines by the Infectious Diseases Society of America and the American Thoracic Society. *Clin Infect Dis* 2016; 63 (5):e61–e111.

32. Avdic E, Cushinotto LA, Hughes AH, et al. Impact of an antimicrobial stewardship intervention on shortening the duration of therapy for community-acquired pneumonia. *Clin Infect Dis* 2012; 54 (11):1581–1587.

33. Li DX, Ferrada MA, Avdic E, Tamma PD, Cosgrove SE. Sustained impact of an antibiotic stewardship intervention for community-acquired pneumonia. *Infect Control Hosp Epidemiol* 2016; 37 (10):1243–1246.

34. Haas MK, Dalton K, Knepper BC, et al. Effects of a syndrome-specific antibiotic stewardship intervention for inpatient community-acquired pneumonia. *Open Forum Infect Dis* 2016; 3(4):ofw186.

35. Nicolle LE, Bradley S, Colgan R, et al. Infectious Diseases Society of America guidelines for the diagnosis and treatment of asymptomatic bacteriuria in adults. *Clin Infect Dis* 2005; 40(5):643–654.

36. Shapiro DJ, Hicks LA, Pavia AT, Hersh AL. Antibiotic prescribing for adults in ambulatory care in the USA, 2007–09. *J Antimicrob Chemother* 2014; 69 (1):234–240.

37. Gossius G and Vorland L. A randomised comparison of single-dose vs. three-day and ten-day therapy with trimethoprim-sulfamethoxazole for acute cystitis in women. *Scand J Infect Dis* 1984; 16 (4):373–379.

38. Trienekens TA, Stobberingh EE, Winkens RA, Houben AW. Different lengths of

treatment with co-trimoxazole for acute uncomplicated urinary tract infections in women. *BMJ* 1989; 299(6711):1319–1322.

39. Warren JW, Abrutyn E, Hebel JR, et al. Guidelines for antimicrobial treatment of uncomplicated acute bacterial cystitis and acute pyelonephritis in women. Infectious Diseases Society of America (IDSA). *Clin Infect Dis* 1999; 29(4):745–758.

40. Counts GW, Stamm WE, McKevitt M, et al. Treatment of cystitis in women with a single dose of trimethoprim-sulfamethoxazole. *Rev Infect Dis* 1982; 4 (2):484–490.

41. Tolkoff-Rubin NE, Weber D, Fang LS, et al. Single-dose therapy with trimethoprim-sulfamethoxazole for urinary tract infection in women. *Rev Infect Dis* 1982; 4 (2):444–448.

42. Schultz HJ, McCaffrey LA, Keys TF, Nobrega FT. Acute cystitis: a prospective study of laboratory tests and duration of therapy. *Mayo Clin Proc* 1984; 59 (6):391–397.

43. Leibovici L, Laor A, Alpert G, Kalter-Leibovici O. Single-dose treatment of urinary tract infection in young women: data indicating a high rate of recurrent infection during a short follow-up. *Isr J Med Sci* 1984; 20(3):257–259.

44. Prentice RD, Wu L, Gehlbach SH, et al. Treatment of lower urinary tract infections with single-dose trimethoprim-sulfamethoxazole. *J Fam Pract* 1985; 20 (6):551–557.

45. Fihn SD, Johnson C, Roberts PL, Running K, Stamm WE. Trimethoprim-sulfamethoxazole for acute dysuria in women: a single-dose or 10-day course: a double-blind, randomized trial. *Ann Intern Med* 1988; 108(3):350–357.

46. Saginur R and Nicolle LE. Single-dose compared with 3-day norfloxacin treatment of uncomplicated urinary tract infection in women: Canadian Infectious Diseases Society Clinical Trials Study Group. *Arch Intern Med* 1992; 152 (6):1233–1237.

47. Arav-Boger R, Leibovici L, Danon YL. Urinary tract infections with low and high

colony counts in young women. Spontaneous remission and single-dose vs. multiple-day treatment. *Arch Intern Med* 1994; 154(3):300–304.

48. Iravani A, Tice AD, McCarty J, et al. Short-course ciprofloxacin treatment of acute uncomplicated urinary tract infection in women: the minimum effective dose. The Urinary Tract Infection Study Group [corrected]. *Arch Intern Med* 1995; 155 (5):485–494.

49. Iravani A. Multicenter study of single-dose and multiple-dose fleroxacin versus ciprofloxacin in the treatment of uncomplicated urinary tract infections. *Am J Med* 1993; 94(3A):89S–96S.

50. Hooton TM, Johnson C, Winter C, et al. Single-dose and three-day regimens of ofloxacin versus trimethoprim-sulfamethoxazole for acute cystitis in women. *Antimicrob Agents Chemother* 1991; 35(7):1479–1483.

51. Leelarasamee A and Leelarasamee I. Comparative efficacies of oral pefloxacin in uncomplicated cystitis. Single dose or 3-day therapy. *Drugs* 1995; 49(Suppl 2):365–367.

52. The Inter-Nordic Urinary Tract Infection Study Group. Double-blind comparison of 3-day versus 7-day treatment with norfloxacin in symptomatic urinary tract infections: the Inter-Nordic Urinary Tract Infection Study Group. *Scand J Infect Dis* 1988; 20(6):619–624.

53. Neringer R, Forsgren A, Hansson C, Ode B. Lomefloxacin versus norfloxacin in the treatment of uncomplicated urinary tract infections: three-day versus seven-day treatment. The South Swedish Lolex Study Group. *Scand J Infect Dis* 1992; 24 (6):773–780.

54. Fang LS, Tolkoff-Rubin NE, Rubin RH. Efficacy of single-dose and conventional amoxicillin therapy in urinary-tract infection localized by the antibody-coated bacteria technic. *N Engl J Med* 1978; 298 (8):413–416.

55. Raz R, Rottensterich E, Boger S, Potasman I. Comparison of single-dose administration and three-day course of amoxicillin with those of clavulanic acid for

treatment of uncomplicated urinary tract infection in women. *Antimicrob Agents Chemother* 1991; 35(8):1688–1690.

56. Savard-Fenton M, Fenton BW, Reller LB, Lauer BA, Byyny RL. Single-dose amoxicillin therapy with follow-up urine culture: effective initial management for acute uncomplicated urinary tract infections. *Am J Med* 1982; 73(6):808–813.

57. Rubin RH, Fang LS, Jones SR, et al. Single-dose amoxicillin therapy for urinary tract infection: multicenter trial using antibody-coated bacteria localization technique. *JAMA* 1980; 244(6):561–564.

58. Greenberg RN, Sanders CV, Lewis AC, Marier RL. Single-dose cefaclor therapy of urinary tract infection: evaluation of antibody-coated bacteria test and C-reactive protein assay as predictors of cure. *Am J Med* 1981; 71(5):841–845.

59. Iravani A, Richard GA. Single-dose cefuroxime axetil versus multiple-dose cefaclor in the treatment of acute urinary tract infections. *Antimicrob Agents Chemother* 1989; 33(8):1212–1216.

60. Pitkajarvi T, Pyykonen ML, Kannisto K, Piippo T, Viita P. Pivmecillinam treatment in acute cystitis: three versus seven days study. *Arzneimittelforschung* 1990; 40(10):1156–1158.

61. Gupta K, Hooton TM, Naber KG, et al. International clinical practice guidelines for the treatment of acute uncomplicated cystitis and pyelonephritis in women: a 2010 update by the Infectious Diseases Society of America and the European Society for Microbiology and Infectious Diseases. *Clin Infect Dis* 2011; 52(5): e103–120.

62. Kavatha D, Giamarellou H, Alexiou Z, et al. Cefpodoxime-proxetil versus trimethoprim-sulfamethoxazole for short-term therapy of uncomplicated acute cystitis in women. *Antimicrob Agents Chemother* 2003; 47(3):897–900.

63. Gupta K, Hooton TM, Roberts PL, Stamm WE. Short-course nitrofurantoin for the treatment of acute uncomplicated cystitis in women. *Arch Intern Med* 2007; 167(20):2207–2212.

64. Christiaens TC, De Meyere M, Verschraegen G, et al. Randomised controlled trial of nitrofurantoin versus placebo in the treatment of uncomplicated urinary tract infection in adult women. *Br J Gen Pract* 2002; 52(482):729–734.

65. Iravani A, Klimberg I, Breifer C, et al. A trial comparing low-dose, short-course ciprofloxacin and standard 7 day therapy with co-trimoxazole or nitrofurantoin in the treatment of uncomplicated urinary tract infection. *J Antimicrob Chemother* 1999; 43(Suppl A):67–75.

66. Stein GE. Comparison of single-dose fosfomycin and a 7-day course of nitrofurantoin in female patients with uncomplicated urinary tract infection. *Clin Ther* 1999; 21(11):1864–1872.

67. Huttner A, Verhaegh EM, Harbarth S, et al. Nitrofurantoin revisited: a systematic review and meta-analysis of controlled trials. *J Antimicrob Chemother* 2015; 70(9): 2456–2464.

68. Talan DA, Stamm WE, Hooton TM, et al. Comparison of ciprofloxacin (7 days) and trimethoprim-sulfamethoxazole (14 days) for acute uncomplicated pyelonephritis pyelonephritis in women: a randomized trial. *JAMA* 2000; 283(12):1583–1590.

69. Klausner HA, Brown P, Peterson J, et al. A trial of levofloxacin 750 mg once daily for 5 days versus ciprofloxacin 400 mg and/or 500 mg twice daily for 10 days in the treatment of acute pyelonephritis. *Curr Med Res Opin* 2007; 23 (11):2637–2645.

70. Peterson J, Kaul S, Khashab M, Fisher AC, Kahn JB. A double-blind, randomized comparison of levofloxacin 750 mg once-daily for five days with ciprofloxacin 400/ 500 mg twice-daily for 10 days for the treatment of complicated urinary tract infections and acute pyelonephritis. *Urology* 2008; 71(1):17–22.

71. Jernelius H, Zbornik J, Bauer CA. One or three weeks' treatment of acute pyelonephritis? A double-blind comparison, using a fixed combination of pivampicillin plus pivmecillinam. *Acta Med Scand* 1988; 223(5):469–477.

72. de Gier R, Karperien A, Bouter K, et al. A sequential study of intravenous and oral Fleroxacin for 7 or 14 days in the treatment of complicated urinary tract infections. *Int J Antimicrob Agents* 1995; 6(1):27–30.

73. Kyriakidou KG, Rafailidis P, Matthaiou DK, Athanasiou S, Falagas ME. Short-versus long-course antibiotic therapy for acute pyelonephritis in adolescents and adults: a meta-analysis of randomized controlled trials. *Clin Ther* 2008; 30 (10):1859–1868.

74. Hecker MT, Fox CJ, Son AH, et al. Effect of a stewardship intervention on adherence to uncomplicated cystitis and pyelonephritis guidelines in an emergency department setting. *PLoS One* 2014; 9(2):e87899.

75. Collins CD, Kabara JJ, Michienzi SM, Malani AN. Impact of an antimicrobial stewardship care bundle to improve the management of patients with suspected or confirmed urinary tract infection. *Infect Control Hosp Epidemiol* 2016; 37 (12):1499–1501.

76. Mazuski JE, Sawyer RG, Nathens AB, et al. The Surgical Infection Society guidelines on antimicrobial therapy for intra-abdominal infections: evidence for the recommendations. *Surg Infect (Larchmt)* 2002; 3(3):175–233.

77. Solomkin JS, Mazuski JE, Baron EJ, et al. Guidelines for the selection of anti-infective agents for complicated intra-abdominal infections. *Clin Infect Dis* 2003 37 (8):997–1005.

78. Sawyer RG, Claridge JA, Nathens AB, et al. Trial of short-course antimicrobial therapy for intraabdominal infection. *N Engl J Med* 2015; 372(21):1996–2005.

79. Lennard ES, Dellinger EP, Wertz MJ, Minshew BH. Implications of leukocytosis and fever at conclusion of antibiotic therapy for intra-abdominal sepsis. *Ann Surg* 1982; 195(1):19–24.

80. Hedrick TL, Evans HL, Smith RL, et al. Can we define the ideal duration of antibiotic therapy? *Surg Infect (Larchmt)* 2006; 7 (5):419–432.

81. Solomkin JS, Mazuski JE, Bradley JS, et al. Diagnosis and management of complicated intra-abdominal infection in adults and children: guidelines by the Surgical Infection Society and the Infectious Diseases Society of America. *Clin Infect Dis* 2010; 50(2):133–164.

82. Popovski Z, Mercuri M, Main C, et al. Multifaceted intervention to optimize antibiotic use for intra-abdominal infections. *J Antimicrob Chemother* 2015; 70(4):1226–1229.

83. Jenkins TC, Sabel AL, Sarcone EE, et al. Skin and soft-tissue infections requiring hospitalization at an academic medical center: opportunities for antimicrobial stewardship. *Clin Infect Dis* 2010; 51 (8):895–903.

84. Hepburn MJ, Dooley DP, Skidmore PJ, et al. Comparison of short-course (5 days) and standard (10 days) treatment for uncomplicated cellulitis. *Arch Intern Med* 2004; 164(15):1669–1674.

85. Prokocimer P, De Anda C, Fang E, Mehra P, Das A. Tedizolid phosphate vs. linezolid for treatment of acute bacterial skin and skin structure infections: the ESTABLISH-1 randomized trial. *JAMA* 2013; 309 (6):559–569.

86. Duong M, Markwell S, Peter J, Barenkamp S. Randomized, controlled trial of antibiotics in the management of community-acquired skin abscesses in the pediatric patient. *Ann Emerg Med* 2010; 55 (5):401–407.

87. Macfie J, Harvey J. The treatment of acute superficial abscesses: a prospective clinical trial. *Br J Surg* 1977; 64(1):264–266.

88. Llera JL and Levy RC. Treatment of cutaneous abscess: a double-blind clinical study. *Ann Emerg Med* 1985; 14(1):15–19.

89. Rutherford WH, Hart D, Calderwood JW, Merrett JD. Antibiotics in surgical treatment of septic lesions. *Lancet* 1970; 1 (7656):1077–1080.

90. Schmitz GR, Bruner D, Pitotti R, et al. Randomized controlled trial of trimethoprim-sulfamethoxazole for uncomplicated skin abscesses in patients at risk for community-associated methicillin-resistant *Staphylococcus aureus* infection. *Ann Emerg Med* 2010; 56(3):283–287.

91. Stevens DL, Bisno AL, Chambers HF, et al. Practice guidelines for the diagnosis and management of skin and soft tissue infections: 2014 update by the infectious diseases society of America. *Clin Infect Dis* 2014; 59(2):147–159.

92. Holmes L, Ma C, Qiao H, et al. Trimethoprim-sulfamethoxazole therapy reduces failure and recurrence in methicillin-resistant *Staphylococcus aureus* skin abscesses after surgical drainage. *J Pediatr* 2016; 169:128–134 e1.

93. Talan DA, Mower WR, Krishnadasan A, et al. Trimethoprim-sulfamethoxazole versus placebo for uncomplicated skin abscess. *N Engl J Med* 2016; 374 (9):823–832.

94. Jenkins TC, Knepper BC, Sabel AL, et al. Decreased antibiotic utilization after implementation of a guideline for inpatient cellulitis and cutaneous abscess. *Arch Intern Med* 2011; 171 (12):1072–1079.

95. Rice LB. The Maxwell Finland Lecture: for the duration-rational antibiotic administration in an era of antimicrobial resistance and *Clostridium difficile*. *Clin Infect Dis* 2008; 46(4):491–496.

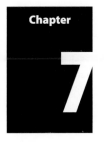

Measurement in Antibiotic Stewardship

Elizabeth S. Dodds Ashley and Edward A. Stenehjem

Introduction

Measuring the quality of healthcare and using the measurements to improve healthcare delivery are commonplace in hospitals across the country. Many measures that are used today are robust, with tight, evidence-based links between process performance and patient outcomes. As antibiotic stewardship (AS) requirements enter the regulatory arena, measurement of antibiotic prescribing appropriateness and measurement of the effectiveness of antibiotic stewardship programs (ASPs) will be critical to assess the need and the impact of ASPs in hospitals, long-term care, and ambulatory care settings.

ASPs are not a new phenomenon;[1] however, the new AS standards from The Joint Commission come with challenges in measuring the effectiveness of ASPs. Defining quality measures to assess antibiotic prescribing appropriateness and the effectiveness of ASPs will be critical to the evolution of AS acceptance and public reporting of measures. The primary objective of antibiotic prescribing and ASPs is to ensure patients receive the right antibiotic, at the right time, at the right dose, via the right route, and for the right duration to treat or prevent infection. All of these steps (or processes) are necessary to optimize patient outcomes, reduce unintended consequences (e.g., *Clostridium difficile* infection [CDI] and adverse drug events) and to minimize the emergence of antibiotic resistance.[2] Stated more simply, the role of the ASP is to ensure patients receive the highest quality of care in the management (i.e., diagnosis and treatment) and prevention of infections using coordinated interventions designed to improve antibiotic use and patient outcomes. The science of measurement surrounding antibiotic prescribing and AS is focused on assessing these processes and outcomes.

The quality measures of antibiotic prescribing and infection management can be grouped into three general categories based on the Donabedian quality measures model:[3] structure measures, process measures, and outcome measures (Table 1).

Structure quality measures of ASPs evaluate what the program does and how it is structured. Structure measures assess the characteristics of the ASP members, the commitment of the hospital leadership to AS, and the components and activities of the ASP. Typically, structure measures assess the state of ASPs within a hospital and are used for epidemiologic purposes as they do not directly measure the effectiveness of a program. Structure measures are often used by regulatory bodies (e.g., The Joint Commission).

Process measures are used to describe the results of a patient and provider interaction. The measures make up the components of appropriate infectious diseases management such as performing blood cultures or prescribing antibiotics. Performing chest imaging in patients with pneumonia and repeating blood cultures to document clearance for *Staphylococcus aureus* bacteremia are two examples of process measures. Antibiotic

Table 1 Examples of Quality Measures Used by Antibiotic Stewardship Programs

Quality Measures in Antibiotic Stewardship

Structure Measures	Leadership commitment to antibiotic stewardship ASP leader designated Pharmacy leader with drug expertise Implements policies and interventions to improve antibiotic use Tracks antibiotic use Report on prescribing and resistance patterns Antibiotic related education ASP provide education to patients and families Organization uses approved multidisciplinary protocols	
Process Measures	Patient Management	Appropriateness: adherence to guidelines Duration of antibiotic therapy Antibiotic de-escalation IV to PO conversion Double anaerobic therapy Time to appropriate therapy Diagnostic utilization Duration and indication included in antibiotic orders Antibiotic free days Infectious diseases consult performed
	Stewardship Program	Antibiotic courses reviewed by the ASP Electronic alerts acknowledged by ASP Interventions or recommendations made by ASP Types of and quantity of interventions/recommendations made by ASP Approval rate of requests for restricted antibiotics
	Consumption	Days of therapy per 1,000 days present or patient days Defined daily doses per 1,000 patient days Length of therapy Doses dispensed Antibiotic starts Excess drug use Other resource use: ventilator days, urinary and intravenous catheters days, intensive care unit days
Outcome Measures	Clinical	Mortality: overall and infection related Length of stay Readmission rates: all-cause and related to infectious diagnosis C. difficile rates Antibiotic related adverse drug events Antibiotic resistance rates Cure rates: clinical and microbiologic response Proportion of patients with clinical failure Length of stay: overall, intensive care unit, following start of antibiotics Hospital-acquired infection rates
	Financial	Drug costs Hospitalization costs Overall cost of therapy Cost per patient per day Cost attributable to infection Cost per unit of quality (i.e., quality adjusted life year)

consumption measures are also process measures, as they are the result of the encounter between a provider and a patient (i.e., providers decide what antibiotic to use and for how long). Given the complexities and the extensive literature available on consumption measures, we will consider these measures separately. If process measures are to be credible quality measures, they must demonstrate that variations in the attribute they measure lead to differences in outcomes.[4]

Outcome measures are the ultimate assessments of program effectiveness. Outcome measures refer to the patient's subsequent health status and the end-result of the provider-patient encounter such as mortality or adverse events as a result of antibiotic prescribing. If outcome measures are to be valid, differences in outcomes will be found if the processes under the control of providers are altered.[4]

Financial measures are outcome measures and must be considered in today's healthcare environment. Changes in financial measures are typically the result of a change in process (e.g., using different antibiotics), a change in outcome (e.g., reducing length of stay), or a structure change (e.g., antibiotic acquisition costs are changed due to a negotiated contract). Financial measures will be discussed separately from clinical outcome measures.

Structure Measures

Structure quality measures assess the characteristics of a care setting and ASP, including the personnel, capacity, and/or policies related to providing high-quality care. Structure measures are often used for epidemiologic and regulatory purposes. Epidemiologic studies use structure measures to assess the status of a specific program as a means of monitoring progress in development and dissemination. Regulators often use structure measures to determine whether a program has the capacity needed to deliver high-quality care. Ideally, structure measures will have been previously evaluated and shown to directly improve the quality of care.

Although structure measures provide essential information about the foundation of a program, it is important to note that these measures do not assess the ability of a program to perform certain functions, do not capture whether these functions actually occur, and do not capture whether those functions improve patient care or clinical outcomes. Structure measures should be considered among many quality measures but should not be relied upon as the sole measure of quality.

Structure measures, as they pertain to ASPs, assess staffing, training, disciplines, and responsibilities of team members, the commitment of hospital leadership, and the implementation of ASP-led activities. The CDC's Core Elements of Hospital Antibiotic Stewardship Programs (www.cdc.gov/getsmart/healthcare/implementation/core-elements.html) are a collection of structure measures that can be used to evaluate ASPs in the United States.[5]

The Joint Commission is a United States based organization that accredits health care organizations and programs in the United States. The Joint Commission accreditation and certification is meant to be a symbol of quality that reflects an organization's commitment to meeting certain performance standards. The Joint Commission standards on inpatient ASPs went into effect on January 1, 2017 (www.jointcommission.org/assets/1/6/New_Anti microbial_Stewardship_Standard.pdf). These standards assess hospital-based ASPs against multiple structure quality measures and is the first regulatory agency to evaluate ASPs. The Joint Commission standards overlap significantly with the CDC's core elements but expands requirements in a number of areas. The Joint Commission has made the use of organization-approved multidisciplinary protocols or guidelines outlining appropriate antibiotic use an individual standard.

For individual ASPs attempting to assess antibiotic prescribing and infection management appropriateness, structure measures will have little utility. Structure measures, however, will likely remain a focus of regulatory bodies and may provide motivation to hospital administrators to ensure ASPs are appropriately staffed and funded. It will remain the responsibility of ASP leadership to perform regular gap analyses to assess their hospitals ability to meet such national standards.

Process Measures

To define quality measures for the process of optimizing the management and prevention of infections, one has to understand what is meant by "the process." The management of infectious diseases begins with making the appropriate diagnosis, which may be the most critical aspect of appropriate management. After a diagnosis is made, the prescriber must choose empiric therapy, proceed with the most appropriate evaluation, alter antibiotic regimens as more information becomes available, choose the most appropriate route for antibiotics, and finally, decide on a duration of therapy. National infectious diseases guidelines, such as those from the Infectious Diseases Society of America (IDSA), assist with determining what is considered optimal infectious diseases care based on available evidence. However, many of the steps in the process are loosely defined, include all possible options (not just optimal choices), and appropriateness is based on expert opinion or minimal clinical evidence. Defining the measures that surround each step in the process will provide information on the appropriateness of management of patients with infectious diseases.

Process measures are the specific steps within the process that leads, either positively or negatively, to a particular health outcome (e.g., cure, mortality, length of stay, etc.). Given the rarity of severe infectious diseases related outcomes (e.g., the mortality rate of uncomplicated cystitis is very low), process measures are often employed as surrogates for clinical outcome endpoints. Process measures can assess tasks that are accomplished (e.g., was a chest x-ray performed when considering the diagnosis of pneumonia?) or the behavior of a prescriber (e.g., how often were broad spectrum antibiotics prescribed for certain conditions?). Process measures can be influenced by ASPs. Changes in process measures after the implementation of an ASP is a common method of measuring the impact an ASP has on the appropriateness of management of patients with infectious diseases.

As their primary goal, ASPs aim to improve the appropriateness of antibiotic prescribing and infection management. Unfortunately, due to a lack of standardized definitions of antibiotic prescribing appropriateness, there is considerable variability in measuring appropriateness.[6] Research into the development of clear, objective, and validated measures of appropriateness is a priority for national societies.[2] CDC has developed assessment tools that can help facilities explore potential opportunities for improving antibiotic use. The forms can be found at www.cdc.gov/getsmart/healthcare/implementation.html. The forms were designed to be used as quality improvement tools intended to highlight situations where providers may be deviating from recommended practices. Areas with considerable variation from established recommendations could present opportunities for further exploration.

The following are examples of process measures commonly used to assess the appropriateness of antibiotic prescribing and infectious diseases management.

Adherence to hospital-specific guidelines Many ASPs develop hospital-specific guidelines for common infection syndromes to define the most appropriate empiric antibiotics based on local epidemiology. Lower respiratory tract, urinary tract, and skin and soft tissue infections typically account for over 50% of the indications for which patients receive antibiotic treatment [7] and are the most common guidelines developed. Reviewing the empiric therapy of patients with these syndromes allows the ASP to assess adherence to institutional guidelines. This review can be done retrospectively on regular intervals or ongoing as part of a prospective audit and feedback program (Chapter 4). Dichotomizing empiric therapy as adherent or not adherent and graphing the results can show significant trends in antibiotic prescribing quality and the impact of integrating institutional guidelines into ASPs.

Duration of antibiotic therapy Measurement of syndrome specific duration of antibiotic therapy is one aspect of treatment that is easily quantifiable and is associated with clinical outcomes.[8] As such, duration of antibiotic therapy is an excellent process measure to assess. As discussed in Chapter 6, community-acquired pneumonia (CAP), urinary tract infections, S. aureus bacteremia, and intra-abdominal infections all have significant evidence to guide clinicians on the most appropriate duration of antibiotic therapy. To assess duration of antibiotic therapy for a specific condition, the AS team must identify the patient population they wish to study (e.g., pyelonephritis patients) in real time via prospective audit or retrospectively via an electronic data pull. Duration of antibiotic therapy is calculated by adding the number of days that the patient received antibiotics as an inpatient and the prescribed outpatient duration according to the discharge summary. Avdic et al. [9] provide an example of measuring baseline duration of antibiotic therapy for CAP and the impact an ASP can have on reducing duration of antibiotic therapy. S. aureus bacteremia is a condition with high morbidity where duration of antibiotic treatment has been shown to be predictive of clinical relapse.[10] ASPs can assess the appropriateness of the planned treatment duration for S. aureus bacteremia to ensure an effective duration of therapy and to ensure appropriate referral to infectious diseases.[11]

Length of antibiotic therapy is an antibiotic consumption metric that will be discussed later in the chapter. Length of therapy is an aggregated usage metric that is not condition specific and is used to assess inpatient antibiotic prescribing.

Antibiotic de-escalation Prescribers initiate broad spectrum empiric antibiotics in an attempt to treat the majority of potential pathogens that are involved in an infection. Antibiotic de-escalation strategies identify patients on broad spectrum empiric regimens to change therapy to a narrower spectrum agent as soon as possible. This strategy is recommended in the surviving sepsis campaign guidelines to ensure appropriate treatment while attempting to minimize the potential of emergence of multidrug-resistant pathogens.[12] Unfortunately, antibiotic de-escalation strategies do not have a consistent definition in the literature making measurement of de-escalation challenging. In their systematic review of antibiotic de-escalation, Tabah et al. outline the multiple definitions used in de-escalation studies.[13] In general, antibiotic de-escalation is the act of changing a broad spectrum antibiotic to a more narrow spectrum antibiotic (e.g., changing meropenem to ceftriaxone), decreasing the number of antibiotics used (e.g., discontinuing vancomycin after 3 days of therapy and negative cultures), or shortening/ceasing antibiotic therapy (e.g., stopping antibiotic therapy at 72 hours when cultures are negative and an alternative diagnosis made).

Assessment of antibiotic de-escalation is typically performed on or before a specified day of therapy or when culture results are available. The measurement of antibiotic de-escalation in clinical practice is typically dichotomous (yes/no) using a ranking system based on spectrum of activity or subjective assessment.[14, 15] More sophisticated tools to quantitatively assess antibiotic de-escalation exist but have not been used to assess de-escalation in single center ASPs.[16]

ASPs can encourage antibiotic de-escalation by integrating a provider- or pharmacist-initiated 48–72 hour antibiotic reassessment into routine clinical practice (e.g., antibiotic time out) and/or a prospective audit with feedback strategy lead by the AS team (Chapter 4).

Conversion of intravenous (IV) to oral (PO) antibiotics One of the simplest AS initiatives is the recommendation to switch from IV to PO antibiotic therapy for pre-designated antibiotics with 100% bioavailability. The effectiveness of these programs initiatives have been shown repeatedly [17, 18] and are discussed in Chapter 4. Measurement of IV to PO conversion can be accomplished in a number of ways. Institutional specific IV to PO guidelines typically designate specific antibiotics that are eligible for IV to PO conversion and provide strict inclusion and exclusion criteria. Compliance with institution specific IV to PO guidelines can be assessed prospectively or retrospectively by evaluating antibiotics included in the guidelines. The number of patients successfully converted from IV to PO antibiotics within a designated time period (e.g., day 3 of antibiotics) divided by the total number of patients meeting the pre-specified IV to PO requirements can be graphed monthly for specific antibiotics and/or hospital units. Alternatively, the total days of PO therapy for a specific antibiotic can be divided by the total days of therapy given by either route (IV or PO). This method is less specific as it does not distinguish IV antibiotic days that were eligible for PO conversion. However, obtaining total usage and route of administration data is often easier than reviewing patients for eligibility for IV to PO conversion. Route of administration and days of therapy are available in the National Healthcare Safety Network (NHSN) Antimicrobial Use (AU) Option per month and per unit. Using these data, an ASP can graph the proportion of PO vs total antibiotic usage. Figure 1 is an example of a graph that displays the proportion of PO levofloxacin versus total use over time for a hospital participating in the Duke Antimicrobial Stewardship Outreach Network. Regardless of method used, a time series analysis can allow ASPs to assess the impact of their IV to PO conversion strategy over time for specific units.

Duplicative antibiotic coverage – double anaerobic therapy Simultaneous use of multiple antibiotics with overlapping spectrum contribute to the inappropriate use of antibiotics. One clear example of duplicative antibiotic coverage is the practice of double coverage for anaerobic pathogens. It is commonly accepted that there is no indication to combine metronidazole with another anti-anaerobic agent with rare exceptions. IDSA guidelines recommend adding metronidazole to other anti-anaerobic agents for the treatment of certain biliary infections, but this is rarely done in clinical practice.[19] Identifying patients receiving double anaerobic coverage is straightforward when done prospectively and does not require time intensive chart review. Manual chart review or automated electronic alerts can alert AS teams to duplicative use. Prospectively evaluating cases of double anaerobic coverage will allow the AS team to identify the total number of cases with duplicative coverage and the number of cases in which the duplicative therapy was successfully discontinued. These data can be expressed as count data and tracked monthly (e.g., number of cases of duplicative therapy identified per month) or expressed as a

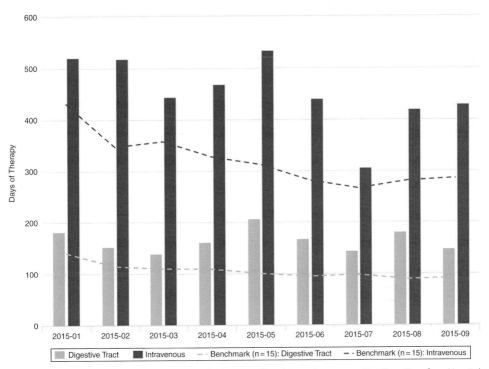

Figure 1 Proportion of Levofloxacin Given Via the Digestive Tract Versus Intravenous Use Over Time for a Hospital Participating in the Duke Antimicrobial Stewardship Outreach Network

proportion to assess the effectiveness of the ASP (e.g., cases of duplicative therapy discontinued divided by the total cases of duplicative therapy). More sophisticated methods to track duplicative anaerobic coverage using patient-level electronic data have been developed.[20]

Measurement of double anaerobic therapy is commonly done as a process measure; however, the link between double anaerobic therapy and clinical outcomes has not been firmly established.

Time to appropriate antibiotic therapy Time can be used as a process measure to assess multiple aspects of antibiotic prescribing. Time to initiation of effective antibiotic therapy, time to de-escalation of antibiotic therapy once bacterial cultures have been reported, and time to directed therapy for specific organisms (e.g., methicillin-sensitive *S. aureus*, *Acinetobacter*, etc.) are all examples of time dependent process measures. Time to appropriate antibiotic therapy has been linked to mortality for a variety of conditions making it a valid process measure.[21, 22] With the development of rapid diagnostic tests for blood culture specimen identification, time to modification in antibiotic therapy has received new focus. Multiple studies have assessed the impact of rapid diagnostic tests on the time to appropriate antibiotic therapy and the resultant change in clinical outcomes.[23–26] Many of these studies show significant changes in time to antibiotic therapy utilizing rapid diagnostic tests but with varying clinical outcome results.

Measuring time as a process measure is challenging for ASPs and requires significant manual data entry and/or sophisticated electronic data capture tools. If the resources and

Table 2 Clinical Examples of Diagnostic Stewardship and Safety Monitoring That Can Be Measured by Antibiotic Stewardship Programs

Category	Example
Imaging	Echocardiography is performed in all cases of *S. aureus* bacteremia Chest imaging is performed in all cases of suspected pneumonia Computed tomography is not routinely used in the assessment of skin and soft tissue infection
Microbiology	Cultures are obtained prior to antibiotic administration Cultures obtained from reliable sources Urine cultures only obtained from patients with urinary symptoms
Laboratory	A urinalysis is obtained for suspected cases of urinary tract infection Urine pneumococcal and legionella antigens are obtained in patients admitted to the intensive care unit with pneumonia *C. difficile* testing only performed on patients with liquid stools and not on laxatives Serum creatinine obtained at routine intervals while on nephrotoxic antibiotics Creatine phosphokinase obtained for patients receiving extended courses of daptomycin

technology are available to assess time dependent measures, they should be used to assess antibiotic prescribing appropriateness and the impact of integrating rapid diagnostic testing into ASPs.

Appropriate diagnostic testing Rapid and accurate diagnosis of infection is critical to ensure appropriate antibiotic therapy initiation and optimal subsequent management. Without the correct diagnosis, the ability for ASPs to ensure appropriate antibiotic prescribing is limited and could result in erroneous recommendations by the AS team. In addition to ensuring patients receive the most appropriate antibiotic, AS teams should also ensure patients receive the correct diagnostic testing for the suspected/confirmed infection. Infectious diseases diagnostic stewardship focuses on three main categories: Imaging, microbiology, and laboratory. Measuring the proportion of patients receiving the optimal diagnostic modalities for a given condition will allow ASPs to focus interventions where they are needed most and track the impact of their interventions. Similar monitoring of laboratory testing can be conducted to ensure the appropriate safety testing is being performed for patients receiving antibiotics. Table 2 provides examples of metrics for diagnostic stewardship.

Duration and indication included in antibiotic orders Documentation of antibiotic indications and duration of therapy is recommended in the CDC's Core Elements of Hospital Antibiotic Stewardship Programs and is considered best practice by most healthcare institutions. Providing an indication and planned duration of therapy at the time of ordering allows for frontline pharmacy staff and the ASP to review the appropriateness, dose, route, and frequency of the antibiotic in a prospective fashion. Requiring these components for antibiotic orders can be accomplished through mandatory order fields in electronic medical records (EMRs), antibiotic order forms, or manual entry when antibiotic orders are hand written. Measuring compliance with ordering standards can easily be audited electronically or via monthly chart reviews in facilities without electronic ordering. In facilities with mandatory antibiotic ordering fields in the EMR, measuring the distribution of indication types and durations of therapy can be done to ensure clinicians are not entering erroneous information to bypass requirements.

In addition to process measures that assess the clinician–patient interaction and define appropriateness, process measures have been defined that assess tasks that are accomplished by the AS team. The following are examples of common process measures that assess the tasks performed by an AS team:

1. Number of antibiotic courses reviewed by the AS team
2. Number of electronic alerts acknowledged by the AS team (i.e., when using real-time electronic AS software)
3. Number of interventions/recommendations made by the AS team
4. Type of interventions/recommendations made by the AS team (e.g., stop antibiotics, alter antibiotic therapy, broaden antibiotic therapy) and percent accepted by the treatment team
5. Approval rate of requests for restricted antibiotics

These measures can be used to evaluate the process of an ASP and the types of interventions most commonly implemented. These types of data are best used in conjunction with clinical process and consumption measures to validate the causal relationship between the AS teams' interventions and the changes observed in clinical practice.

All of the above process measures assess individual components of the process that make up optimal antibiotic prescribing and infectious diseases management. Quantification of appropriateness remains challenging as no standardized measurement exists and national benchmarks have not been established. Measuring baseline appropriateness via point prevalence surveys or medication use evaluations utilizing the measures described above will allow ASPs to identify areas of prescribing and/or management that may warrant further attention and intervention. Measuring the change in appropriateness after an ASP intervention will provide a useful assessment of the effectiveness of the intervention. Defining and measuring appropriateness via process measures and evaluating their impact on clinical outcomes will create a stronger link between the process and outcome.[27]

Process Measures: Antibiotic Consumption

Measuring antibiotic consumption in a meaningful way remains a source of discussion, debate, and significant research efforts focusing on feasibility, comparability, and ideal targets. Complexities arise from tracking drug use across healthcare delivery systems, relying on data from platforms designed for other uses (such as documentation or dispensing of medications), and obtaining accurate measures to account for patient complexity. Despite these challenges, there are many metrics that have been successfully used by ASPs to quantify antibiotic use.

Numerators

Defined daily dose (DDD) and days of therapy (DOT) are the two numerator measures most commonly used. The DDD uses a normalized reference standard developed by the World Health Organization (WHO) of the assumed average maintenance dose per day for a drug.[28] For example, the DDD of vancomycin is 2 grams and piperacillin/tazobactam is 14 grams (of the piperacillin component). These standards are intended to equate to a total daily exposure of an antibiotic. To estimate antibiotic use in a hospital, the total number of grams of each antibiotic used during the period of interest (e.g., per month) are divided by the assigned DDD for that drug. Dividing total grams of use by the DDD (grams/day) yields an estimate of the number of days of antibiotic therapy. DDD can be calculated from many sources of antibiotic data (e.g., purchased, dispensed, or administered), does not require significant computer programming effort, and easily allows comparisons between institutions that calculate DDD similarly.

DOT is the metric adopted by the CDC for implementation in the NHSN AU option for reporting and tracking antibiotic consumption on a national level.[29] One DOT is the result of administration of a single agent on a given day regardless of the number of doses or dosage strength. If the first exposure to an antibiotic is documented one minute before midnight on a given day, this is still considered one full DOT for the purposes of this metric. In addition, antibiotic dosing has no impact on the DOT measure. A single 2-gram pre-operative dose of cefazolin counts as 1 DOT as does 2 grams given every eight hours. DOT is typically calculated from an electronic measure of drug administration (e.g., electronic medication administration record) and is a direct measure of how many days a specific drug is actually administered to a patient. With the dramatic rise in implementation of EMRs over the past decades, many institutions are now able to track DOT more easily than ever before and are moving to this as the preferred measure of antibiotic use; however, the most recent ASP guidelines endorse DDD as an acceptable alternative if DOT is not feasible.[30]

On the surface, it may seem that DDD and DOT could be used somewhat interchangeably. These measures, however, take different approaches to defining drug exposure which leads to slightly different results, even when applied to the same data set. Generally, measures of DOT tend to exceed DDD totals, with the exception of drugs administered only once daily, in which case the two track very closely together.[31] It is worth noting that DDD is not a valid measure of pediatric antibiotic usage or usage in patients with altered renal function due to dosing that is not consistent with the WHO defined standards.

There are other measures of antibiotic consumption that have been used by ASPs. Antibiotic starts, antibiotic doses dispensed, and length of antibiotic therapy are just a few. Antibiotic starts is a summation of all of the unique inpatient encounters that were started on an antibiotic during a defined time period. This measure is often used to quantify the overall exposure of a population of patients in a given facility to a specific antibiotic or any antibiotic. Antibiotic starts can be obtained from the medical record or via pharmacy data, but does not provide significant actionable AS data aside from monitoring usage of high value antibiotic agents (e.g., daptomycin).

Antibiotic doses dispensed is a measure of all antibiotic doses that leave the pharmacy, regardless of strength. Doses dispensed can be calculated from pharmacy data reports. Total antibiotic doses dispensed provides a slightly better summary of overall antibiotic exposure at a facility because it captures all doses dispensed and can therefore provide some estimate of the overall drug exposure or duration compared to just the number of individuals who received a given agent. It should be noted, however, that not all antibiotic doses dispensed from the pharmacy actually reach a patient, with many doses being returned to the pharmacy.

Length of antibiotic therapy has also been proposed as a way to measure use in inpatient facilities. Length of therapy can be calculated for individual antibiotics or as a summary measure of all, or a specific group, of antibiotics. Assessing the overall inpatient length of antibiotic therapy quantifies the number of days that any antibiotic was given to an inpatient for a given condition. This captures initial empiric therapy choices, therapies that have been streamlined based on susceptibilities and any transitions to oral treatment as appropriate. Length of therapy can be calculated for individual drugs as well, particularly those used as empiric agents that are targeted for de-escalation by the AS team (e.g., vancomycin). Length of antibiotic therapy is different than duration of therapy as was discussed earlier in the chapter. Duration of therapy is syndrome specific and assesses both inpatient and outpatient antibiotic therapy. Length of therapy can be challenging to calculate due to pharmacy order entry conventions that typically result in a new start date each time an interval, dose and/or formulation change is made to the order. As such, determining length of therapy is a calculation that often requires the assistance of computer programming in tandem with knowledge from AS providers regarding how individual drug orders should be combined for appropriate interpretation.

Denominators

Normalizing antibiotic consumption data to patient volumes is equally as important as accurate measurement of antibiotic consumption. Numerous denominators have been proposed that capture hospital occupancy volumes. The metrics most commonly used with antibiotic use data are defined in Table 3. Understanding the subtle differences in these data will enhance the understanding of the metric ultimately reported.

All clinical areas contributing antibiotic use data to the numerator should also be included in the denominator. This may dictate, in part, which denominator is selected for a given data set based on which data are available. If antibiotic use is only available at the facility level, then hospital-level data that captures all patients must be used. This may require using a facility-level denominator source such as total admissions (encounters) or total patient days. Using facility-level data does not allow for refinement to specific care locations or patient populations.

The denominator used in the CDC NHSN AU option is days present. Days present are defined as the aggregate number of patients housed to a patient care location or facility for any portion throughout a day during the defined time period, typically one month. Obtaining days present data for the NHSN AU option requires an electronic admission, discharge, transfer (ADT) feed for calculating patient volume. The "days present" denominator should be contrasted with the "patient days" denominator used for reporting healthcare-associated infections data to NHSN. Patient days are most often calculated manually by taking a total count of each patient in a facility at a given time of day and subtracting specific populations that are excluded from the measure. For some smaller facilities, the entire process of capturing patient days includes a daily manual determination of patient days and data capture corresponds with capturing device utilization at the same time. The underlying complexities of automated ADT data capture drive the need for manual capture of patient days at many facilities. In addition, these complexities present challenges to using these feeds for calculating days present. These issues highlight the need for robust and continual data validation protocols.

Some metrics of antibiotic use cross the continuum of patient care. This approach, taken by many European nations requires a more global denominator to fully define the population. In this case, the number of inhabitants of a region or country per day or year are often used (normalized to 100s or 1,000s) to describe overall antibiotic use.[32]

Table 3 Metrics of Antibiotic Consumption

Metric	Definition	How is it calculated?	Advantages	Disadvantages	Data Source
Numerators					
Costs [63]	The amount paid for antibiotics in aggregate for facility	Sum of all expenditures for antibiotic class	Easy to obtain Often tracked by administration and can be used to justify programs	Not sensitive to what is given to patients (there are many other reasons for purchasing antibiotics that may never reach inpatients) Often cannot track where antibiotics are used based on purchasing data Cost data greatly influenced by different purchasing patterns and contracting that can change frequently	Pharmacy purchasing software, but be sure to include all sources as often products such as frozen antibiotics are obtained from outside sources
Charges [63]	The amount a facility charges for antibiotics. Most institutions use a standard cost-to-charge ratio for this.[52]	Sum of all charges through the hospital billing system	Should be relatively easy to obtain Obtained at the individual patient level Does not run the risk of revealing contract pricing	Like cost data, often subject to changes in pricing depending on the local charge practices	Hospital billing department data
Defined Daily Doses (DDD)	Assumed average maintenance dose per day for a drug used for its main indication in adults	A total quantity of drug (in grams) is tallied. This total is divided by the reference standard published by the WHO.[28] Using the	Can be calculated from any data source (purchasing, dispensing, administration)	Reference standards not valid in pediatric patients May underestimate use in patients with renal failure	Various sources- can be calculated from pharmacy purchasing data dispensing data or administration data (all of these need to be

142

Metric	Definition		Advantages	Disadvantages	Data source
			...ference standard makes data comparable between facilities	Limited by quality of data source	...nverted to grams of drug)
Days of Therapy (DOT) [64]	The number of days that an antibiotic agent is given	Counted as each calendar day in which a patient received a given antibiotic	Reflects actual drug administration data. Difficult to measure without electronic medication administration records. Standard adopted by the CDC for the NHSN AU Option	A DOT does not necessarily reflect a full effective day of treatment. Combination therapy can result in higher DOT estimates when data are totaled between agents	Electronic medication administration record (eMAR)
Antibiotic starts [65]	The sum of all new antibiotic orders/prescriptions during a given time period	All new orders are compiled and each therapy is counted as a new start	May be easier to calculate when eMAR data are not available. Recommended as a measure of antibiotic use for long-term care facilities	Does not measure overall exposure (length of therapy)—therefore, chronic therapy and single dose prophylaxis regimens are counted the same. Have to develop a method for tracking formulation changes that may result in a new "order" without changes in therapy	Pharmacy dispensing data; ordering data; eMAR data
Antibiotic doses dispensed	Sum of all individual antibiotic doses dispensed from the pharmacy department	Total of all individual antibiotic doses dispensed	Does not require eMAR data. Most pharmacy software programs capture doses	Subject to variations in pharmacy dispensing model. Between 30–50% of all dispensed doses are	Pharmacy dispensing data; eMAR data

Table 3 (cont.)

Metric	Definition	How is it calculated?	Advantages	Disadvantages	Data Source
			dispensed per each order Can be used to estimate DOT data if needed	never administered to patients so may over estimate use	
Length of Therapy	Sum of all days in which an antibiotic is administered	Sum of DOT for a given treatment course in a given patient care setting (inpatient)	Looks at total therapy for a treatment course and not just for a given agent	Can be difficult to combine step-down therapy (either through de-escalation or IV to oral conversion) without double counting overlap day	Agent specific- eMAR data
Overall Length of Therapy	Overall duration of both inpatient and outpatient antibiotic treatment for a given infection/ treatment course	Sum of DOT for inpatient treatment and planned outpatient duration	Better descriptor of overall antibiotic exposure	Inpatient use is measured in DOT so captures drug actually administered to patients. There is no verification that outpatient medication administration and therefore, this portion of calculation is simply an estimate	eMAR data in addition to discharge prescription data
Denominators					
Patient Days	The number of occupied patient bed days- calculated at a single time each day	At a given time each day, a count is made of each patient in a given location	Same measure that is used for HAI data Readily available in most facilities	May not count patients where actually receiving antibiotics if use is started after transfer/ admission May not count discharge day	Administrative databases and/or manual calculation

Term	Definition	Measurement	Advantages	Disadvantages	Data source
Days Present	Time period during which a given patient is at risk for antibiotic[33] exposure for a given patient location	Count of the number of patients who were present for any portion of day in a given location	Quantifies risk of exposure accurately for each unit. Allows a more granular description of patient movement	New metric that relies on electronic data capture so validation is needed	Hospital admission, discharge, transfer (ADT) data
Inpatient admission	An encounter when a patient is admitted to a facility [66]	Count of the number of patients with inpatient status	Readily available. In theory captures patient areas most influenced by AS team	Does not count observation patients who may be large consumer of antibiotics. May be inflated by certain patient populations such as inpatient psychiatry and rehabilitation not likely to use antibiotics	Administrative databases
Patient encounter	An interaction between a patient and healthcare participant for the purpose of providing services [66]	Count of all patient interactions with the health system. Can be limited to type (inpatient encounter)	Denominator that captures inpatient and outpatient visits. Used by NHSN for laboratory identification events	Not very specific for type of encounter	Billing data
Inhabitants	The census of a given region under study	Captured through census data		Not specific to healthcare setting	Government census data

The following are key questions to ask about denominator data:

What units are included? The patient volume denominator must include patient volume data for all units where antibiotic use is measured. If facility-level antibiotic use is measured, administrative measures of patient volume must include the same units from which antibiotic usage data was obtained. It is important to note that not all administrative measures of patient volumes include the entire facility. This confusion is compounded by NHSN HAI module definitions such as "FACWIDE" that imply all beds are included when in fact there are very specific definitions of what should be included in these measures.[33] Observation units, inpatient psychiatry units, and inpatient rehabilitation units are units that need special attention. These units may be contributing data to overall antibiotic use, but patient days may not be included in hospital-wide measures of patient days, particularly if data are generated by the Infection Prevention Department.

Are admission and discharge days captured? Some methods of capturing patient days do not include the day of admission or the day of discharge in their calculation, as these do not represent full calendar days. Previous studies have demonstrated that estimates of antibiotic use can differ by up to 25% when the day of admission and discharge are omitted from calculations.[32] The NHSN AU option includes both admission and discharge days in the patient day's calculation.

How are observation patients handled? Admitting patients to the hospital under observation status is steadily increasing with some estimates reaching 10% of hospital admissions now being observation status.[34] The way observation admissions are handled differs between facilities and needs to be understood when determining a denominator for antibiotic use. For the purposes of NHSN reporting, units that care primarily for observation patients (e.g., 80% of patients admitted under observation status) are identified as outpatient areas and therefore are not included in calculation of inpatient days. Observation patients are included in unit-based calculations if they account for a minority of patient encounters in the unit. Similarly, if tracking overall patient admissions, depending on the administrative source, observation encounters may not be included in the overall hospital totals.

Applying Antibiotic Use Data

Benchmarking

Benchmarking can be a powerful tool to drive improvement when appropriately used. Benchmarking is the process of gathering data from large numbers of hospitals to allow for inter-hospital comparisons of processes and outcomes after risk adjustment. An ideal benchmarking system would include targets that are replicable, scalable, validated as quality measures, risk adjusted, representative, and provide actionable data.[35] The experience and evidence of benchmarking antibiotic use is evolving but has yet to meet the requirements of an ideal system.

Numerous efforts have been launched throughout the world to track and report comparative antibiotic use between facilities and different levels of care;[36] however, some of the most meaningful benchmarking occurs at the local or regional level.[37] In recent years, several local, regional, and statewide collaboratives have formed and facilitate sharing of information that can be used to drive improvement in antibiotic use at the local level. Seeking out such a group in your local area can be a valuable tool to gain access to expertise in tracking and reporting antibiotic use.

Using antibiotic consumption data for benchmarking purposes can be a powerful AS tool. The NSHN AU option is the first step in allowing hospitals to compare themselves to national standards in a methodologically consistent manner. If hospitals are using data outside of the NHSN AU option for benchmarking purposes, it is essential to ensure methods used to obtain antibiotic use data are consistent across all benchmarking facilities to ensure valid comparisons.

One of the key aspects of benchmarking antibiotic use is risk adjustment. Not all hospitals care for the same acuity of patients and, therefore, adjustments must be made for inter-facility comparisons. These adjustments can be made at the patient or facility level and several methods have been used. The case-mix index (CMI) is one method to adjust for clinical acuity/severity of patients admitted to a hospital. Every hospital discharge is assigned to a diagnosis related group (DRG). Each DRG is then assigned a weight based on charge data collected. The CMI is calculated by summing the weights of the DRGs of all the encounters and dividing the sum by the number of encounters.[38] This can be done for all encounters or just federally funded beneficiaries. CMI is calculated at the facility level and is used for several adjustments in healthcare. CMI has been shown to correlate with facility-level antibiotic use and has been proposed as a risk adjustment tool for inter-facility comparisons.[39]

CDC has implemented a standardized measure for antibiotic use called the Standardized Antibiotic Administration Ratio (SAAR). The SAAR is calculated from the antibiotic use data captured through the NHSN AU module. The SAAR is currently captured for five different categories of antibiotics and is stratified by level of care. The ratio is a comparison of observed to expected antibiotic use based on initial data on AU from early adopters of the module. Reporting AU to the CDC has had limited uptake secondary to technical challenges in preparing and submitting data in an environment of competing priorities for information technology resources.

The SAAR is risk adjusted for facility-level indicators reported to the CDC but does not include CMI. Concerns have been raised that hospital-level indicators do not adequately address case-mix differences, but early experience with the SAAR have shown that these hospital-level indicators perform similarly as patient-specific adjustment tools. More data are needed to further assess the utility of the SAAR and its impact on antibiotic prescribing practices. Neither the SAAR measure nor other benchmarking tools assess the appropriateness of antibiotic use but, rather, serve as a starting point to identify areas of potential variance in antibiotic use.

Lack of Antibiotic Use

Other measures of antibiotic use focus on avoiding drug use and counting the absence of antibiotics. Two such measures are antibiotic free days and antibiotic days avoided. It is easier to measure antibiotic free days as a simple count of days that patients remain free from antibiotic exposure. This has been done for specific disease states such as ventilator-associated pneumonia. This measure is sometimes used to justify that earlier discontinuation of therapy did not result in subsequent need for prolonged treatment due to failure of a regimen.[40, 41] Antibiotic days avoided is a more difficult measure. A common example of how this might be calculated is to track a stewardship intervention that is targeting a common infectious condition such as community-acquired pneumonia. If there is a stewardship intervention to stop antibiotic treatment at 5 days when providers are initially ordering 10 days of treatment, then the antibiotic days that were prevented by the intervention would be considered avoided antibiotic days.[42]

Outcome Measures

If the primary goal of ASPs is to optimize patient outcomes, reduce unintended consequences (e.g., CDI and adverse drug events) and to minimize the emergence of antibiotic resistance, ASPs must measure and track these outcomes to determine whether an ASP has achieved its goal. As stated by Donabedian, "outcomes will remain the ultimate validators of the effectiveness and quality of medical care."[43] Using outcomes data to assess antibiotic prescribing quality and the impact of an ASP can be challenging. In the United States, many clinical outcomes are relatively rare events (e.g., death) and many patients will improve even when they do not receive the most appropriate care. In addition, clinical outcomes are confounded by patient-level factors (e.g., comorbidities) that more strongly influence the outcome than process measures of antibiotic prescribing.

The following are examples of outcome measures commonly used to assess both ASP interventions and infectious diseases management.

Overall mortality Mortality is something that is easily measured and is considered the ultimate outcome measure for many prospective clinical trials. There are several concerns, however, with using mortality as a metric to determine the effectiveness of a particular AS intervention or ASP overall. First, most AS interventions are not designed to effect the overall treatment outcome but rather limit unnecessary antibiotic use. In these instances, overall mortality is better used as a balancing measure to ensure that overall outcomes are not worsened by an ASP instead of targeting a reduction in mortality related to AS activities.[42] This is supported in a meta-analysis of 10 studies that included overall mortality as part of an ASP assessment. In these trials, there was no significant difference in mortality, although this analysis may have been limited by the study design of the included studies.[44]

Infection-related mortality Infection-related mortality has been proposed as a more direct measure of AS activities compared to overall mortality. There are several challenges, however, that limit the utility of infection-related mortality as a routine metric for assessing activities of the ASP. First, it can be very difficult to assess the true cause of death for many patients and the role the infection had in the cause of death is quite subjective. Second, to ensure adequate statistical power for infection-related mortality measurements, a large number of patients and deaths are required. Lastly, mortality metrics are best assessed in prospective, randomized trials which are, typically, beyond the capacity of frontline stewards. For these reasons, infection-related mortality has largely been reserved for large scale AS studies. Even in these settings, overall differences have been difficult to demonstrate.[44]

Length of stay Measuring the duration of an entire hospital stay, the duration of a hospital stay following an infection diagnosis, the duration of an admission in a particular level of care (e.g., intensive care unit), or the duration of a hospital stay following receipt of antibiotics can all be used as outcome measures related to AS interventions. Length of stay metrics are attractive in that overall length of hospital stay is readily available, is accepted as a quality metric by hospital leadership, and is a surrogate for overall resource utilization and cost. This measure, like all outcome measures associated with AS interventions, is dependent on many factors beyond the presence or absence of an appropriately treated infection. Therefore, it can be difficult to attribute changes in this measure directly to AS activities even with appropriately designed studies. The interventions most closely tied to shortening overall length of hospital stay include interventions targeting intravenous antibiotics for conversion to oral administration.[18] and rapid diagnostic tests integrated into ASPs.[45, 46]

Readmission rates Reducing unnecessary hospital readmissions has been a focus of significant intervention throughout the United States for the past decade. Through this work, it has become clear that the reasons for readmission to the hospital are complex and often multifactorial.[47] Using 30-day readmission rates for patients with designated infections (e.g., community-acquired pneumonia), whether or not related to the initial infection treated, has been proposed as an AS related outcome. This is an attractive clinical outcome due to the financial incentives applied in reducing these rates and the clinical importance of readmissions. In addition, readmission data are often readily available from existing administrative data sources. The true clinical impact that an ASP can have on infection-related readmission rates via antibiotic and diagnostic optimization has yet to be determined.

C. difficile infection (CDI) In theory, improved antibiotic prescribing should result in decreased collateral damage associated with antibiotic use. The main outcome measure associated with collateral damage from antibiotics is CDI. ASPs have been shown to reduce CDI when antibiotics such as fluoroquinolones, third-generation cephalosporins, and clindamycin have been targeted, making CDI a valuable outcome measure.[48, 49] Antibiotic prescribing by itself, however, is not enough to impact CDI rates as infection prevention and control programs are also critical. Studies that have shown a reduction in CDI often have strict infection control programs, making the association between an ASP and the reduction in CDI challenging as both programs need to be in place. Both hospital-onset and healthcare-associated but community-onset CDIs can be counted when evaluating an ASP. Hospital-onset CDIs occur > 3 days after admission to the hospital but prior to discharge. Community-onset, healthcare-associated CDI are diagnosed as an outpatient but the patient had been in a hospital < 4 weeks prior to the date of the diagnosis. Ideally, an ASP would monitor both incident infection types; however, detecting community-onset infections can be more difficult due to significant IT resources required.

Antibiotic resistance rates Overuse of antibiotics is an important driver of antibiotic resistance. One of the primary goals of ASPs is to prevent the occurrence of and/or improving existing rates of antibiotic resistant bacteria. With antibiotic resistance being such a prominent outcome of ASPs, it should be measured, tracked, and reported regularly. Factors associated with antibiotic resistance are multifactorial and include infection prevention, antibiotic use outside of the facility, colonization status of the patient population, geography, new outbreaks of drug resistance, and patient comorbidities and immune status. In addition, it may take years for the impact of an AS intervention on resistance rates to be recognized. Regardless of these challenges, many studies have demonstrated the impact ASPs can have on resistance.[50, 51]

Defining the antibiotic resistance patterns (e.g., extended-spectrum beta-lactamase producing *Enterobacteriaciae*) to be targeted and structuring AS interventions to specifically address those forms of resistance are essential first steps in planning and executing a successful intervention. In addition, working closely with the microbiology laboratory to determine how resistance is defined (e.g., phenotypically or genotypically) and how microbiologic cultures are counted are essential in determining how resistance changes over time. There are also national efforts to track antibiotic resistance and multi-drug resistant organisms via the NHSN.

Financial Measures

The focus of ASPs should not be continual reduction in cost; however, evaluating costs can help programs identify areas for improved use and cost reduction. Reducing cost can be accomplished by evaluating the formulary for high cost antibiotics, altering guidelines to favor less costly, yet equally effective antibiotics, and implementing restriction criteria for high cost drugs. These interventions will likely reduce antibiotic cost without influencing overall utilization rates.

Many ASPs are initially justified based upon the potential to reduce antibiotic costs.[44] There are two main types of financial measures used by most ASPs, costs and charges. Often, these terms are confused or used interchangeably but reflect two distinct measures (Table 3). An understanding of the differences and knowing how they are used is critical for any discussion regarding financial measures related to antibiotic stewardship.

Cost is the amount that a hospital or healthcare network pays for a drug and is the metric that can be modified by AS efforts. Cost is influenced by many factors including contract changes, rebate offerings, patent changes, drug shortages, and overall changes in purchasing patterns (e.g., changing from powder vials to frozen pre-made bags). Charge, in contrast, is the amount that a hospital bills for an antibiotic. The advantage of charge data is that it can be used as a measure of antibiotic consumption. Charge data indicate that an antibiotic was directly dispensed to an individual patient and subsequently billed to that patient's account. Cost-to-charge ratios are routinely published and updated by the US Federal Government through the Healthcare Cost Utilization Project (HCUP).[52] Using these simple ratios, which are published for each individual hospital, you can convert charge data to estimated cost data allowing for comparisons between facilities. This method, however, does not address any of the previously described challenges that are encountered when using cost data.

There are several limitations with using financial data in describing antibiotic use. The biggest limitation of using financial data is that it does not reflect the true goals of an ASP, improving antibiotic prescribing quality to improve patient outcomes.[53, 54] However, in the complex healthcare system of today, programs do need to be conscious of financial resources and tracking financial measures related to antibiotic prescribing is a necessity for most.[54, 55] In a survey of ASPs, only 10% of respondents reported that financial outcomes were an important outcome of an ASP; however, 73% of respondents reported that they tracked antibiotic costs routinely.[55] Another limitation of using financial data in assessing ASPs is that financial savings plateau with time. Typically, an ASP will show a reduction in antibiotic expenditures over the first 2 – 3 years of a program and then savings will plateau. It is important to clearly articulate to administration that the savings obtained from the ASP will quickly be lost with the removal of a successful ASP.[56]

When measured as part of an ongoing ASP, financial measures should only be one element of the program that is tracked. Programs tracking these data longitudinally should be sure to account for factors such as inflation and changing drug contracts in order to realize the true financial gains of a program despite appearing to have plateaued with time.[57]

Measurement Challenges

Currently, there are no standard, universally accepted quality measures for assessing the effectiveness of an ASP.[51] As regulatory bodies adopt ASP accreditation standards for all acute care hospitals and states increasingly pass AS legislation, defining quality measures to assess the impact of an ASP will become increasingly important. The structure measures currently assessed by The Joint Commission are an important first step in evaluating the state of AS in acute care hospitals; however, these measures fall short in assessing the true effectiveness of ASPs.[5, 58] In addition, the stated goals of an ASP, to ensure appropriate antibiotic therapy and improve clinical outcomes, are often not aligned with the quality metrics that are typically tracked.[55, 59] Defining and validating quality measures in antibiotic stewardship remains a research priority.[2, 60–62] Ideally, these measures would be reproducible, objective, accessible, linked to clinical outcome data, and applicable to all acute care facilities regardless of size. Ultimately, the choice of measures used to evaluate antibiotic prescribing and the effectiveness of ASPs at individual hospitals will be directly related to data and resource availability and the goals of the hospital administration and the ASP.

References

1. McGowan JE, Jr., Finland M. Infection and antibiotic usage at Boston City Hospital: changes in prevalence during the decade 1964–1973. *J Infect Dis* 1974; 129(4): 421–428.

2. American Society for Healthcare Epidemiology, Infectious Diseases Society of America, and Society of Pediatric Infectious Diseases. Policy statement on antimicrobial stewardship by the Society for Healthcare Epidemiology of America (SHEA), the Infectious Diseases Society of America (IDSA), and the Pediatric Infectious Diseases Society (PIDS). *Infect Control Hosp Epidemiol* 2012; 33(4):322–327.

3. Donabedian A. The quality of care: how can it be assessed? *JAMA* 1988. 260(12):1743–1748.

4. Brook RH, McGlynn EA, Cleary PD. Quality of health care. Part 2: measuring quality of care. *N Engl J Med* 1996; 335(13):966–970.

5. Pollack LA, van Santen KL, Weiner LM, et al. Antibiotic stewardship programs in U.S. acute care hospitals: findings from the 2014 National Healthcare Safety Network Annual Hospital Survey. *Clin Infect Dis* 2016; 63(4):443–449.

6. DePestel DD, Eiland EH III, Lusardi K, et al. Assessing appropriateness of antimicrobial therapy: in the eye of the interpreter. *Clin Infect Dis* 2014; 59 (Suppl 3):S154–161.

7. Magill SS, Edwards JR, Beldavs ZG, et al. Prevalence of antimicrobial use in US acute care hospitals, May–September 2011. *JAMA* 2014; 312(14):1438–1446.

8. Stevens V, Dumyati G, Fisher SG, van Wijngaarden E. Cumulative antibiotic exposures over time and the risk of *Clostridium difficile* infection. *Clin Infect Dis* 2011; 53(1):42–48.

9. Avdic E, Cushinotto LA, Hughes AH, et al. Impact of an antimicrobial stewardship intervention on shortening the duration of therapy for community-acquired pneumonia. *Clin Infect Dis* 2012; 54(11):1581–1587.

10. Chong YP, Moon SM, Bang K-M, et al. Treatment duration for uncomplicated *Staphylococcus aureus* bacteremia to prevent relapse: analysis of a prospective observational cohort study. *Antimicrob Agents Chemother* 2013; 57(3):1150–1156.

11. Paulsen J, Solligard E, Damas JK, et al. The Impact of infectious disease specialist consultation for *Staphylococcus aureus* bloodstream infections: a systematic review. *Open Forum Infect Dis* 2016; 3(2): ofw048.

12. Dellinger RP, Levy MM, Rhodes A, et al. Surviving sepsis campaign: international guidelines for management of severe sepsis and septic shock: 2012. *Crit Care Med* 2013; 41(2):580–637.

13. Tabah A, Cotta MO, Garnacho-Montero J, et al. A systematic review of the definitions, determinants, and clinical outcomes of

antimicrobial de-escalation in the intensive care unit. *Clin Infect Dis* 2016; 62(8):1009–1017.

14. Leone M, Bechis C, Baumstarck K, et al. De-escalation versus continuation of empirical antimicrobial treatment in severe sepsis: a multicenter non-blinded randomized noninferiority trial. *Intensive Care Med* 2014; 40(10):1399–1408.

15. Stenehjem E, Hersh AL, Sheng X, et al. Antibiotic use in small community hospitals. *Clin Infect Dis* 2016;36(10):1273-1280.

16. Madaras-Kelly K, Jones M, Remington R, et al. Development of an antibiotic spectrum score based on veterans affairs culture and susceptibility data for the purpose of measuring antibiotic de-escalation: a modified Delphi approach. *Infect Control Hosp Epidemiol* 2014; 35(9):1103–1113.

17. Goff DA, Bauer KA, Reed EE, et al. Is the "low-hanging fruit" worth picking for antimicrobial stewardship programs? *Clin Infect Dis* 2012; 55(4):587–592.

18. Sallach-Ruma R, Phan C, Sankaranarayanan J. Evaluation of outcomes of intravenous to oral antimicrobial conversion initiatives: a literature review. *Expert Rev Clin Pharmacol* 2013; 6(6):703–729.

19. Solomkin JS, Mazuski JE, Bradley JS, et al. Diagnosis and management of complicated intra-abdominal infection in adults and children: guidelines by the Surgical Infection Society and the Infectious Diseases Society of America. *Surg Infect (Larchmt)* 2010 11(1):79–109.

20. Huttner B, Jones M, Madaras-Kelly K, et al. Double trouble: how big a problem is redundant anaerobic antibiotic coverage in Veterans Affairs medical centres? *J Antimicrob Chemother* 2012; 67(6):1537–1539.

21. Kumar A, Roberts D, Wood KE, et al. Duration of hypotension before initiation of effective antimicrobial therapy is the critical determinant of survival in human septic shock. *Crit Care Med* 2006; 34(6):1589–1596.

22. Kumar A, Ellis P, Arabi Y, et al. Initiation of inappropriate antimicrobial therapy results in a fivefold reduction of survival in human septic shock. *Chest* 2009; 136(5):1237–1248.

23. Wenzler E, Goff DA, Mangino JE, et al. Impact of rapid identification of Acinetobacter Baumannii via matrix-assisted laser desorption ionization time-of-flight mass spectrometry combined with antimicrobial stewardship in patients with pneumonia and/or bacteremia. *Diagn Microbiol Infect Dis* 2016; 84(1):63–68.

24. Perez KK, Olsen RJ, Musick WL, et al. Integrating rapid diagnostics and antimicrobial stewardship improves outcomes in patients with antibiotic-resistant Gram-negative bacteremia. *J Infect* 2014; 69(3):216–225.

25. Emonet S, Charles PG, Harbarth S, et al. Rapid molecular determination of methicillin resistance in staphylococcal bacteraemia improves early targeted antibiotic prescribing: a randomized clinical trial. *Clin Microbiol Infect* 2016; 22(11):946.e0–946.e15.

26. Vardakas KZ, Anifantaki FI, Trigkidis KK, Falagas ME Rapid molecular diagnostic tests in patients with bacteremia: evaluation of their impact on decision making and clinical outcomes. *Eur J Clin Microbiol Infect Dis* 2015; 34(11):2149–2160.

27. Khadem TM, Dodds Ashley E, Wrobel MJ, Brown J. Antimicrobial stewardship: a matter of process or outcome? *Pharmacotherapy* 2012; 32(8):688–706.

28. Methodology, W.C.C.f.D.S. ATC classification index with DDDs. 2015. (Accessed April 27, 2016, at www.whocc.no/atc_ddd_index/.)

29. Fridkin SK, Srinivasan A. Implementing a strategy for monitoring inpatient antimicrobial use among hospitals in the United States. *Clin Infect Dis* 2014; 58(3):401–406.

30. Barlam TF, Cosgrove SE, Abbo LM., et al. Implementing an antibiotic stewardship program: guidelines by the Infectious Diseases Society of America and the Society for Healthcare Epidemiology of America.

Clinical Infectious Diseases 2016;62(10): e51–77.

31. Polk RE, Fox C, Mahoney A, Letcavage J, MacDougall C. Measurement of adult antibacterial drug use in 130 US hospitals: comparison of defined daily dose and days of therapy. Clin Infect Dis 2007; 44(5):664–670.

32. Kuster SP, Ruef C, Ledergerber B, et al. Quantitative antibiotic use in hospitals: comparison of measurements, literature review, and recommendations for a standard of reporting. Infection 2008; 36(6):549–559.

33. National Healthcare Safty Network (NHSN). (Accessed November 1, 2017, at www.cdc.gov/nhsn.)

34. Sheehy AM, Graf B, Gangireddy S, et al. Hospitalized but not admitted: characteristics of patients with "observation status" at an academic medical center. JAMA Intern Med 2013; 173(21):1991–1998.

35. Reddy SC, Jacob JT, Varkey JB, Gaynes RP. Antibiotic use in US hospitals: quantification, quality measures and stewardship. Expert Rev Anti Infect Ther 2015; 13(7):843–854.

36. McNeil V, Cruickshank M, Duguid M. Safer use of antimicrobials in hospitals: the value of antimicrobial usage data. Med J Aust 2010; 193(Suppl 8):S114–117.

37. Bhavnani SM. Benchmarking in health-system pharmacy: current research and practical applications. Am J Health Syst Pharm 2000; 57(Suppl 2):S13–20.

38. Fetter RB, Shin Y, Freeman JL, Averill RF, Thompson JD. Case mix definition by diagnosis-related groups. Med Care 1980; 18(Suppl 2):iii, 1–53.

39. Kuster SP, Ruef C, Bollinger AK, et al. Correlation between case mix index and antibiotic use in hospitals. J Antimicrob Chemother 2008 62(4):837–842.

40. Fagon JY, Chastre J. Management of suspected ventilator-associated pneumonia. Ann Intern Med 2000; 133(12):1009.

41. Chastre J, Wolff M, Faygon JY, et al., Comparison of 8 vs 15 days of antibiotic therapy for ventilator-associated pneumonia in adults: a randomized trial. JAMA 2003; 290(19):2588–2598.

42. Morris AM. Antimicrobial Stewardship Programs: appropriate measures and metrics to study their impact. Curr Treat Options Infect Dis 2014; 6(2):101–112.

43. Donabedian A. Evaluating the quality of medical care. Milbank Mem Fund Q 1966; 44(3):Suppl:166–206.

44. Karanika S, Paudel S, Frigoras C, Kalbasi A, Mylonakis E. Systematic review and meta-analysis of clinical and economic outcomes from the Implementation of Hospital-Based Antimicrobial Stewardship Programs. Antimicrob Agents Chemother 2016; 60(8):4840–4852.

45. Timbrook TT, Morton JB, McConeghy KW, et al. The effect of molecular rapid diagnostic testing on clinical outcomes in bloodstream infections: a systematic review and meta-analysis. Clin Infect Dis 2017;64(1)15–23.

46. Huang AM, Newton D, Kunapuli A, et al. Impact of rapid organism identification via matrix-assisted laser desorption/ionization time-of-flight combined with antimicrobial stewardship team intervention in adult patients with bacteremia and candidemia. Clin Infect Dis 2013; 57(9):1237–1245.

47. Srivastava R, Keren R. Pediatric readmissions as a hospital quality measure. JAMA 2013; 309(4):396–398.

48. Kallen AJ Thompson A, Ristaino P, et al. Complete restriction of fluoroquinolone use to control an outbreak of Clostridium difficile infection at a community hospital. Infect Control Hosp Epidemiol 2009; 30(3):264–272.

49. Aldeyab MA, Kearney MP, Scott MG, et al. An evaluation of the impact of antibiotic stewardship on reducing the use of high-risk antibiotics and its effect on the incidence of Clostridium difficile infection in hospital settings. J Antimicrob Chemother 2012; 67(12):2988–2996.

50. Septimus E. Antimicrobial stewardship-qualitative and quantitative outcomes: the role of measurement. Curr Infect Dis Rep 2014; 16(11):433.

51. Akpan MR, Ahmad R, Shebl NA, Ashiru-Oredope D. A review of quality measures for assessing the impact of antimicrobial stewardship programs in hospitals. *Antibiotics (Basel)* 2016; 5(1).

52. Agency for Healthcare Research and Quality. Cost-to-Charge Ratio Files. Healthcare Cost and Utilization Project (HCUP). (Accessed November 1, 2017, at www.hcup-us.ahrq.gov/db/state/costtocharge.jsp.)

53. Dellit TH, Owens RC, McGowan JE, et al. Infectious Diseases Society of America and the Society for Healthcare Epidemiology of America guidelines for developing an institutional program to enhance antimicrobial stewardship. *Clin Infect Dis* 2007; 44(2):159–177.

54. Dodds Ashley ES, Kaye KS, Depestel DD, Hermsen ED. Antimicrobial stewardship: philosophy versus practice. *Clin Infect Dis* 2014; 59 Suppl 3:S112–121.

55. Bumpass JB, McDaneld PM, DePestel DD, et al. Outcomes and metrics for antimicrobial stewardship: survey of physicians and pharmacists. *Clin Infect Dis* 2014; 59 Suppl 3:S108–111.

56. Standiford HC, Chan S, Tripoli M, Weekes E, Forrest GN. Antimicrobial stewardship at a large tertiary care academic medical center: cost analysis before, during, and after a 7-year program. *Infect Control Hosp Epidemiol* 2012; 33(4):338–345.

57. Beardsley JR, Williamson JC, Johnson JW, et al. Show me the money: long-term financial impact of an antimicrobial stewardship program. *Infect Control Hosp Epidemiol* 2012; 33(4):398–400.

58. The Joint Commission. Prepublication standards – new antimicrobial stewardship standard 2016. (Accessed August 4, 2016, at www.jointcommission.org/standards_ information/prepublication_standards.aspx.)

59. Van Parys J, Stevens MP, Moczygemba LR, Pakyz AL. Antimicrobial stewardship program members' perspectives on program goals and national metrics. *Clin Ther* 2016; 38(8):1914–1919.

60. McGowan JE. Antimicrobial stewardship – the state of the art in 2011: focus on outcome and methods. *Infect Control Hosp Epidemiol* 2012; 33(4):331–337.

61. Morris, AM, Brener S, Dresser L, et al. Use of a structured panel process to define quality metrics for antimicrobial stewardship programs. *Infect Control Hosp Epidemiol* 2012; 33(5):500–506.

62. Pollack LA, Plachouras D, Sinkowitz-Cochran R, et al. A concise set of structure and process indicators to assess and compare antimicrobial stewardship programs among EU and US hospitals: results from a multinational expert panel. *Infect Control Hosp Epidemiol* 2016; 37(10):1201–1211.

63. Finkler SA. The distinction between cost and charges. *Ann Intern Med* 1982; 96(1):102–109.

64. Schwartz DN, Evans RS, Camins BC, et al. Deriving measures of intensive care unit antimicrobial use from computerized pharmacy data: methods, validation, and overcoming barriers. *Infect Control Hosp Epidemiol* 2011; 32(5):472–480.

65. Centers for Disease Control and Prevention. Core elements of hospital antibiotic stewardship programs. 2014. (Available at www.cdc.gov/getsmart/healthcare/e/implementation/core-elements.html.)

66. www.hl7.org.

Chapter 8

What Every Steward Should Know About Pharmacokinetics and Pharmacodynamics

Jason M. Pogue and Marc H. Scheetz

Introduction to Pharmacokinetic and Pharmacodynamic Principles and Terminology

At the outset, the antibiotic steward might wonder why pharmacokinetics and pharmacodynamics (PK/PD) are important to antibiotic stewardship. Antibiotic stewardship focuses not only on prescribing the correct drug (i.e., antibiotic) but also prescribing the optimal dose. The dose of an antibiotic is specific to the individual; a fixed dose of an antibiotic is unlikely to be efficacious for all just as a fixed amount of food is unlikely to satiate each member of a population. Appropriately stewarding antibiotics requires a fundamental understanding of how each antibiotic works best (i.e., is most efficacious and least toxic). The skilled steward can leverage PK/PD strategies to decrease overall antibiotic consumption, better target individual pathogens (in contrast to using broad and unselective coverage), and provide optimal outcomes for patients at the individual and population level through the creation of rationally designed policy.

Pharmacokinetics describes the disposition of a drug in the body.[1, 2] Major processes of interest are absorption, distribution, metabolism, and elimination. The summation of these processes can be distilled into a concentration-time curve, which is displayed graphically (Figure 1). It is common for the pharmacokinetics of an antibiotic to be described relative to a central compartment that is easily measurable (e.g., blood prepared as heparinized blood, serum, plasma, etc.) Other distributions and metabolisms can then be described relative to the change in the central compartment concentration. Figure 1 displays a typical concentration-time graph of a drug in the blood, where drug concentration is displayed on the y-axis and time is on the x-axis. PK parameters are either observed or imputed through modeling, the latter is well summarized elsewhere.[3, 4] Pharmacokinetic parameters of interest include the maximal concentration in the plasma (C_{max}), area under the concentration curve for 24 hours (AUC_{0-24}), the time that the drug concentration exceeds a certain value ($T>$concentration), and the minimum concentration during a dosing interval (C_{min}).

Most antibiotics follow first-order elimination. First-order elimination is a mathematic principle defining a log-linear clearance from the central compartment. Because of this, a half-life (i.e., $T_{1/2}$) can be calculated. The half-life of a drug is the time that elapses when the concentration halves because of elimination, distribution, or metabolism. For instance, if a drug has a C_{max} of 100 mg/L and a half-life of 2 hours, the concentration from the central compartment will be 50 mg/L after 2 hours, and then 25 mg/L after 4 hours (i.e., 4 hours after the C_{max}). Antibiotics that follow first-order elimination also reach a "steady-state" if administered in the same fashion (same dose, interval, etc.) for a period of time that is at least 3-fold greater than the half-life as long as the patient remains clinically stable. This

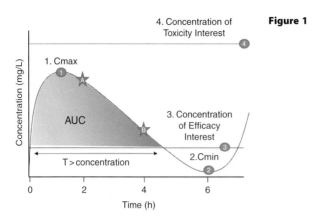

Figure 1

means that the antibiotic will reach a terminal maximal and minimal concentration according to the dosing scheme. That is, identical steady-state C_{max} and C_{min} waveforms will be achieved for consistent dosing if elimination (e.g., renal function) and distribution characteristics (e.g., ascites) do not change. Log-linear elimination counter-intuitively leads most anti-infectives to be classified as "linear" drugs. Linear drugs are so termed because changes to drug dosing made at steady-state will result in a linear and proportional change to drug exposure. For instance, if 1,000 mg of vancomycin results in a C_{max} of 30 mg/L and a C_{min} of 5 mg/L in a given patient that has reached steady state, a 2,000-mg dose at the same interval will result in a C_{max} of 60 mg/L and a C_{min} of 10 mg/L.

Zero-order elimination results in a different pharmacokinetic exposure profile, though fewer anti-infectives, such as voriconazole,[5] display this type of elimination within therapeutic concentrations of the drug. Zero-order elimination is a linear elimination per unit of time and is more common for drugs that are primarily hepatically metabolized. A common and well-understood example is that of ethyl alcohol. Here, the average individual is able to metabolize approximately 0.015 g/dL (i.e., %) per hour, which is equivalent to one "drink" per hour.[6, 7] A subject that has a blood alcohol concentration of 0.08% (i.e., the legal limit for most states in the United States) will have a blood alcohol concentration of 0.05% after 2 hours (i.e., a 37.5% elimination from initial) and a concentration of 0.02% after another 2 hours (60% elimination at 2 hours from the time point). Hence the elimination amount is a fixed amount per time period, rather than a fixed percentage. This leads zero-order elimination drugs to be termed "non-linear." Fixed dosing schemes will not reach a steady state though will eventually decrease in rate of gain. Practical implications are as follows. If a patient achieves a voriconazole trough of 1 mg/L when receiving a dose of 200 mg twice daily, achieving a trough of 2 mg/L is likely to occur with a dose less than 400 mg twice daily. The antibiotic steward can assist with small dose adjustments, such as a 50-mg incremental increase (i.e., 250 mg twice daily) unless complex modeling is undertaken. Understanding these differences allows the trained clinician the ability to manipulate dosing schemes to achieve desired pharmacodynamic endpoints as described below.

Pharmacodynamics is defined as the effect of a drug, manifested as efficacy and toxicity. [8, 9] For antibiotics, efficacy begins at the cellular level for the pathogen. Each clinically utilized antibiotic has specific mechanisms of action that particularly target and have higher affinity for non-mammalian cells compared to mammalian cells. In Figure 1, efficacy begins when concentration labeled at point 3 is exceeded. While multiple concentration targets could be used for any antibiotic:pathogen pair, the most commonly utilized reference point is the Minimum Inhibitory Concentration (MIC). The MIC is the *in vitro* antibiotic concentration required for net-bacterial stasis; i.e., to prevent visual antibiotic growth at 16–20 hours.[10] Though net bacterial stasis exists at the MIC for fixed antibiotic concentrations, killing is maximized at different concentrations relative to the MIC for individual antibiotic classes (as further described below under Antibacterial Susceptibility). For instance, β-lactam killing of bacteria is maximized when the free concentration of the drug exceeds the MIC (i.e., fT>MIC) for a given period of time. Achieving high C_{max} does not generally increase killing, and optimal goals are for the concentration at the site of the infection to exceed the MIC for 100% of the dosing interval. Alternatively, other drugs such as aminoglycosides and fluoroquinolones achieve maximal killing when the maximum concentration exceeds the MIC of the bacteria by a high multiple of the MIC.

The interfacing between necessary drug exposures and rates of killing is often termed PK/PD and is necessary for all antibiotic stewards to understand. As noted above, drug exposure is most frequently described relative to the MIC as the PD endpoint. Certain conditions, such as meningitis and endocarditis may require bactericidal rather than the bacteriostatic drug concentrations defined by the MIC.[11] Minimum bactericidal concentrations (MBCs) are defined as a 99.9% bacterial killing at 24 hours.[12] In the case of a suggested starting inoculum of 5×10^5 colonies/mL, this equates to a terminal number of colonies of 5×10^2 colonies/mL. These methods utilize a very similar testing procedure to the MIC with an added step at 24 hours of plating and colony counting resultant solutions. The extra process requires an additional day of technical work. Since few clinical studies have demonstrated improved outcomes with the knowledge of MBCs and lack of availability, PK/PD endpoints rarely focus on MBCs.

Clinicians wishing to optimize efficacy often design individual drug regimens for patients and create drug policy for populations of patients. Many sites now employ alternative dosing strategies (i.e., dosing schemes other than US Food and Drug Administration [FDA] approved dosages) to maximize efficacy. The approaches presented in this chapter are vetted in the literature, though one must always consider toxicity of alternative approaches. A balance exists, and mathematic thresholds can commonly be defined for both efficacy (i.e., pathogen toxicity) and toxicity (i.e., human toxicity or adverse drug events). In Figure 1, the concentration at which toxicity occurs is labeled point 4. In this simplified example, whenever the threshold concentration is exceeded, toxicity can be predicted as a universal event. However, much like complexities of PK/PD for efficacy, the interface between pharmacokinetics and toxicodynamics (termed PK/TD) occurs at dynamic thresholds. This is demonstrated with Figure 2, where concentration predicts a probability event for both efficacy (e.g., for a fixed MIC pathogen) and toxicity.[13]

Fitting the mathematic function is less important for the antibiotic steward than understanding the components of the equation that describes efficacy/toxicity. That is, when concentration is set to zero, there is an intercept term that defines activity in the absence of the drug. It is important for the steward to understand that efficacy occurs even in the absence of antibiotic. Efficacy is often additive. For instance, if 10,000 people receive an antibiotic for otitis media, we might expect 9,000 patients to have improved constitutional symptoms by day 7. If a separate group of 10,000 people received no antibiotic for otitis media, the improvement of constitutional symptoms at day 7 still might occur in 8,000 people. Thus, the absolute benefit of antibiotic therapy is best described as a 1,000/10,000 or 10% benefit as opposed to 90% efficacious. In an infection, adaptive and innate

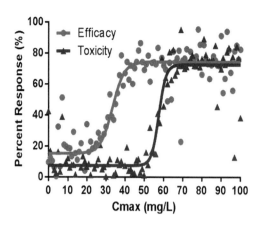

Figure 2 Percent Response of Efficacy and Toxicity According to C_{max}

immune mechanisms are responsible for baseline efficacy (i.e., the efficacy that is expected without drug). Additionally, maximal efficacy (or toxicity) rarely reaches 100% within the doses given to patients. The net benefit of antibiotics for most infections have been estimated at ~30% (as calculated by a likely efficacy of 90% for susceptible bacteria and a likely efficacy of 60% for resistant bacteria). This phenomenon has been termed the 90:60 rule.[14] While some untreated infections were universally fatal prior to the age of antibiotics (e.g., endocarditis), the treatment effect explained by antibiotics against conditions such as skin and soft tissue infections [15] and pneumonias [16] follow the 90:60 rule. Also of high relevance, these equations help to define the therapeutic window. The therapeutic window is the gap (concentration or PK parameter) between which efficacy is first achieved and incremental toxicity is observed. This is graphically displayed for the individual in Figure 1 as the span of concentrations between points 3 and 4. In Figure 2, the area between the two curves is an example of the span of concentrations in the therapeutic window.

Alternatives to FDA approved dosing strategies discussed later in this chapter are generally well vetted and are not known to create additional toxicity, though thresholds likely exist and clinicians utilizing strategies that have less supportive evidence should guide therapy with therapeutic drug monitoring whenever possible and carefully monitor for adverse events. For instance, neurotoxicity is one of the dose-limiting side effects of β-lactams, specifically cefepime. The PK/TD driver for cefepime has been suggested as a trough concentration of ≥ 22 mg/L.[17] However, clinical experience and mathematical modeling have not supported this (as aggressive dosing strategies commonly used often exceed this threshold, without a significantly increased incidence in this adverse event). [18] Thus, PK/PD efficacy is well defined for cefepime [19–24] and the commonly utilized prolonged infusion strategies appear effective and safe in small studies.[25–28] However, little is known about the driver of toxicity, and antibiotic stewards should exercise prudence in pushing the doses beyond those which have been well studied.

Pharmacokinetic and Pharmacodynamic Targets

Common Metrics

As described above, antibiotics are generally classified with PK/PD metrics. The three most common metrics are: C_{max}/MIC, T>MIC, and AUC/MIC (Figure 1). As a drug that is free of protein binding (i.e., "free drug") is the only drug that is generally active against bacterial pathogens,[29, 30] these metrics are commonly termed with "f" to indicate when free drug was modeled or imputed (i.e., fC_{max}/MIC, fT>MIC, and fAUC/MIC).[31] In Figure 1, C_{max}/MIC would be defined by dividing the maximum serum concentration (point 1) by the MIC of the pathogen (point 3). Both values are in mass/volume (e.g., mg/L) and therefore cancel to give a single multiplier of the MIC (e.g., 4× the MIC). T>MIC is calculated by determining the amount of time that the concentration exceeds the MIC of the pathogen. In Figure 1, this corresponds to the time in hours that the concentration exceeds the MIC (i.e., the number of hours that are represented by the shaded portion) divided by the total number of hours of the dosing interval. The dosing interval is not given in Figure 1, but one can surmise from the illustration that a subsequent dose was given after the Cmin. Thus, in Figure 1 if the shaded portion represents 4.5 hours of time and the patient is dosed every 6 hours, then the T>MIC is equal to 4.5hours/6hours = 75%. Again, the units cancel and the result is reported as a fraction or a percentage of the dosing interval. Finally, the AUC/MIC is defined by the total area under the concentration curve. It is either integrated or more simply calculated by the trapezoidal rule when sufficient data points are present. The trapezoidal rule is simply an extension of basic geometric calculations where:

$$Area\ of\ Trapezoid = \frac{base1 + base2}{2} \times (height)$$

Application to the concentration time profile (Figure 1) is as follows:

$$Area\ under\ the\ curve\ (hour\ 2\ to\ hour\ 4) = \frac{Concentration(A) + Concentration(B)}{2} \times (elapsed\ time\ between\ A\ and\ B)$$

Since the calculation is concentration in a weight per volume (e.g., mg/L) multiplied by time (e.g., hours), the resultant value is expressed in multiplicative fashion (mg/L × hr). Convention is to define these per 24-hour period by summing all of the trapezoids that make up the curve. Thus, AUC_{0-24h} / MIC is generally described as a relative value. It should be noted that as the MIC <1 approaches values closer to zero, the AUC_{0-24h} / MIC becomes infinite. Thus, many of the calculations for AUC_{0-24h}/MIC with low MICs are not true area ratios.

Target Identification

Once calculations are performed as above, each of the metrics (i.e., fC_{max}/MIC, fT>MIC, and fAUC/MIC) are compared to a set of outcomes. PK/PD interactions that are described by T>MIC are considered "time dependent." Drugs that are described by C_{max}/MIC are considered "concentration dependent." Drugs that are best described by AUC/MIC are generally a hybrid of concentration and time dependent activity.

To date, animal work has been considered the pre-clinical standard [32, 33] as strictly mathematic simulation approaches have been unable to completely classify in-vivo activity, though significant progress has been made with in vitro simulation strategies such as the hollow fiber model (HFM) system.[34, 35] Of high importance, pre-clinical animal PK/PD identified metrics have a high level of agreement with human PK/PD outcomes.[21, 22, 24, 36–39] The standard model employed for discernment of PK/PD targets is murine. In murine models, various infections can be studied (including pneumonia, thigh infection, and others).[8] The murine model and HFM both allow investigation of systematic permutations to antibiotic dose and frequency of antibiotic infusion. The HFM model further allows the investigator additional controls, such as modification of infusion scheme, which is possible with animal models but more technically complicated because of faster clearance mechanisms for species with smaller body surface area.[40] Outcomes studied include change in bacterial burden, emergence of bacterial resistance, and (less frequently in today's environment) animal mortality. The latter has been substituted with pre-lethal illness by many investigators.

In the murine model, mice are generally rendered neutropenic in order to get the best assessment of the contribution of the antibiotic to pathogen death; however, even in profound neutropenia models, innate mechanisms of bacterial killing exist in the mouse.[41] This provides a "worst case scenario" for humans. Various doses and infusion schedules are modeled to create a heterogenous dispersion of the PK/PD parameter of interest. That is, doses are allometrically scaled with the goal that the fC_{max}/MIC, $f T>MIC$, and $fAUC/MIC$ are varied from high to low with minimal collinearity. Some level of collinearity is unavoidable, yet the exposure for a single animal can be classified with each PK/PD metric and compared to the desired outcome. In an ideal example, a single dosing scheme will isolate one PK/PD metric. For instance, a dose that allows a high C_{max}/MIC with low T>MIC and AUC/MIC allows one to discern if the outcome for the animal was favorable or not favorable on the basis of high C_{max}/MIC. In Figure 3 below, each animal and their corresponding PK/PD is represented by a single data point in each of the three simulated graphs. The fictitious drug simulated in Figure 3 would be considered time dependent and best explained by %T>MIC where maximal response is seen when %T>MIC exceeds 60%.

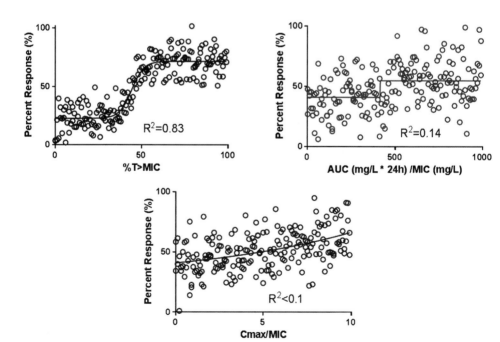

Figure 3 Simulation of Exposure Metrics and Efficacy Response Rates.
Simulation 02/23/16 Using Four Parameter Hill-Type Equations

Antibiotic Susceptibility: What Does It Mean, Where Does It Come From, and How Do We Utilize It

Once PK/PD targets are identified, the next step is to utilize that information to understand whether or not an antibiotic, at a given dose, can be expected to lead to a positive clinical response (i.e., a clinical or microbiological cure). Antibiotic susceptibility, in its purest form, should do just that. If an organism is susceptible to an antibiotic, clinicians should feel confident that they are giving their patient the best likelihood of a cure. On the other hand, if an organism is resistant to a given agent, clinicians should avoid its use if possible. In actuality, however, it is a much more complex scenario with up to three different drivers of susceptibility breakpoints, with various governing bodies in the United States and Europe independently setting different breakpoints (e.g., CLSI vs. EUCAST)[42]. Perhaps even more frustratingly, different agencies within the same country can also have different breakpoints (i.e., FDA vs. CLSI), which can significantly complicate how automated susceptibility testing methodologies (which must be FDA cleared) can report susceptibility.

Ultimately, and ideally, susceptibility breakpoints are driven by clinical data. That is, at a target drug exposure verified by patient level pharmacokinetic data and a verified MIC, a favorable response was seen in patients, and at a higher MIC with the same drug exposure, an unfavorable response was seen. While there are select data that do just this, the application can in some instances be limited by the fact that these data are often in the form of Phase II and III trials as these are often the only well-controlled studies where serum concentrations of antibiotics are available. Unfortunately, these patient populations can be much different than critically ill, immunosuppressed, or otherwise more complicated patients that often have infections with more resistant organisms, and Phase IV trials that can address these questions are often not funded/conducted.

In the absence of robust clinical data, susceptibility breakpoints are derived by a combination of PK/PD modeling, as described above, and epidemiological MIC distributions of a particular organism to the antibiotic of interest. Epidemiological cutoffs separate the MIC distributions of wild type organisms that lack any resistance mechanisms to a given agent from those that possess resistance mechanisms for that same agent, such as a common β-lactamase (e.g. bla_{TEM-1} in *E. coli*). Ideally, pharmacokinetic exposures with commonly used dosing regimens will achieve pharmacodynamic targets for the susceptible isolates and the majority of intermediate isolates. As resistance continues to evolve and as strategies are developed to dose optimize exposures of different antibiotic classes, often the PK/PD breakpoint (i.e., the highest MIC in which PK/PD targets can reliably be expected to be achieved for a given dosing strategy) will split through the distribution of "resistance" as defined from the epidemiological standpoint.

There is much debate about how to handle these increasingly common scenarios, and governing bodies and experts disagree with how to best utilize all of these data, in addition with available clinical data, to best set susceptibility breakpoints. Unfortunately, but not surprisingly, the beliefs about which factor should have the highest importance in determining breakpoints are often driven by the specialty of the expert (e.g., clinical microbiologists will prefer epidemiological cutoffs whereas those intimately involved with developing and determining PK/PD exposures associated with outcomes in models will favor this method). While we believe that the order of importance should ultimately start with clinical data, followed by optimized PK/PD exposure data, and then finally epidemiological breakpoints, it is important to understand that all three viewpoints are valid and all need to be incorporated into breakpoint decisions. While epidemiological cutoff data (i.e., breakpoints that differentiate wild type phenotypes with those possessing resistance mechanisms) are difficult to interpret for the practicing clinician focused on the likelihood of efficacy, it is important for antibiotic stewards to appreciate why microbiologists often prioritize epidemiological breakpoints. Within a susceptible or resistant phenotype there are a range of MICs that are seen. Unfortunately, while there is good categorical reproducibility in MICs, there is poor reproducibility of a given MIC.[43] For most antibiotic:pathogen pairs, the range of MICs seen are ±log base 2. For example, one can envision that an *E. coli* producing a β-lactamase (e.g., a "resistant" phenotype) can have MICs range from 2–8 mcg/mL for a given cephalosporin. In this example, the *E. coli* has a measured cephalosporin MIC of 4 mcg/mL. Also in this example, PK/PD supports that with a common optimized dosing regimen, target exposures can be reached for MICs up to 4 mg/L. The concern from the epidemiological standpoint is that while this scenario suggests that success could be seen with this antibiotic, there really is "no difference" between an MIC of 4 and an 8 mcg/mL from a microbiological standpoint, and therefore there is risk in assuming that the MIC of 4 mcg/mL is correct. However, a very easy solution exists. PK/PD modelers can incorporate the additional variability of MICs into their calculations, or breakpoints can be set one dilution lower (i.e., MIC/2) than the best PK/PD target attainment predictions.

Additionally, from a PK/PD standpoint there is much debate about what the target exposure should be when considering non-clinical and surrogate endpoints. Is net bacterial stasis in animal modeling sufficient? Is a 1-log or 2-log kill preferred? Depending on which of these targets is selected, a different PK/PD breakpoint will be identified. This further underscores the importance of eventually linking surrogate endpoints with hard clinical outcomes. From a clinical standpoint, it is likely that different PK/PD targets are necessary for different infection types, as patients will vary with regards to infection type, severity of illness, bacterial burden, and immune status. For example, a skin infection in an outpatient may only require a static effect while an immunosuppressed ICU patient with ventilator-associated pneumonia may require a 2- or 3-log kill. Ultimately it is a combination of clinical data, PK/PD exposures, and epidemiological cutoffs that dictate breakpoints; but these nuances are important for the antibiotic steward to understand in order to individualize stewardship recommendations based on the clinical scenario.

Determining PK/PD Breakpoints: How It Is Done

Pharmacodynamic targets, as described above, are initially derived from in vitro studies and animal modeling, and as noted above are ideally supported by clinical data. Clinical data to support these targets are more commonly seen with agents coming to market today due to robust pre-clinical in vitro and animal modeling and the increasing requirement of clinical trials to include pharmacokinetic data allowing post hoc PK/PD analyses of outcomes.

In the absence of robust clinical data showing exposures associated with clinical or microbiological cure, clinicians can utilize population pharmacokinetic analyses in order to predict whether or not they are likely to see a positive outcome. Unfortunately, there are rarely robust pharmacokinetic data in target populations to drive these analyses. Clinicians often only have access to small pharmacokinetic dose ranging Phase I studies that show key pharmacokinetic exposures with commonly used dosing regimens. While ideally the data from these dose ranging studies can be utilized to predict how many patients would hit their PK/PD targets (e.g., $fT > MIC$ of ~50%) at a range of doses, this is inappropriate due to the homogeneity of Phase I patients and the known high interpatient variability in more typical patients.[44] Other factors seen in critically ill patients such as highly variable protein binding (more free drug for both distribution and clearance), volume of distribution (due both to acute illness and fluid resuscitation), as well as clearance (either decreased clearance due to acute kidney injury or increased clearance due to augmented renal function due to hypermetabolic states), all make population estimates "best guesses" that are frequently not representative of the individual patient.[45]

In order to account for known and unknown variabilities, a mathematical modeling technique called Monte Carlo simulations can be employed. Simply put, Monte Carlo simulations are a statistical technique where pharmacokinetic data from a smaller sample of patients are utilized to simulate a larger population of patients (e.g., 10,000 patients).[45] This can be completed parametrically by using mean and standard deviation data (and thus the interpatient variability) from the small analysis to randomly simulate a large number of patient variables according to the underlying statistical distribution or it can be completed semi-parametrically with non-normal distributions of the covariates. Once these simulations are complete, concentration versus time exposures can be created for simulated patients in order to assess the likelihood the PK/PD target of interest is achieved with a given dosing regimen/strategy. For example, let us assume that our Monte Carlo simulation is trying to assess the likelihood of reaching the target $fAUC/MIC_{(0-24)}$ exposure of ciprofloxacin of ~75 with differing dosage regimens (Figure 4). The first simulated patient with dosing strategy 2 in the simulation achieves a total $AUC_{(0-24)}$ exposure of 40 mg×h/L. When taking into account the ~30% protein binding of the drug, this leaves a fAUC of 28 mg × h/L. This value is then divided by increasing MICs, showing that the highest MIC that will allow us to hit our target of 75 is a value of 0.25 mg/L (28/0.25 = 112; 28/0.5 = 56). This same process is then repeated for the rest of the 5,000 simulated patients. Once complete, data will have been generated showing the likelihood of hitting the target

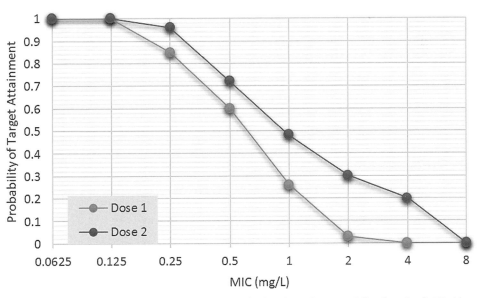

Figure 4 Simulated Probability of Target Attainment, i.e., $fAUC/MIC_{(0-24)}$ Exposure of Ciprofloxacin of ~75 with Differing Dosage Regimens

exposure (fAUC/MIC of 75) at increasing MIC distributions. The percentage of patients who hit the target at various MICs is then calculated; this is called the probability of target attainment or PTA. For example, if 4,800 of the simulated patients in this example hit the target exposure at an MIC of 0.25 mg/L, this gives us a PTA of 96% (4,800/5,000 × 100), whereas at an MIC of 0.5 mg/L only 3,600 patients hit the target for a PTA of 72% (Figure 4 dose 2). The PTA that is considered "acceptable" as a cutoff is 90%,[19] and therefore in this example (as is true in actuality for ciprofloxacin) the PK/PD breakpoint where we can expect to have ≥90% PTA with our dosing strategy 2 is at an MIC of 0.25 mg/L. As you can see in the example, dosing regimen 1 does not hit a PTA of 90% at that MIC, and therefore the PK/PD breakpoint with that dosing regimen would be at an MIC of 0.125 mg/L. It is important to note that the 90% cutoff, while generally accepted, is arbitrary, and there might be a clinical scenario where there is no alternative therapy and you cannot safely increase the dose. In that circumstance, a 72% chance of a successful outcome is your best option. We occasionally encounter these scenarios in clinical practice and would recommend combination therapy in this setting.

Another term that stewards will find in the literature surrounding Monte Carlo simulations and PTA is cumulative fraction of response or CFR. Simply put, CFR takes the above methodology for determining susceptibility and incorporates MIC distributions of a particular pathogen or pathogens to describe how a particular agent (often at different dosing regimens) performs against a clinical sample of isolates. These data will ultimately tell you the percentage of time that PK/PD targets will be reached with an agent against this clinically relevant sample of organisms to help support empiric or definitive therapy in this clinical scenario with an agent. This can be a very useful strategy if resources are available at your own institution to understand, for example, which anti-pseudomonal β-lactam will best achieve PK/PD target exposures against all Gram-negative bacilli causing pneumonia in the ICUs in order to optimize empiric therapy.

Stewardship Applications: Applying PK/PD Understanding to Optimize Patient Exposures and Outcomes

Table 1 displays which PK/PD indices are associated with efficacy for different antibiotic classes.[19, 36, 45] Depending on what the ideal PK/PD target is, there are different strategies to optimize exposure in patients while minimizing the chance of toxicity with those agents. This section gives three well-described opportunities for stewards to optimize

Table 1 Target PK/PD indices for commonly used antibacterials

Time Dependent (T>MIC)	Concentration Dependent (C_{max}/MIC)	Concentration and Time dependent (AUC/MIC)
Penicillins	Aminoglycosides	Aminoglycosides
Cephalosporins	Fluoroquinolones	Vancomycin
Carbapenems		Fluoroquinolones
Aztreonam		Daptomycin
Linezolid		Polymyxins
		Tigecycline
		Linezolid
		Tetracyclines
		Macrolides

these exposures and describes a blueprint for utilizing the same principles for lesser-understood antibiotic scenarios that will come up in practice.

β-lactams

β-lactam antibiotics are the representative class of antibiotics with time dependent activity. In other words, at a certain exposure, which is generally considered to be 4× the MIC, further increasing the concentration does not increase the bactericidal activity of these agents;[36] however, it does increase the likelihood that these agents will be at toxic levels. The PK/PD parameter associated with in vitro activity as well as clinical cure in both animal models and clinical analyses is fT>MIC. The actual fT>MIC target can slightly differ based on agent, organism of interest, and degree of killing desired; however, the generally accepted targets for the pencillins are a fT>MIC of 50%, for the cephalosporins are fT>MIC of 60–70%, and for the carbapenems are a fT>MIC of ~35–40%. The fT>MIC goals are more poorly defined for aztreonam but exposures of fT>MIC of 50–60% are commonly targeted. It is also important to reiterate, that as previously described, breakpoints take into account more than just PK/PD targets and therefore the exposures desired by a clinician and those that go into breakpoint setting might differ.

Since these agents display time dependent activity, dosing strategies for these antibiotics need to target optimizing the duration rather than the magnitude of the exposure. A key variable in this equation is that β-lactams in general (but with notable exceptions like ceftriaxone and ertapenem) have very short half-lives, often ranging from 1 to 2 hours. Because of this, bolus-dosing regimens that consist of high doses given infrequently are suboptimal. Boluses and short infusions result in higher peak levels (which do not enhance the efficacy and could potentially increase the toxicity) followed by rapid decreases (due to the short half-life) that can leave the serum concentration below the MIC for a significant amount of the dosing interval.

There are several strategies to optimize β-lactam exposures. The first, and simplest is to give the same daily dose but divide it more frequently. Due to the smaller amount of time between doses there is less time for the concentration to drop below the MIC and therefore, the fT>MIC is greater. An application of this concept has also been utilized in the past as a cost-savings approach. One notable example of this was with meropenem. Standard dosing of meropenem was 1,000 mg every 8 hours; however, PK/PD data showed similar PTA with regimens of 500 mg every 6 hours. Therefore institutions were able to decrease acquisition costs by ~33% but still able to "hit PK/PD targets."[46] While this is true, we would caution the practitioner against these types of practices. As described above, PK/PD targets are often derived in healthy volunteers and therefore as meropenem is not routinely used in healthy volunteers there is concern that this smaller daily dose, when combined with altered pharmacokinetic parameters might lead to suboptimal exposures, particularly at higher MIC values. Therefore, while dividing the drug out more frequently still makes sense, we would recommend still utilizing the same daily dose. This ensures optimal PK principles are being utilized but minimizes the chance for suboptimal exposures that could lead to failure or resistance development. It is important that clinicians utilize PK/PD to optimize maximal exposures rather than as a cost-savings initiative, given the delicate balance between drug exposure, response, and resistance development.

In addition to smaller, more frequent doses, there are infusion strategies that can further optimize exposures of β-lactams. Ideally, all β-lactams would be given as a continuous infusion. That is, a bolus dose would be given to get the concentration above the target MIC (or susceptible MIC range), and then a maintenance infusion would be given at the same rate of elimination of the drug from the body, to keep a consistent concentration and have a $fT>MIC$ of 100%. While this is ideal from a pharmacokinetic standpoint, it is not practical for important members of the provider team, most notably the nursing staff who might need to access the line for other reasons (e.g., giving other medications) as well as the patient who will now be inconvenienced by being tethered to an intravenous pump around the clock. For these reasons, we recommend limiting continuous infusions to critically ill patients with multiple vascular access points or patients infected by organisms with elevated MICs where PK/PD targets can only be met via a continuous infusion.

Because of the limitations described with continuous infusion, the "happy medium" for optimal β-lactam exposure that is clinically achievable is administration of these agents via an extended infusion (each dose usually over 3–4 hours) rather than as a standard bolus administration (usually 30 minutes) (Figure 5). The reason this serves as a "happy medium" is because it minimizes the concerns above for the patient and the nursing staff, while still limiting the amount of time in between doses for concentrations to rapidly drop, given the short half-lives of the β-lactams. In a seminal publication on this topic, Lodise and colleagues showed that if targeting a $fT>MIC$ of 50% for piperacillin, a smaller daily dose (3.375 g of piperacillin/tazobactam every 8 hours) given as a 4-hour infusion was able to have a PTA of 100% for piperacillin MICs of ≤16 mg/L, whereas higher doses of 3.375 every 4–6 hours as a standard infusion (30 minute bolus) only achieved a PTA $\geq$ 90% for MIC's of 4mg/L or less (the current MIC breakpoint is 16 mg/L).[47]

Similar to the story with meropenem, these findings have led many to utilize extended infusion of β-lactams as a cost savings measure (3 times a day instead of 4–6 times a day can decrease daily expenditures). However, much like in the above example, we would highlight that these strategies should ultimately be used to increase or improve exposures of these agents and hopefully clinical outcomes rather than to get similar exposures with less drug. In the study by Lodise and colleagues, the authors demonstrated the extended-infusion dosing approach translated into clinical benefit. Critically ill patients (defined as those with APACHE II scores ≥17) who received extended infusion piperacillin/tazobactam had lower 30-day mortality rates than patients who received standard infusions (12.2% vs. 31.6%, respectively; $p = 0.04$).

Importantly, in this study the MIC distributions of the *Pseudomonas* isolates were not described and no patients received higher daily doses via extended infusion (common dosing strategies for piperacillin/tazobactam are up to 18 g/day). Whether higher dosing

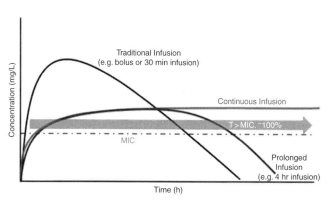

Figure 5 Concentration Time Profiles of Various Infusion Schemes

could achieve better results or whether a population with higher, but susceptible MICs, would respond the same way to 3.375 grams every 8 hours as an extended infusion is unclear. Despite that caveat, as the β-lactams have a wide therapeutic index, these dosing strategies have the opportunity to both improve outcomes, allow PK/PD targets to be hit at higher MICs, and hopefully, with higher doses, minimize the development of resistance. For all of the above reasons, while we are strong proponents of extended infusions of β-lactams, most notably the anti-pseudomonal agents given their propensity to be prescribed in sicker patients and to be targeting less susceptible isolates, we would recommend maximal doses as extended infusions in order to truly optimize the exposures in a given patient for the reasons described in this section.

One final practical consideration for implementation and utilization of extended infusions of β-lactams is handling patients with renal insufficiency. It is likely that in this population, due to extended half-lives from decreased elimination, that the impact of extended infusions is marginalized. Therefore, the question arises of whether or not to limit extended infusions to those with "normal" renal function. While this is logical, and might make sense at a given institution, we have chosen not to omit extended infusions in renal insufficiency at our institutions. The concern is that it can cause confusion among practitioners regarding when to give these agents as standard or prolonged infusions. As education required with alternate infusion schemes is substantial, we felt it easier to not complicate the matter by trying to instruct practitioners to treat renally insufficient patients differently. However, these decisions are institution specific.

Aminoglycosides

Aminoglycosides, most notably gentamicin, tobramycin, and amikacin, remain important antibiotics in the armamentarium, whether it is for synergy in serious, life threatening Gram-positive infections (i.e., gentamicin) or empiric, and sometimes definitive therapy for troublesome multidrug resistant Gram-negative organisms (i.e., tobramycin and amikacin). Aminoglycosides remain one of the most well-described antibiotic classes from a PK/PD standpoint, with a good correlation seen between both AUC/MIC and C_{max}/MIC exposures and activity.[36] Clinically, there are data to support C_{max}/MIC targets, and given the ease by which peak concentrations can be measured in clinical practice, C_{max}/MIC remains the preferred target for these agents. In a key publication, Moore and colleagues looked at the impact of C_{max}/MIC ratio on clinical response in patients with Gram-negative infections. Response rate gradually increased from 55% in patients with C_{max}/MIC ratios of 2:1 to a maximal impact of 83–92% when the ratios were 8–12:1.[48] These data served as the basis for recommending peak/MIC ratios of ~10:1 for Gram-negative infections. These data, while encouraging, led to issues with traditional dosing strategies of aminoglycosides. While these doses of 1–2 mg/kg every 8 hours can hit this target when the MICs are low (0.5–1 mg/mL) they fail to reach peak targets when the MICs reach the upper end of the susceptibility breakpoint (2 mg/L) commonly seen in multidrug resistant pathogens requiring aminoglycosides. Therefore, alternative dosing strategies were investigated and led to the development of high-dose extended interval dosing of the aminoglycosides. In this strategy, patients receive a higher, one-time dose of the target aminoglycoside (for example 5–7 mg/kg × 1 of tobramycin) to achieve a C_{max} in the range of 20 mg/L. The mg/kg dose can be modified based on expected volume of distribution of the patient as initial concentration (mg/L) = Dose (mg/kg)/Volume of Distribution (L/kg). If targeting a C_{max} of 20 mg/L (to have a 10:1 ratio for an organism with an MIC of 2 mg/L), the mg/kg dose would simply be reflective of the expected volume of distribution. For example, if this is a critically ill patient with fluid overload, one might assume a higher volume of distribution of tobramycin of 0.35 L/kg. Therefore, you would want to give 7 mg/kg for a C_{max} of ~20 mg/L (7/0.35 = 20). The dosing interval with this method is dependent on clearance rate and can range from every 24 to 72 hours. Multiple nomograms are available to help guide interval selection, or two concentrations can be drawn and patient specific kinetics can be determined. In our experience, critically ill and even some stable patients have volumes of distribution that can vary significantly therefore patient specific kinetics are ideal and can be easily calculated by obtainment of a 2- and 12-hour level. However, as is often the case clinically, tobramycin (or amikacin) is often being given empirically to cover for potential resistant pathogens and therefore, by the time a second dose is due, the patient may be unlikely to continue therapy. Therefore, clinicians may hold off on obtaining levels until continuation is confirmed. If continuation occurs, two levels are then obtained and an individualized regimen is developed.

In addition to allowing clinicians to optimize peak exposures, extended interval dosing also takes advantage of two additional features of this class of antibiotics. First, the aminoglycosides display time dependent toxicity as well. Binding and subsequent uptake into renal cells and cochlear and vestibular membranes is generally saturable; that is continually increasing peak concentrations do not linearly increase the amount of toxicity. Furthermore, if patients can have an aminoglycoside free interval, the damaged cells can often regenerate, mitigating the damage.[49] Therefore, in addition to high peaks, clinicians should target drug free intervals. The concern for failure or resistance development is lessened because despite these sub-MIC exposures occuring near the end of the dosing interval, the aminoglycosides, like other concentration-dependent antibiotics, exhibit a post-antibiotic effect. Nicalou and colleagues proved this concept by showing lower rates of nephrotoxicity with the implementation of extended interval dosing when compared to traditional dosing strategies.[50]

Importantly, however, not all patients require high exposures and traditional dosing still serves a role for urinary tract infections (where high degrees of urinary elimination lead to concentrations of aminoglycosides in the urine of >100 mg/L,[51] even with minimal serum peak concentrations [3–5 mg/L]). Although definitive data are lacking, it appears traditional dosing is also an appropriate dosing strategy when the aminoglycosides (namely gentamicin) are being used for Gram-positive synergy in combination with a β-lactam.

Vancomycin

Vancomycin, like most antibiotics, is a hybrid of concentration and time dependent killing where the PK/PD index that is best associated with activity is AUC/MIC.[36, 45] In this setting, total daily drug exposure relative to the MIC is the driver of efficacy with the antibiotic, and the same total daily dose, regardless of how it is divided, would be expected to have the same impact on therapy.

Vancomycin has an interesting history that contributes to the confusion surrounding optimal dosing, which still today, remains a significant challenge for clinicians. Vancomycin was originally introduced over 50 years ago prior to the modern drug development process. Originally produced with many impurities, vancomycin was associated with high rates of acute kidney injury and thus was minimally utilized as β-lactams retained good activity against clinically relevant Gram-positive organisms. With the introduction and subsequent explosion of methicillin-resistant *Staphylococcus aureus*, and to a lesser degree penicillin-resistant *Streptococcus pneumoniae*, vancomycin's role as an anti-infective became paramount. Thankfully, at this time the impurities in the manufacturing process had been improved and vancomycin, unless given with another nephrotoxic agent like the aminoglycosides,[52] was rarely associated with acute kidney injury. However, optimal dosing was unknown, and while therapeutic drug monitoring of standard doses of 1 gram every 12 hours occurred, there was poor standardization of this practice and minimal if any literature to support the practices. Interestingly, the initial push for higher trough targets of 15–20 mg/L were actually guideline driven recommendations for bacterial meningitis [53] and nosocomial pneumonia.[54] These recommendations were based on data showing poor penetration into lung tissue and cerebral spinal fluid and the desire to hit fT>MIC targets at the site of infection, as the thought at the time was that vancomycin was best described as a time dependent antibiotic.

In 2004, clinical data began to emerge suggesting that AUC/MIC was the PK/PD exposure of interest. In the first such analysis, Moise-Broder and colleagues showed that in a population of 90 patients with MRSA pneumonia that patients with AUC/MIC exposures ≥400 had higher rates of clinical and microbiological cure compared with those who did not achieve this target.[55] In the same analysis the authors also showed a lack of association between T>MIC and either outcome. When these data were taken with emerging evidence that suggested vancomycin failures were more likely when vancomycin MICs were >1 mg/mL, vancomycin consensus guidelines were developed in 2009 that recommended that for "serious infections" clinicians consider a one-time loading dose followed by maintenance dosing strategies to target a trough value of 15–20 mg/L as a surrogate marker of an AUC/MIC of ≥400 for MIC values of ≤1 mg/L. Additionally, increased failures were thought to be due to limitations with vancomycin's ability to target this AUC/MIC ratio when the MIC was >1 mg/L.[56] Since the publication of these guidelines, further evidence has supported AUC/MIC ratios as being predictors of positive outcomes, including mortality in MRSA bacteremia ± infective endocarditis. The exact AUC/MIC target in these studies has ranged from 211 to 650,[57–61] and interpretation of the true target is further complicated by the fact that investigations have utilized different techniques for estimating AUC exposures as well as for determining the vancomycin MIC. Both of these measures are known to vary as a function of the testing mechanism making the best target unclear, but a target AUC/MIC ratio of ~400–600 is reasonable for invasive MRSA infections. Additionally, and importantly, recent evidence has suggested that troughs are a poor surrogate for AUC exposures and simply utilizing trough targets of 15–20 mg/L can lead to potential over or under exposure depending on what range of the 400–600 ratio you are targeting.[62] This finding should not be overlooked as a recent meta-analysis has shown that trough values >15mg/L increase the risk of acute kidney injury 3.1 fold over trough values <15 mg/L [63] and while the exact AUC exposure associated with acute kidney injury is poorly described to date, select evidence suggests that there is not an increased risk at the AUC targets suggested above.[64]

Based on these findings we recommend that where it is feasible, stewards should make every attempt to move away from trough only targets for vancomycin and to targeting AUC exposures of ~400–600 mg*h/L. When possible, trough targets to reach this AUC should be kept between 10 and 15 mg/L to minimize excessive troughs and the risk for acute kidney injury. Although there are dosing strategies that would allow reaching this AUC target with even lower troughs, given that select data suggests that trough values <10 mg/L can increase the development of resistance [56] we would recommend keeping troughs between 10–15 mg/L. At one of our institutions where vancomycin AUCs are routinely targeted, AUCs in the ~500 mg × h/L range have usually been achieved with trough values in the 12–13 mg/L range.

There are important practical considerations to these advancements in vancomycin dosing that the clinician must consider. First off, depending on resources at an institution, obtaining multiple vancomycin concentrations to calculate AUCs might not be feasible. Encouragingly however, Bayesian estimation of AUC can be completed with few levels, and these programs are becoming increasingly available to the clinician. A few examples of these programs available at the time of writing of this chapter can be found at www.lapk.org, www.pkpdcompass.com, and www.tdmx.eu.

An additional consideration is that these targets have been identified clinically for the treatment of invasive infections. It is reasonable to conclude, based on clinical trial data that show high success rates, that a more simplistic and less aggressive dosing of vancomycin of 1,000 mg (or 15 mg/kg) every 12 hours with renal dosing adjustments is sufficient for the treatment of skin and soft tissue infections. Furthermore, the clinician is encouraged to remember that these targets (AUC/MIC ~ 400–600) for vancomycin are with MRSA. They cannot be extrapolated to coagulase negative staphylococci or enterococcus spp. where MIC distributions are routinely higher and an AUC/MIC ratio of 400–600 will not be routinely hit. It is our recommendation that until more information is available for those organisms, or that data suggest that AUCs of 400–600 are associated with higher rates of toxicity, that these same values are targeted for invasive infections due to these other pathogens and be considered a "maximal tolerable dose." Finally, given significant penetration issues and a lack of data to support any recommendation it is reasonable for clinicians to continue to target troughs of 15–20 mg/L for the treatment of meningitis.

PK/PD Stewardship Opportunities for Other Antibiotics

While the agents discussed so far offer common opportunities for all stewards to optimize outcomes by optimizing the exposure of those agents, the same opportunities exist for all antibiotics. When stewards are given a scenario where they are employing an agent they are less familiar with for treatment of a target pathogen due to resistance or intolerance, they should follow the same process for determining how (and if) they can optimize the agent. While the susceptibility breakpoint is a starting point, as described in this chapter, it is important to remember that many factors go into the breakpoint, and that information alone might not answer the question of whether or not a positive outcome can be expected. The first place the clinician should look in this scenario is to identify if there are clinical, patient level data that suggest a given PK/PD exposure is associated with favorable clinical outcomes. If these exist, the next step is to determine if exposures that can be expected with the doses that are tolerable for a patient will hit these targets at the MIC of the infecting organism. Patient specific pharmacokinetic assays of the drug of interest are ideal. In the absence of this, Monte Carlo simulations and PTA will drive this decision (due to taking into account the large degree of interpatient variability); however, if those data are not available, mean exposures in healthy volunteers can be used as a rough guide from an exposure standpoint. In the absence of clinical data, which will often be the case, animal data supporting exposure/effect should be the next choice. While there is much debate over what the target should be (bacteriostasis, 1 log kill, 2 log kill, etc), the clinical scenario should help dictate that decision. In an uncomplicated infection in a patient with an intact immune system, bacteriostasis might be sufficient. For most patients, a 1-log kill (90% reduction bacterial burden) is a reasonable target. However, for some patients, most notably critically ill or immunosuppressed patients, further killing might be warranted and in general the maximal tolerable dose (and optimal administration method) should be employed. If there is concern that such targets cannot be met, the clinician is encouraged to consider combination therapy. Additionally, clinical response, or lack thereof should help dictate further steps.

Conclusion

Antibiotic stewards have a unique opportunity to take the principles discussed in this chapter and make interventions both on the healthcare system–wide level (such as extended infusions) as well as for optimizing exposures in individual patients treated with MDR or XDR pathogens. It is extremely important that they understand the underpinnings and complexity of applying pharmacokinetics and pharmacodynamic principles to optimize patient outcomes and minimize antibiotic toxicity.

References

1. Winter ME. *Basic Clinical Pharmacokinetics*. 5th ed. Philadelphia: Lippincott, Williams, and Wilkins, 2010.

2. Shargel L, Wu-Pong S, Yu A. *Applied Biopharmaceutics and Pharmacokinetics*. 6th ed. New York: McGraw Hill, 2012.

3. Jelliffe RW, Schumitzky A, Van Guilder M, et al. Individualizing drug dosage regimens: roles of population pharmacokinetic and dynamic models, Bayesian fitting, and adaptive control. *Ther Drug Monit* 1993; 15 (5):380–393.

4. Bonate P. Pharmacokinetic-Pharmacodynamic Modeling and Simulation. 2nd ed. Springer, 2011.

5. Pfizer. VFEND® IV (voriconazole) for injection, VFEND® tablets, VFEND® for oral suspension. (Accessed February 18, 2016, at www.accessdata.fda.gov/drugsatfda_docs/label/2010/021266s0321bl.pdf.)

6. Cederbaum AI. Alcohol Metabolism. *Clinics in Liver Disease* 2012; 16 (4):667–685.

7. National Institute on Alcohol Abuse and Alcoholism. Alcohol alert: alcohol metabolism. No. 35, PH 371. Bethesda, MD: 1997. (Accessed February 18, 2016, at http://pubs.niaaa.nih.gov/publications/aa35.htm.)

8. Craig WA. Pharmacokinetic/pharmacodynamic parameters: rationale for antibacterial dosing of mice and men. *Clin Infect Dis* 1998; 26(1):1–10; quiz 1–2.

9. Scheetz MH, Hurt KM, Noskin GA, Oliphant CM. Applying antibiotic pharmacodynamics to resistant gram-negative pathogens. *Am J Health Syst Pharm* 2006; 63(14): 1346–1360.

10. Clinical and Laboratory Standards Institute. *Methods for dilution antibiotic susceptibility tests for bacteria that grow aerobically; approved standard*. 10th ed. CLSI document M07-A10. Wayne, PA: Clinical and Laboratory Standards Institute, 2015.

11. Finberg RW, Moellering RC, Tally FP, et al. The importance of bactericidal drugs: future directions in infectious disease. *Clin Infect Dis* 2004; 39(9): 1314–1320.

12. National Committee for Clinical Laboratory Standards. Methods for determining bactericidal activity of antibiotic agents. Approved Guideline M26-A. NCCLS, Wayne, PA, 1999.

13. Goutelle S, Maurin M, Rougier F, et al. The Hill equation: a review of its capabilities in pharmacological modelling. *Fundam Clin Pharmacol* 2008; 22(6):633–648.

14. Rex JH, Pfaller MA. Has antifungal susceptibility testing come of age? *Clin Infect Dis* 2002; 35(**8**): 982–989.

15. Spellberg B, Talbot GH, Boucher HW, et al. Antibiotic agents for complicated skin and skin-structure infections: justification of noninferiority margins in the absence of placebo-controlled trials. *Clin Infect Dis* 2009; 49(**3**):383–391.

16. Spellberg B, Talbot GH, Brass EP, et al. Position paper: recommended design features of future clinical trials of antibacterial agents for community-acquired pneumonia. *Clin Infect Dis* 2008; 47(Suppl 3):S249–265.

17. Lamoth F, Buclin T, Pascual A, et al. High cefepime plasma concentrations and neurological toxicity in febrile neutropenic patients with mild impairment of renal function. *Antimicrob Agents Chemother* 2010; 54(**10**):4360–4367.

18. Rhodes NJ, Kuti JL, Nicolau DP, Neely MN, Nicasio AM, Scheetz MH. An exploratory analysis of the ability of a cefepime trough concentration greater than 22 mg/L to predict neurotoxicity. *J Infect Chemother* 2016; 22(**2**):78–83.

19. Dudley MN, Ambrose PG, Bhavnani SM, et al. Background and rationale for revised clinical and laboratory standards institute interpretive criteria (breakpoints) for Enterobacteriaceae and Pseudomonas aeruginosa: I. Cephalosporins and Aztreonam. *Clin Infect Dis* 2013; 56 (**9**):1301–1309.

20. Crandon JL, Nicolau DP. In vivo activities of simulated human doses of cefepime and cefepime-AAI101 against multidrug-resistant Gram-negative Enterobacteriaceae. *Antimicrob Agents Chemother* 2015; 59(**5**):2688–2694.

21. Crandon JL, Bulik CC, Kuti JL, Nicolau DP. Clinical pharmacodynamics of cefepime in patients infected with Pseudomonas aeruginosa. *Antimicrob Agents Chemother* 2010; 54(**3**):1111–1116.

22. Rhodes NJ, Kuti JL, Nicolau DP, et al. Defining clinical exposures of cefepime for Gram negative bloodstream infections that are associated with improved survival.

Antimicrob Agents Chemother 2015 60 (3):1401–1410.

23. Kim A, Kuti JL, Nicolau DP. Probability of pharmacodynamic target attainment with standard and prolonged-infusion antibiotic regimens for empiric therapy in adults with hospital-acquired pneumonia. *Clin Ther* 2009; 31(**11**):2765–2778.

24. MacVane SH, Kuti JL, Nicolau DP. Clinical pharmacodynamics of antipseudomonal cephalosporins in patients with ventilator-associated pneumonia. *Antimicrob Agents Chemother* 2014; 58(**3**):1359–1364.

25. Bauer KA, West JE, O'Brien JM, Goff DA. Extended-infusion cefepime reduces mortality in patients with Pseudomonas aeruginosa infections. *Antimicrob Agents Chemother* 2013; 57(**7**):2907–2912.

26. Nicasio AM, Ariano RE, Zelenitsky SA, et al. Population pharmacokinetics of high-dose, prolonged-infusion cefepime in adult critically ill patients with ventilator-associated pneumonia. *Antimicrob Agents Chemother* 2009; 53(**4**):1476–1481.

27. Nichols KR, Karmire LC, Cox EG, Kays MB, Knoderer CA. Implementing extended-infusion cefepime as standard of care in a children's hospital: a prospective descriptive study. *Ann Pharmacother* 2015; 49(**4**):419–426.

28. Cheatham SC, Shea KM, Healy DP, et al. Steady-state pharmacokinetics and pharmacodynamics of cefepime administered by prolonged infusion in hospitalised patients. *Int J Antimicrob Agents* 2011; 37(**1**):46–50.

29. Schmidt S, Rock K, Sahre M, et al. Effect of protein binding on the pharmacological activity of highly bound antibiotics. *Antimicrob Agents Chemother* 2008; 52 (**11**):3994–4000.

30. Heuberger J, Schmidt S, Derendorf H. When is protein binding important? *J Pharm Sci* 2013; 102(**9**):3458–3467.

31. Mouton JW, Dudley MN, Cars O, Derendorf H, Drusano GL. Standardization of pharmacokinetic/pharmacodynamic (PK/PD) terminology for anti-infective drugs: an update. *J Antimicrob Chemother* 2005; 55(**5**):601–607.

32. US Department of Health and Human Services. Food and Drug Administration, Center for Drug Evaluation and Research, and Center for Biologics Evaluation and Research. Product development under the animal rule guidance for industry. 2015.

33. US Department of Health and Human Services. Food and Drug Administration, Center for Drug Evaluation and Research, and Center for Biologics Evaluation and Research. Guidance for Industry S6 Preclinical Safety Evaluation of Biotechnology-Derived Pharmaceuticals. 1997.

34. Velkov T, Bergen PJ, Lora-Tamayo J, Landersdorfer CB, Li J. PK/PD models in antibacterial development. *Curr Opin Microbiol* 2013; 16(5):573–579.

35. Bulitta JB, Landersdorfer CB, Forrest A, et al. Relevance of pharmacokinetic and pharmacodynamic modeling to clinical care of critically ill patients. *Curr Pharm Biotechnol* 2011; 12(12):2044–2061.

36. Ambrose PG, Bhavnani SM, Rubino CM, et al. Pharmacokinetics-pharmacodynamics of antibiotic therapy: it's not just for mice anymore. *Clin Infect Dis* 2007; 44(1):79–86.

37. D'Agostino C, Rhodes NJ, Skoglund E, Roberts JA, Scheetz MH. Microbiologic clearance following transition from standard infusion piperacillin-tazobactam to extended-infusion for persistent Gram-negative bacteremia and possible endocarditis: a case report and review of the literature. *J Infect Chemother* 2015; 21(10):742–746.

38. Defife R, Scheetz MH, Feinglass JM, Postelnick MJ, Scarsi KK. Effect of differences in MIC values on clinical outcomes in patients with bloodstream infections caused by gram-negative organisms treated with levofloxacin. *Antimicrob Agents Chemother* 2009; 53(3):1074–1079.

39. Esterly JS, Wagner J, McLaughlin MM, Postelnick MJ, Qi C, Scheetz MH. Evaluation of clinical outcomes in patients with bloodstream infections due to Gram-negative bacteria according to carbapenem MIC stratification.

Antimicrob Agents Chemother 2012; 56(9):4885–4890.

40. US Department of Health and Human Services and Center for Drug Evaluation and Research. Guidance for Industry. Estimating the maximum safe starting dose in initial clinical trials for therapeutics in adult healthy volunteers. 2005.

41. Guo B, Abdelraouf K, Ledesma KR, Chang KT, Nikolaou M, Tam VH. Quantitative impact of neutrophils on bacterial clearance in a murine pneumonia model. *Antimicrob Agents Chemother* 2011; 55(10):4601–4605.

42. Labreche MJ, Graber CJ, Nguyen HM. Recent updates on the role of pharmacokinetics-pharmacodynamics in antibiotic susceptibility testing as applied to clinical practice. *Clin Infect Dis* 2015; 61(9):1446–1452.

43. Turnidge J, Paterson DL. Setting and revising antibacterial susceptibility breakpoints. *Clin Microbiol Rev* 2007; 20(3):391–408, Table of Contents.

44. Bradley JS, Garonzik SM, Forrest A, Bhavnani SM. Pharmacokinetics, pharmacodynamics, and Monte Carlo simulation: selecting the best antibiotic dose to treat an infection. *Pediatr Infect Dis J* 2010; 29(11):1043–1046.

45. Roberts JA, Abdul-Aziz MH, Lipman J, et al. Individualised antibiotic dosing for patients who are critically ill: challenges and potential solutions. *Lancet Infect Dis* 2014; 14(6):498–509.

46. Perrott J, Mabasa VH, Ensom MH. Comparing outcomes of meropenem administration strategies based on pharmacokinetic and pharmacodynamic principles: a qualitative systematic review. *Ann Pharmacother* 2010; 44(3):557–564.

47. Lodise TP, Jr., Lomaestro B, Drusano GL. Piperacillin-tazobactam for Pseudomonas aeruginosa infection: clinical implications of an extended-infusion dosing strategy. *Clin Infect Dis* 2007; 44(3):357–363.

48. Moore RD, Lietman PS, Smith CR. Clinical response to aminoglycoside therapy: importance of the ratio of peak concentration to minimal inhibitory

concentration. *J Infect Dis* 1987; 155 (1):93–99.

49. Craig WA. Once-daily versus multiple-daily dosing of aminoglycosides. *J Chemother* 1995; 7(Suppl 2):47–52.

50. Nicolau DP, Freeman CD, Belliveau PP, Nightingale CH, Ross JW, Quintiliani R. Experience with a once-daily aminoglycoside program administered to 2,184 adult patients. *Antimicrob Agents Chemother* 1995; 39(3):650–655.

51. Wood MJ, Farrell W. Comparison of urinary excretion of tobramycin and gentamicin in adults. *J Infect Dis* 1976; 134:S133–136.

52. Rybak MJ, Abate BJ, Kang SL, Ruffing MJ, Lerner SA, Drusano GL. Prospective evaluation of the effect of an aminoglycoside dosing regimen on rates of observed nephrotoxicity and ototoxicity. *Antimicrob Agents Chemother* 1999; 43 (7):1549–1555.

53. Tunkel AR, Hartman BJ, Kaplan SL, et al. Practice guidelines for the management of bacterial meningitis. *Clin Infect Dis* 2004; 39(9):1267–1284.

54. American Thoracic S, Infectious Diseases Society of A. Guidelines for the management of adults with hospital-acquired, ventilator-associated, and healthcare-associated pneumonia. *Am J Respir Crit Care Med* 2005; 171 (4):388–416.

55. Moise-Broder PA, Forrest A, Birmingham MC, Schentag JJ. Pharmacodynamics of vancomycin and other antibiotics in patients with *Staphylococcus aureus* lower respiratory tract infections. *Clin Pharmacokinet* 2004; 43(13):925–942.

56. Rybak M, Lomaestro B, Rotschafer JC, et al. Therapeutic monitoring of vancomycin in adult patients: a consensus review of the American Society of Health-System Pharmacists, the Infectious Diseases Society of America, and the Society of Infectious Diseases Pharmacists. *Am J Health Syst Pharm* 2009; 66(1):82–98.

57. Lodise TP, Drusano GL, Zasowski E, et al. Vancomycin exposure in patients with methicillin-resistant *Staphylococcus aureus* bloodstream infections: how much is enough? *Clin Infect Dis* 2014; 59(5):666–675.

58. Jung Y, Song KH, Cho J, et al. Area under the concentration-time curve to minimum inhibitory concentration ratio as a predictor of vancomycin treatment outcome in methicillin-resistant *Staphylococcus aureus* bacteraemia. *Int J Antimicrob Agents* 2014; 43(2): 179–183.

59. Holmes NE, Turnidge JD, Munckhof WJ, et al. Vancomycin AUC/MIC ratio and 30-day mortality in patients with *Staphylococcus aureus* bacteremia. *Antimicrob Agents Chemother* 2013; 57(4):1654–1663.

60. Brown J, Brown K, Forrest A. Vancomycin AUC24/MIC ratio in patients with complicated bacteremia and infective endocarditis due to methicillin-resistant *Staphylococcus aureus* and its association with attributable mortality during hospitalization. *Antimicrob Agents Chemother* 2012; 56(2):634–638.

61. Kullar R, Davis SL, Levine DP, Rybak MJ. Impact of vancomycin exposure on outcomes in patients with methicillin-resistant *Staphylococcus aureus* bacteremia: support for consensus guidelines suggested targets. *Clin Infect Dis* 2011; 52 (8):975–981.

62. Neely MN, Youn G, Jones B, et al. Are vancomycin trough concentrations adequate for optimal dosing? *Antimicrob Agents Chemother* 2014; 58 (1):309–316.

63. van Hal SJ, Paterson DL, Lodise TP. Systematic review and meta-analysis of vancomycin-induced nephrotoxicity associated with dosing schedules that maintain troughs between 15 and 20 milligrams per liter. *Antimicrob Agents Chemother* 2013; 57(2):734–744.

64. Lodise TP, Patel N, Lomaestro BM, Rodvold KA, Drusano GL. Relationship between initial vancomycin concentration-time profile and nephrotoxicity among hospitalized patients. *Clin Infect Dis* 2009; 49(4):507–514.

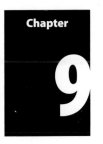

Collaborating with the Microbiology Laboratory

Graeme N. Forrest and Denise Kirsch

The clinical microbiology laboratory plays a vital role in any antibiotic stewardship program (ASP) and are strongly recommended in the Infectious Disease Society of America Antimicrobial Stewardship Implementation guidelines.[1, 2] The communication between microbiology laboratories and ASPs are necessary to ensure timely and accurate reporting of results as well as the implementation of new guidelines and technologies. The laboratory provides many essential services to ASPs including ensuring susceptibility testing and reporting are consistent with Clinical and Laboratory Standards Institute (CLSI) guidelines, selective susceptibility reporting of antibiotics, development of accurate antibiograms, and identification of technologies that may support ASPs. Antibiotic stewards must understand what platforms are being used for susceptibility testing (i.e., Kirby Bauer versus automated systems) and ensure antibiotic susceptibility reporting reflects what is available in the institutional formulary.[1, 3] Communication between the microbiology laboratory and ASPs has become more important with the introduction of new rapid molecular diagnostic technologies.[4] With increasing regulations, complexity of testing and the costs of maintaining microbiology laboratories, many hospitals are now outsourcing these services to either a central laboratory within their system or to a corporation.[3] This has made collaboration more challenging, but it remains critically important for the ASP to work closely with microbiology.

This chapter will review the critical elements of the clinical microbiology laboratory that are necessary for a successful ASP. This includes the following: specimen suitability, selective susceptibility testing and reporting of culture results, antibiogram development, provider and ASP communication, rapid molecular testing from blood cultures and other specimens, and direct molecular methods without culturing.

Specimen Management The microbiology laboratory receives specimens from many wards within healthcare facilities. The impact of processing inadequate or contaminated specimens on patient care is enormous.[5] Poor-quality specimens, inappropriate testing of specimens, and requests for ineffectual "drug-bug" combinations can impact therapeutic decisions and lead to adverse patient outcomes including increased hospital costs and length of stay or serious adverse drug events.[5] The "ten commandments" of specimen processing as recommended in the combined Infectious Disease Society of America (IDSA) and American Society of Microbiology Guidelines on how to utilize the microbiology laboratory to diagnose infectious diseases are just as important for antibiotic stewardship as they are for the microbiology laboratory.[5] They include the following:

a) Rejection of poor-quality specimens: processing saliva, urine with mixed flora, formed stool, and specimens with unsealed containers or inadequate volume have been shown to result in contaminated specimens. This could lead to unnecessary antibiotic therapy or delays in the diagnosis of true infections.

b) Judicious reporting of microorganisms and susceptibility results: over-reporting, for example, yeast in sputum or low quantities of bacteria in urine, can lead to unnecessary therapy. Also, requests for antibiotic susceptibility testing on bacteria which are known to be intrinsically resistant (e.g., tigecycline susceptibility requests on *Pseudomonas aeruginosa*) are an unnecessary use of laboratory resources.[6]

c) Care in reporting results from non-sterile sites: "background noise" from specimens from non-sterile sites (sinuses, sputum, superficial wounds) can yield multiple non-clinically significant organisms.

d) Avoiding processing of swabs: re-education of providers to provide actual fluid, tissue, or aspirate and not swabs for evaluation for microbial growth.

e) Avoiding "test of cure" for certain scenarios. More is not always better. Repeated blood cultures for *Staphylococcus aureus* endocarditis is important; however, daily sputum specimens from a patient on a ventilator are not helpful. Similarly, tests of cure for urinary tract infections or *Clostridium difficile* infection should be discouraged.

f) Specimens should be collected before starting antibiotics. Whenever possible, all cultures should be obtained prior to starting anti-infective therapy to increase organism recovery.

g) Specimens should be labeled accurately. Coagulase-negative staphylococci from a superficial wound is not the same as from a deep prosthetic joint site. Poor labeling means erroneous reporting and potentially unnecessary therapy.

h) Focused susceptibility testing: for commonly recovered organisms, only antibiotics on the hospital formulary should be reported to clinicians.[7] For example, reporting imipenem susceptibility when meropenem is the formulary carbapenem confuses providers and makes the ASP's work more difficult.

i) Develop an algorithm for unexplained or inaccurate results. If a result is contrary to what is normally observed for the organism isolated or its susceptibility profile (e.g., an *E. coli* resistant to cefepime but sensitive to ceftriaxone), a member of the microbiology laboratory should communicate with an infectious diseases specialist prior to reporting results. This is particularly the case if the microbiologist does not have formal clinical infectious diseases training.

j) Compliance with regulations: the ASP should work with the clinical microbiology laboratory to understand necessary regulations the laboratory must abide by.

Antibiograms

A crucial component of an effective ASP is the knowledge of evolving local antibiotic resistance patterns. Cumulative antibiograms which summarize the annual susceptibility rates at local and even regional institutions can be developed. These antibiograms support clinical decision-making and provide valuable information for empirical selection of anti-biotics.[8] As these data are critical to both physicians providing patient care and the ASP, precision and standardization are essential in antibiogram creation.[8]

The CLSI recognizes that antibiograms utilized by clinical laboratories were developed in varied and inconsistent ways which make it difficult to compare susceptibility statistics between institutions and often result in overestimating drug-resistance rates. In response, consensus guidelines (CLSI M39–4A) were developed to provide direction for the construc-tion and use of antibiograms.[7]

Antibiogram Development

It is expected that antibiograms are accurate and current. The guidelines recommend that antibiograms should be published at least annually and include data collected during one calendar year. At least 30 isolates are required to generate antibiograms, as smaller numbers may inaccurately characterize the population. Of note, these isolates should not be collected from surveillance cultures.[7, 8] The first clinical isolate from a patient contributing multiple isolates of the same pathogen is preferred.[7, 8] Using repeat isolates from patients may falsely elevate the percentage of resistant strains within a hospital setting and result in the selection of broader, more toxic agents for empiric therapy agents than necessary. For example, if one patient contributes 20 carbapenem-resistant *P. aeruginosa* isolates out of 50 total isolates, this could lead to requests for colistin for presumed pseudomonal infections, where less toxic and more effective therapies could be selected. Approaches to managing repeat isolates include: a) patient-based algorithms (each patient contributes equally to the calculation), b) episode-based algorithms (each episode contributes equally to the calculation; differing definitions of episodes such as the site of the infection or interval between the infections), or c) resistance phenotype-based algorithms (each phenotypic strain, i.e., specific resistance patterns, contribute equally to the calculation).[7, 8] Both episode-based and resistance phenotype-based algorithms are less standardized and more difficult to compare due to being easily influenced by institutional practices, such as frequency of specimen collection in which antibiotics are tested for resistance and lack of consensus definitions for either episodes or phenotypes of resistance.[8] As a result, it is recommended that calculating susceptibility is based on the first isolate per patient.[8–10]

The guidelines recommend that antibiograms should include both quantitative (inhibition zone diameters for disk diffusion and minimal inhibitory concentration values) and qualitative data (i.e., whether the isolate is classified as resistant, intermediate, or susceptible).[7] This is based on the premise of changing breakpoints over time, however, in reality adds to the complexity of interpreting antibiograms. Therefore, most institutions simplify the data into a percentage of isolates that are susceptible to each antibiotic and whether they change from year to year.[7] This allows the ASP to determine if there is an emergence of antibiotic resistance that might alter empiric therapy recommendations.

Many automated susceptibility machines (e.g., VITEK2, Microscan) use fixed panels of antibiotics, some of which may not be on a hospital's formulary, may be less effective than other agents for a specific site of infection, or may be more costly or toxic than alternative agents. Reporting susceptibility data for every antibiotic that is tested will lead to inappropriate antibiotic requests. For example, reporting imipenem on the antibiogram when meropenem is the formulary choice can result in unnecessary calls to the pharmacy for the non-formulary antibiotic. Similarly, there may not be a benefit in reporting susceptibility data on every quinolone when one will suffice. Close collaboration between the ASP and microbiology laboratory can minimize confusion.[1]

Traditional antibiograms have their limitations. They lack information on combination antibiotic therapy and on different susceptibility patterns in specific patient locations or populations such as intensive care unit (ICU), oncology, pediatric, or ambulatory care patients. Some institutions have developed combination and unit-specific antibiograms to bridge these gaps.

Unit-Specific Antibiograms

A general antibiogram for a large hospital may misrepresent populations of patients in areas where antibiotic resistance is greater such as the ICU or oncology units. The *E. coli* urinary tract infection in a patient in the ICU is likely to be more resistant to standard antibiotics than in a healthy young person in the community. Multiple studies have demonstrated that these location-differentiated populations provide different susceptibility patterns compared to hospital-wide data.[11–14] The unit-specific data can be valuable in guiding empiric therapy choices. Binkley et al. evaluated the differences between the susceptibility patterns reported in unit-specific and hospital-wide antibiograms over a three-year period.[11] They found that the percentages of antibiotic-resistant organisms were significantly higher in the medical and surgical ICUs than in general wards. When ICU data were included in the hospital-wide antibiogram, susceptibility patterns appeared significantly worse than when ICU data were reported separately.[11] Similar to ICUs, antibiotic resistance in community-acquired infections may be overestimated if an inpatient antibiogram is used to guide empiric therapy and lead to the prescribing of excessively broad-spectrum agents.[15, 16] Therefore, many institutions now generate outpatient-specific antibiograms.

Combination Antibiograms

With increasing antibiotic resistance, the selection of empiric therapy has become especially challenging, particularly as delays in appropriate empiric therapy are associated with increased mortality.[17] Combination therapy can be useful in patients who are more likely to have a resistant infection such as those in the ICU or from a nursing home

Combination antibiograms have the advantage over traditional antibiograms because they take into account whether the combination of agents of different antibiotic classes provides additive coverage. Christoff et al. found that when a second agent was added to one of the backbone anti-pseudomonal agents for the treatment of five common gram-negative organisms in critically-ill patients, there was a significant increase in the likelihood that empiric therapy was active against the causative pathogen.[18] Hsu et al. evaluated 175 isolates of carbapenemase-producing Enterobacteriaceae with different combinations of antibiotic agents.[19] They utilized the pharmacokinetic-pharmacodynamic data of high-dose continuous infusion meropenem with breakpoints of ≤ 8 µg/ml and evaluated the percent effectiveness increase when added to other agents. They were able to increase the activity of meropenem from 35% with monotherapy to 91% and 88%, respectively with the addition of amikacin or colistin.[19] The knowledge gained from combination antibiograms can assist both the ASP and providers in better selection of empiric therapy when a carbapenemase-producing Enterobacteriaceae is suspected.

Syndromic Antibiograms

A specific subtype of a unit-based antibiogram is a syndromic combination antibiogram.[20] Syndrome-specific antibiograms have emerged in recent years because cumulative antibiograms have limited utility for guiding empiric therapy for infections where multiple organisms are anticipated, such as intra-abdominal infections.[21] The syndromic antibiogram is designed to provide clinicians with guidance on antibiotic selection for patients with an infectious syndrome rather than for a specific pathogen. In one study, syndromic antibiograms were developed from isolates causing ventilator-associated pneumonias in critical-care patients with and/or catheter-related blood stream infections.[20] These syndromic antibiograms improve empiric coverage by 56% in the first 12 hours of infection compared to monotherapy. However, the study did not demonstrate any mortality difference between ICU patients who received early vs late adequate empirical antibiotic coverage.[20]

Regional Antibiograms

When used longitudinally, antibiograms can identify changes in antibiotic susceptibility patterns within a community. Var et al. showed how a regional antibiogram in Virginia could predict resistance to commonly used antibiotics for community-acquired pneumonia and urinary tract infections.[22] Of note, Moehring et al. in the Duke Network of Community Hospitals in North Carolina showed only 9% of the 38 hospitals had compliance with CLSI guidelines for antibiogram development.[23] They recognized that there needed to be greater outreach from larger facilities to assist these centers in creating and maintaining accurate antibiograms to accurately reflect their region's antibiotic resistance patterns.

In conclusion, an accurate, unit-based antibiogram based on formulary antibiotic agents can assist ASPs in providing optimal empiric antibiotics for patients and updating antibiotic use policies. More specialized antibiograms including combination and syndrome-specific antibiograms may be beneficial in hospitals with complex patients and multidrug-resistant bacteria.

Rapid Molecular Diagnostics

Over the last two decades, there has been an acceleration in the development of rapid diagnostics including non-amplified probe technologies, proteomics, and nucleic acid amplification methods.[24] Most of these technologies are used for blood cultures post Gram-stain and can significantly reduce time to organism identification compared to standard methods.[2, 4, 25] Additionally, a number of newer technologies have been able to identify the presence of genes encoding resistance mechanisms.[4, 24, 25] A summary of the assays and their clinical impacts can be found in Table 1. Direct from blood pre-Gram-stain Rapid microbiologic diagnostics that use multiplex polymerase chain reaction (PCR) to analyze blood cultures directly pre-Gram-stain are already available in Europe. Lastly, there are non-microbiologic diagnostics such as procalcitonin which are being used to distinguish bacterial and viral infections and to guide durations of antibiotic therapy. Incorporation of these assays into clinical practice is most effective when facilitated by education and point-of-care assistance by antibiotic stewardship programs. A timeline of these new technologies is in Figure 1.

Assays for Identification of Pathogens from Positive Blood Cultures

The assays below are listed based on when first described with use and clinical outcomes data. This is to demonstrate the progression of technological advances over the last decade and how it has impacted both laboratory and stewardship activities.

Table 1 Features of Select Rapid Diagnostic Assays Currently Used in Clinical Practice

Technology	Manufacturer	Specimen	Organisms	Resistance Markers	Time Required Following Organism Growth	FDA Cleared
PNA-FISH	AdvanDx, Inc./OpGen Woburn, MA	Blood	S. aureus/Coagulase-negative staphylococci E. faecalis/other Enterococcus species E. coli/K. pneumoniae/P. aeruginosa C. albicans/C. parapsilosis/ C. tropicalis/C. glabrata/C. krusei.	mecA	0.3–1.5 hours	Yes
qPCR	BD GeneOhm, Inc, Sparks MD; Cepheid, Sunnyvale, CA; Roche Molecular Systems, Inc. Indianapolis, IN	Blood, wounds	S. aureus	mecA/ SCCmec	1–2 hours	Yes
MALDI-TOF MS	Bruker Daltonics, Inc. Billerica, MA; bioMerieux, Inc. Durham, NC	All body sites	Large number of organisms including bacteria and yeast	None	0.2 hours	Yes
Nucleic Acid Microarray BC-GP	Nanosphere, Inc. Northbrook, IL	Blood	Staphylococcus spp., S. aureus, S. epidermidis, S. lugdunensis, Streptococcus spp., S. pneumoniae, S. pyogenes, S. agalactiae, S. anginosus group, E. faecalis, E. faecium, Listeria spp.,	mecA, vanA, vanB	2.5 hours	Yes

Test	Manufacturer	Sample	Organisms	Resistance markers	Time	FDA
Nucleic Acid Microarray BC-GN	Nanosphere, Inc. Northbrook, IL	Blood	*Escherichia coli/Shigella* spp., *K. pneumonia, K. oxytoca, P. aeruginosa, S. marcescens, Acinetobacter* spp, *Proteus* spp., *Citrobacter* spp., *Enterobacter* spp.	KPC, NDM, CTX-M, VIM, IMP, OXA.	2.5 hours	Yes
Multiplex Nucleic Acid Amplification Test	Biomerieux, Durham, NC	Blood	*Enterococcus* spp., *L. monocytogenes, Staphylococcus* spp, *S. aureus, Streptococcus* spp., *S agalactiae, S. pyogenes, S. pneumoniae, A. baumannii, H. influenzae, N. meningitides, P. aeruginosa, E. cloacae complex, E. coli, K. oxytoca, K. pneumoniae, S. marcescens, Proteus* spp, *Enterobacteriaceae* spp, *C. albicans, C. parapsilosis, C. tropicalis, C. glabrata, C. krusei*	*mecA, vanA, vanB,* KPC	1 hour	Yes
Beacon-based FISH	Miacom Diagnostics, Inc, Apex, NC	Blood	*Enterococcus* spp., *Staphylococcus* spp, *S. aureus, Streptococcus* spp., *S agalactiae, S. pyogenes, S. pneumoniae, A. baumannii, H. influenzae, P. aeruginosa, E. cloacae complex, E. coli, K. pneumoniae, S. maltophilia, Proteus* spp.,		30 min	Yes

Timeline of Blood Culture Identification Tests

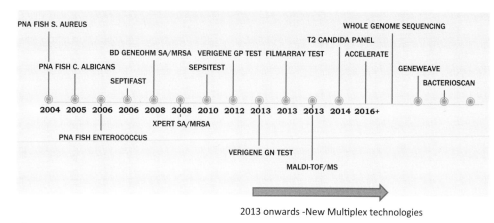

Figure 1

Peptide Nucleic Acid Fluorescence in Situ Hybridization (PNA-FISH)

PNA-FISH (AdvanDx, OpGen, Woburn, MA) was one of the first molecular technologies used to assist clinicians in adjusting antibiotic therapy in real-time. PNA-FISH technology uses fluorescein-labeled DNA mimics that target pathogen-specific 16S rRNA of bacteria or 26S rRNA of yeast. Once a blood culture bottle signals growth and a Gram-stain is performed, the appropriate PNA-FISH probe can rapidly identify several important pathogens.[25] There are currently two PNA-FISH platforms, one that requires a wash stage and takes 90 minutes, and *quick*FISH™, which takes 20 minutes. A summary of the organisms the PNA-FISH probes have been cleared for by the United States Food and Drug Administration (FDA) and European Medicines Agency (EMA) are shown in Table 1.[24]] Other than a recently approved *mec*A testing, PNA-FISH tests do not detect resistance markers.

A number of studies have investigated the utility of PNA-FISH in clinical practice. Forrest et al. utilized the *Staphylococcus aureus* single probe, *Candida albicans* single probe, and probes for *Enterococcus faecalis* and other enterococci in conjunction with ASP interventions. He to demonstrated major clinical benefits associated with combining rapid diagnostic information into strategic antibiotic utilization.[26–28] Before implementing any of the probes, they assessed each probe for accuracy and clinical impact.[25] Initially they showed a significant decrease in median length of hospital stay from 6 to 4 days, a 5% reduction on vancomycin use, and overall hospital cost-savings of $4,000 per patient.[27] The *C. albicans* probe reduced echinocandin usage with a cost-savings of $1,729 per patient. An unexpected finding was that the *C. albicans* probe was more sensitive than the standard germ tube; discordant results found that several isolates that were previously called *C. albicans*, were actually *Candida dubliniensis*.[29] Lastly, a two-year quasi-experimental study with the PNA-FISH *E. faecalis* and other enterococci probes in conjunction with ASP interventions demonstrated a significant reduction in time to effective therapy (1.3 vs. 3.1 days) and 30-day mortality (26% vs. 45%) in patients with *E. faecium* bacteremia.[28]

Ly et al, evaluated the impact of the PNA-FISH *S. aureus*/Coagulase-negative staphylococci (CoNS) dual-probe with ASP in a prospective randomized controlled study on patient outcomes. They showed a reduction in mortality, from 17% to 8%, with the greatest impact on ICU patients. Vancomycin usage was reduced an average of two days.[30] Heil et al. found that when combining the *Candida* PNA-FISH probe with ASP interventions (i.e., calling the clinician with antifungal selection, dosage, and duration recommendations), there were significant decreases in time to targeted therapy (from 2.3 to 0.6 days), time to microbial clearance (from 5 to 4 days), and cost-savings ($415 per patient). However, they were unable to demonstrate a difference in duration of hospital stay or mortality.[31]

Holtzman et al. showed that using the *S. aureus* probe without ASP in a pre-post impact study had no impact on vancomycin usage, hospital length of stay or mortality.[32] Their laboratory batched the testing, ran it overnight and recorded the results in the electronic medical record (EMR). They demonstrated that without education and clear communication, implementing the technology was not beneficial.[32] There have been no published studies evaluating the PNA-FISH probes distinguishing *P. aeruginosa* from *E. coli* and *K. pneumoniae*.[24]

Recently, a beacon-based FISH (bbFISH) test was cleared by the FDA for use for positive blood cultures. The HemoFISH® Masterpanel (Miacom diagnostics, Dusseldorf, Germany) uses molecular beacons to act as a microarray to identify multiple pathogens after blood cultures turn positive. The panel can detect 13 bacterial species (Table 1) from the same blood culture bottle, without separate testing. Similar to PNA-FISH, it offers rapid 30-minute results; however, it has the same limitation of lack of resistance markers. Currently there are no clinical stewardship data on this platform. Despite the pioneering efforts of PNA-FISH in advancing rapid microbiologic testing, its limitations (lack of resistance markers, lack of automation, and need for hands-on time) has resulted in its use being largely replaced by newer molecular technologies.

Real-Time PCR Assays (qPCR)

Real-time PCR assays have been available for many years, mostly as locally developed products. They are relatively simple to use without much preparation time. The results are very sensitive and specific and are usually available within two hours.[33] The two major platforms commercially available in the US focus on *S. aureus* and detection of the *mecA* gene to differentiate methicillin-resistant *S. aureus* (MRSA) from methicillin-sensitive (MSSA); they are the BD GeneOhm Staph SR (BD GeneOhm, Sparks MD) and the Xpert MRSA/SA (Cepheid, Sunnyvale CA).[33] Those platforms can be used for other rapid diagnostic tests, e.g., for pathogens of importance to guide infection control practices such as vancomycin-resistant enterococci, *C. difficile*, respiratory viruses, and *Mycobacterium tuberculosis*.

Carver et al. utilized a local institutional *mecA* PCR test to determine if ASP could improve antibiotic prescribing for *S. aureus* bacteremia.[34] They performed a two-phase study where first they introduced the test without stewardship and a second phase with stewardship. They showed a reduction of 25 hours (from 64 hours pre to 39 hours post) for time to appropriate therapy but did not evaluate outcomes or mortality.[34] Bauer et al. used the Cepheid Xpert SA/MRSA test with ASP in a quasi-experimental analysis of *S. aureus* bacteremia treatment.[35] They demonstrated that post-PCR, patients with MSSA bacteremia were switched from empiric vancomycin to beta-lactam therapy 1.7 day sooner, had a 6.2 day shorter length of stay and lower hospital costs by about $21,000.[35] Nguyen et al. utilized a laboratory developed qPCR assay for MSSA bacteremia that resulted in about a two-day decrease in days of vancomycin therapy and a three-day decrease in length of hospital stay, without any concomitant ASP interventions.[36]

Frye et al. implemented the BD GeneOhm StaphSR PCR assay at their institution without an ASP and reported the results into the EMR.[37] Despite the 13 hour reduction in time to identify the bacteremia, there was an increase of 4 hours to appropriate therapy, no change in vancomycin usage and despite having earlier results, there were patients who continued to receive ineffective therapy.[37] This study reflects the critical importance of an ASP working closely with the clinical microbiology laboratory to determine how to best report results and assist clinicians with point-of-care questions as results become available.

The limitations of these RT-PCR tests are that they only focus on *S. aureus* and CoNS. Also, false-negative results for MRSA with empty *mec* cassettes has resulted in divergent results on occasions and thus the need for monitoring susceptibility results remains important.[38]

Broad-Based Multiplexed Nucleic Acid Assays for Blood Cultures

There are several multi-array platforms that can rapidly identify organisms from blood cultures. There are two FDA-cleared platforms in the United States, the Verigene® Blood Culture Gram Positive (BC-GP) and Negative (BC-GN) Nucleic Acid tests (Luminex Corporation Northbrook, IL) and the Filmarray BCID assay (Biomerieux, Durham, NC). In Europe, there is Prove-it Sepsis (Mobidiag, Esbo, Finland). Each are very similar in that they can rapidly identify up to 60 organisms and some resistance markers.

The Verigene® Blood Culture platform uses a gold nanoparticle microarray to identify 13 pathogenic gram-positive organisms and 8 gram-negative pathogens. (Table 1) It also detects the *mec*A and *van*A and *van*B on the BC-GP test, while the BC-GN test identifies the extended-spectrum beta lactamase $bla_{CTX-M-group}$ and several carbapenemases (bla_{KPC}, bla_{IMP}, bla_{OXA}, bla_{NDM} and bla_{VIM}).[24] It is important to remember that some gram-negative organisms are not included in this panel, such as *Serratia marcescens* and *Stenotrophomonas maltophilia*. The use of this assay is limited to blood cultures and results are available approximately 2.5 hours after Gram-stain identification. The decision to run gram-positive or gram-negative cartridges relies on Gram-stain results. The platform also can be used to perform Influenza virus and *C. difficile* testing.

There has already been a tremendous impact on patient care using the Verigene platform in conjunction with ASP interventions. Sango et al. demonstrated that using the BC-GP platform combined with AS interventions for enterococcal bacteremia resulted in a decrease in time to effective therapy, length of hospital stay (average of 21.7 days) and hospital costs ($60,729), compared with conventional methods.[39] Similarly, Box et al. performed a pre-post-intervention study with the BC-GP platform at 5 hospitals and decreased mean duration of antibiotic therapy for blood culture contaminants by 19 hours and overall hospitalization costs by $7,000.[40] Beal et al. developed a treatment algorithm from the BC-GP platform for patients with MSSA and VRE bacteremia and in a quasi-experimental study showed a 16% increase in optimal initial antibiotic use.[41]

There are currently fewer data on the BC-GN assay. Bork et al. performed a theoretical evaluation of the BC-GN assay with ASP support and estimated a 16 hour reduction in time to receive optimal effective therapy than without.[42] Lastly, Suzuki et al. performed a large multicenter prospective study on the BC-GN assay. They consented every patient in this study before testing with the BC-GN assay. The results of the testing were reported directly to an ID physician who then notified the treating physician to discuss management. There was no pharmacist involvement and they showed improvements in time to optimal therapy, antibiotic cost-savings, and a mortality benefit.[43]

The Filmarray® BCID assay is a multiplex nucleic acid amplification test that can be performed straight from positive blood culture bottles. It identifies 3 genera and 4 species of gram-positive cocci, *Listeria monocytogenes*, 9 gram-negative rods to species level, *Proteus* spp., and 5 species of yeasts (see Table 1). In addition, it detects the following resistance determinants: *mecA, vanA, vanB*, and *bla*$_{KPC}$. The platform can also be used for a respiratory virus panel, a gastrointestinal panel, and a cerebrospinal fluid panel.[44–46] Pardo et al. evaluated the BCID assay. The assay resulted in a shorter duration of empiric vancomycin for patients with MSSA bacteremia while patients with VRE bacteremia received earlier active therapy.[47] A study in children showed that in combination with an ID physician consultation within 24 hours, BCID allowed for 25% earlier de-escalation of antibiotics.[48] A prospective randomized controlled trial found use of the Filmarray assay was associated with less treatment of contaminant blood cultures, less broad-spectrum antibiotic use, and shorter time to appropriate antibiotic escalation and de-escalation.[49] Although the Verigene BC-GN and Filmarray assays can detect only a limited number of gram-negative resistance genes, particularly the Filmarray assay, they may be helpful in escalating therapy but may be less likely to be helpful with de-escalating therapy. For example, either assay can detect *bla*$_{KPC}$ genes but will not identify the ~50% of patients infected with carbapenem-resistant gram-negative organisms caused by non-carbapenemase mediated mechanisms (e.g., carbapenem-specific porin loss or mutation).

Lastly, the Prove-It Sepsis™ array (Mobidiag, Espoo, Finland) is also a microarray technology which can identify 60 bacteria, 13 fungi, and the *mecA* gene in 3.5 hours.[50] It appears to be as accurate as the other technologies. Thus far, there are no publications on the impact of this technology on ASP interventions. Also, Target Enriched Multiplex Polymerase Chain Reaction (TEM-PCR™) by Diatherix (Huntsville, AL) offers direct pathogen testing from multiple different specimens including respiratory, stool, urine, and wound cultures. The technology offers detection of MRSA and Panton Valentin Leukocidin from blood cultures.[51] There is limited clinical data but this technology add further to detection of organisms rapidly in non-blood stream infections.[52]

Matrix-Assisted Laser Desorption Ionization Time of Flight Mass Spectrometry (MALDI-TOF MS)

MALDI-TOF MS has been routinely used throughout Europe for microbial identification and is now becoming more widely used in the US since FDA approval in 2013 of both the Bruker Biotyper (Bruker Daltonics, Inc. Billerica, MA) and the bioMerieux MS (bioMerieux, Inc. Durham, NC). Both systems can identify a large number of organisms including bacteria and yeast recovered from cultures from various body sites within 15–20 minutes of organism growth.[53, 54] MALDI-TOF MS has greatest sensitivity and specificity from pure culture, but techniques have evolved to increase the yield of bacteria directly from blood cultures bottles.[55, 56] However, a study by Clerc et al. using MALDI-TOF MS with pellets of positive blood cultures rather than waiting for pure culture showed that with monomicrobial cultures only 87% of organisms were correctly identified, but this was reduced to 30% in polymicrobial cultures.[57] MALDI-TOF MS impacted antibiotic choices in 33% of cases, generally resulting in broadening therapy.[57]

Perez et al. was able to demonstrate MALDI-TOF MS in conjunction with reporting results to an ID pharmacist 24 hours a day/7 days a week showed a reduction in length of hospital stay (average of 2.6 days) and costs (average of $19,547) but did not impact mortality.[58] Huang et al. also performed a pre-post implementation quasi-experimental study with MALDI-TOF MS combined with real-time ASP interventions in patients with bloodstream infections. The ID pharmacist was notified by both pager (from 6:00 a.m. to 11:30 p.m.) and an email of positive test results. Their program demonstrated decreases in time to organism identification, time to effective therapy, length of ICU stay, 30-day mortality, and recurrent bacteremia compared to a historical control group.[59] There are additional reports in the literature demonstrating MALDI-TOF MS has a positive impact on optimizing antibiotic therapy.[60–62]

Meta-Analysis Data

A summary of the major studies evaluating rapid blood culture technologies are in Table 2. A meta-analysis of the effect of rapid molecular diagnostic technologies on clinical outcomes in blood stream infections reviewed thirty-one studies including 5,920 patients.[63] The authors found that the mortality risk was significantly lower with rapid molecular testing than with conventional microbiology methods (OR, 0.66; 95% CR, 154–0.80), yielding a number needed to treat of 20. The use of ASP and rapid molecular testing had a slightly lower mortality risk (OR, 0.64; 95% CI, 0.51–0.79), while studies without ASP could not demonstrate a significant decrease in mortality risk (0.72; 0.46–1.12). There were significant decreases in mortality risk with both gram-positive (OR, 0.73; 95% CI, 0.55–0.97) and gram-negative organisms (0.51; 0.33–0.78) but not yeast (0.90; 0.49–1.67). Time to effective therapy decreased by a weighted mean difference of −5.03 hours (95% CI, −8.60−−1.45 hours), and length of stay was decreased by −2.48 days (−3.90−−1.06 days). The strength of this data in impacting patient care with ASP and new technologies cannot be understated.

Implementation of New Technologies

There are four important steps that should be taken before selecting and implementing any new rapid diagnostic. Before formally introducing the test, there should be a period to the test and evaluate its performance.

A. Will the test be used enough to offset the costs?

Costs associated with implementing a new rapid diagnostic assay include purchasing equipment, training costs, maintenance costs, reagents, and staff salaries. The volume of cultures sent to the laboratory, the epidemiology of the pathogens identified by the particular rapid diagnostic, and the percentage of resistant isolates should be evaluated prior to deciding on a platform. If an institution very rarely identifies KPC-producing organisms, implementing an assay to detect blaKPCs may not be a good return on investment. If the test can reduce the use of costly, broad-spectrum, or toxic antibiotic agents, or discharge a patient earlier, then working with hospital administration to overcome the compartmentalism of costs between pharmacy and labor.

Technology	Reference	Study Design	Organisms/antibiotic resistance targets	AS-I	Impact on the Antibiotic Therapy	Other Outcomes	Notes
PNA-FISH	Forrest et al., 2006	Retrospective, cost-effective analysis comparing PNA-FISH result combined with AS interventions to historical control in patients with CoNS bacteremia	S. aureus single probe	Yes	Non-significant trend toward less vancomycin use in non-ICU setting (4.9 DDD vs. 6.78 DDD), and only 5% decrease in vancomycin use in ICU setting	Significant reduction in median length of stay (4 vs. 6 days, p<0.05) Decreased hospital costs, ~$4000 per patient	
PNA-FISH	Forrest et al., 2006	Before and after design evaluating potential cost-savings of PNA-FISH result combined with AS in patients with candidemia	Single probe C. albicans	Yes	Significant decrease in DDD/patient usage of caspofungin	Decrease in antifungal costs of $1,729 per patient	Small sample
PNA-FISH	Forrest et al., 2008	Quasi-experimental study, pre- and post-PNA-FISH implementation with AS interventions in patients with GPCPC bacteremia	E. faecalis/other Enterococcus species	Yes	E. faecalis: No difference in time to EAT (0.3 vs. 0 days, p = 1) E. faecium: Significantly shorter in PNA-FISH group (1.3 vs. 3.1, p<0.001)	LOS: no difference Decreased 30-day mortality in PNA-FISH group for patients with E. faecium (26% vs. 45%, p = 0.04), and no difference for E. faecalis	
PNA-FISH	Ly et al., 2008	Prospective, randomized controlled study comparing clinician	S. aureus single probe	No	Antibiotic use was reduced by 2.5 days (p = 0.01) in patients with CoNS, no	LOS: no difference Median charges: $72,932 in PNA-FISH group vs. $92,374 in	Patients in usual care had higher comorbidity index compared to

Table 2 (cont.)

Technology	Reference	Study Design	Organisms/antibiotic resistance targets	AS-I	Impact on the Antibiotic Therapy	Other Outcomes	Notes
		notification of PNA-FISH results in patients with GPCC in blood			difference in patients with *S. aureus*	usual care (p = 0.09). Overall reduced mortality PNA-FISH group (8% vs. 17%, p = 0.05), but no difference when CoNS or *S. aureus* were analyzed individually	PNA-FISH which may be confounder in patient outcomes
PNA-FISH	Holtzman et al., 2011	Retrospective pre- and post-intervention study in patients with CoNS bacteremia	*S. aureus* single probe	No	No significant difference in duration of vancomycin treatment (3.51 vs. 4.15 days, p = 0.49)	Mean LOS: 20.9 days vs. 18.7 days, p = 0.35	
PNA-FISH	Heil et al., 2012	Before and after design comparing PNA-FISH result combined with AS interventions to historical control in patients with candidemia	*C. albicans/ C. parapsilosis, C. tropicalis, C. glabrata/ C. krusei*	Yes	Mean time to TT was significantly shorter in PNA-FISH group (0.6 days vs. 2.3 days, p = 0.0016)	Median time to culture clearance was significantly shorter (4 days vs. 5 days, p = 0.01) LOS: median 12 vs. 25 (p = 0.82) No significant difference hospital mortality	Small sample size

Method	Study	Target/Sample	AS intervention	Results	Secondary outcomes	Comments
qPCR	Carver et al., 2008	Prospective two-phase study. Phase I-results reported only Phase II-results with AS intervention	S. aureus/mecA and SCCmec from blood	Yes	Time to OAT decreased by 25.4 hours		Sample was too small to evaluate other clinical outcomes
qPCR	Nguyen et al., 2010	Retrospective comparative study, comparing qPCR with historical control in patients with MSSA and receiving vancomycin	S. aureus/mecA and SCCmec from blood	No	Decrease in vancomycin usage from 3 to 1 day (p<0.0001) Switch from vancomycin to beta-lactam increased significantly (38.5% to 61.7%, p = 0.004)	Hospitalization days decreased by median of 3 days (5 days vs. 8 days, p = 0.03)
qPCR	Bauer et al., 2010	Nonequivalent study comparing pre-qPCR and post-qPCR with AS intervention	S. aureus/mecA and SCCmec from blood	Yes	Shorter time to switch (1.7 days) from vancomycin to nafcillin/cefazolin for MSSA group (p = 0.02), no difference in MRSA group	Non-significant decrease in mean LOS by 6.2 days (p = 0.07) Mean hospital costs were decreased by $21,387 in rPCR group	qPCR was not independently associated with hospital mortality
qPCR	Parta et al., 2010	Retrospective comparative study, comparing qPCR with historical control	S. aureus/mecA and SCCmec from blood	No	Significant decrease in the use of antistaphylococcal antibiotics for staphylococcus spp. other than S. aureus (24% vs. 45%, p<0.01) Significantly shorter mean time OAT for		

Table 2 (cont.)

Technology	Reference	Study Design	Organisms/ antibiotic resistance targets	AS-I	Impact on the Antibiotic Therapy	Other Outcomes	Notes
qPCR					MSSA (5.2 hours vs. 49.8 hours, p = 0.007) Time to initiation of therapy for MRSA did not differ		
	Frye et al., 2012	Retrospective, interventional cohort study pre-qPCR and post-qPCR	S. aureus/mecA and SCCmec from blood	No	The average time to optimal antibiotic therapy for MRSA was increased by an average of 3.7 h (P > 0.1) as was the time to optimal antibiotic therapy for MSSA was also increased by 2.3 h,	No difference in Mortality (12.7% both groups) or LOS (12.1 days vs. 11.6 days).	More patients received ineffective therapy in qPCR group.
MALDI-TOF MS	Huang et al., 2013	Pre-post quasi-experimental study combined with real-time AS interventions	Gram-positive, gram-negative, yeast from blood	Yes	Time to EAT improved by 10 h in intervention group (20.4 h vs. 30.1 h, p = 0.021) Time to OAT improved by 43 h in intervention group (47.3 h vs. 90.3 h, p<0.001)	Decreased ICU stay in intervention group (14.9 days vs. 8.3 days, p = 0.014) LOS: no difference (14.2 days vs. 11.4 days, p = 0.66) Mortality: 14.5% intervention vs. 20.3% control (p = 0.021)	In multivariate regression analysis acceptance of AS intervention was not associated with reduced mortality

Method	Author, Year	Study design	Target	Intervention	Outcomes	Clinical outcomes	Notes
MALDI-TOF MS	Perez et al., 2013	Pre- and post-intervention study coupled with real-time AS interventions	Gram-negatives from blood	Yes	At 24 hours after bacteremia onset, fewer patients were on inactive therapy in intervention cohort (4.7% vs. 19.6%); Average time to initiation of active therapy was shorter in intervention cohort (36.5 hours vs. 73.2 hours, $p<0.001$)	LOS: significantly lower in the intervention cohort (9.3 vs. 11.9, $p = 0.01$) Mean hospital costs were significantly lower in the intervention group ($26,162 vs. $45,709, $p = 0.009$) Mortality: no difference (5.6% vs. 10.7%)	Active therapy at 48 h and intervention were independently associated with decreased hospitalization
MALDI-TOF MS	Vlek et al., 2012	Pre- and post-intervention study	All positive blood cultures	No	11.3% increase in % of patients receiving appropriate antibiotic therapy 24 hours after blood cultures turned positive (75.3% vs. 64%, $p = 0.01$)		Other clinical outcomes were not evaluated
MALDI-TOF MS	Clerc et al., 2013	Prospective observational study; all patients received ID consultation	Gram-negatives from blood	No	Modifications in empiric therapy occurred in 35.1% patients; most frequent was early broadening of therapy (43.7%)		No comparative group; impact of antibiotic changes on clinical outcomes was not evaluated
qPCR + MALDI-TOF MS	Clerc et al., 2013	Prospective, randomized open study comparing MALDI-TOF MS to MALDI-TOF MS +	S. aureus/mecA and SCCmec from blood	No	Non-significant decrease unnecessary glycopeptides coverage for MSSA		

Table 2 (cont.)

Technology	Reference	Study Design	Organisms/antibiotic resistance targets	AS-I	Impact on the Antibiotic Therapy	Other Outcomes	Notes
		qPCR (results were reported to clinicians in both groups)			(17.1% vs. 29.2%, p = 0.09), when patients with PCN allergy were exclude decrease was significant (8.1% vs. 26.1%, p<0.01)		
Nucleic acid microarray (Verigene BC-GP)	Sango et al., 2013	Pre-post quasi-experimental study	*Enterococcus* spp; vanA, vanB	Yes	Non-significant decrease in time to AAT for VSE (40.2 h vs. 18.6, p = 0.115); Significant decrease in time to AAT for VRE (62.7 h vs. 31.6 h, p<0.0001).	LOS: significantly shorter 21.5 vs. 43.2 days (p = 0.048). Not observed when deceased patients were removed I-LOS: no difference Costs: decrease in hospital costs by $60,729 (p = 0.02) Infection related readmission w/ 90 days: no difference. Attributed mortality: no difference	Patient groups were not matched
Nucleic acid microarray (Verigene BC-GP)	Box et al., 2015	This multicenter, pre-post, quasi-experimental study conducted at five community hospitals	Gram-Positive Panel	Yes	Decreased time to targeted antibiotic therapy by 26 hours (p<0.001) and duration of antibiotic	LOS reduced by 2 days (p = 0.04) and hospitalization costs by $7300 in the intervention group.	Lab testing only done between 7 a.m. and 7 p.m. No discussion overnight specimens.

Test/Platform	Author	Study design	Panel	Consent	Findings	Mortality	Comments
					therapy for blood culture contaminants by 18 hours (p = 0.03).	No difference in mortality	
Nucleic acid microarray (Verigene BC-GP)	Beal et al., 2015	Single center pre-post-intervention study	Gram-Positive Panel	No	Reduced time to optimal antibiotics by 18.9 hours (P = 0.004) overall, with a 20.6-hour reduction (P = 0.009) for patients with MSSA and a 20.7-hour reduction (P = 0.077) for patients with VRE. Increased proportion of patients started on optimal antibiotics from 64% (45/70) pre-BC-GP to 80% (43/54) post-BC-GP.	No difference in mortality (pre 27% vs post 16%, P = 0.16). No change in LOS in VRE or MRSA groups.	Small single center study.
Nucleic acid microarray (Verigene BC-GP and GN)	Suzuki et al., 2015	Multicenter study, six-month pre-period compared to post six month period. Consent obtained	Gram Positive and Negative panel	No	Optimal therapy significantly earlier than the control period (P = 0.001), and most of cases (90%; 79/88) were treated with susceptible antibiotic agents	30-day mortality significantly lower (13% vs 3%, P = 0.02). Greater cost reduction with GP cases (2488 yen vs. 11585 yen, P = 0.002), but not observed in the community-onset GN cases (3797 yen vs. 4272 yen, P = 0.797).	Higher hospital associated infections in control period

Table 2 (cont.)

Technology	Reference	Study Design	Organisms/ antibiotic resistance targets	AS-I	Impact on the Antibiotic Therapy	Other Outcomes	Notes
Filmarray	Banerjee et al., 2015	Single Center, prospective randomized study. 3 arms: standard BC processing, BCID reported with templated comments, or BCID reported with templated comments and antibiotic stewardship (AS) team.	Gram positive, negative and Candida	Yes	Both intervention groups reduced piperacillin-tazobactam vs control (44% vs 56%, P = .01) and had less treatment of contaminants (control 25% vs. BCID alone 11%, vs. BCID +AS 8%; P = .015). Time to change antibiotics was shortest in the BCID +AS group (de-escalation: 21 hours vs. control 34 hours, vs BCID 38 hours, P<.001; escalation: BCID+AS 5 hours, control 24 hours, BCID 6 hours, P = .04).	No difference in mortality (Control 10.6%, BCID 10.1%, BCID+AS 8.6%), LOS (all median 8 days), or cost of test or antibiotic costs.	Largest randomized prospective study of rapid tests. Evaluated multiple variables in large tertiary center.
Filmarray	Pardo et al., 2016	Single center, retrospectively BCID testing period and a matched historical control group before	Gram positive, negative and Candida	Yes	Reduced duration of vancomycin for patients with contaminated blood cultures (P = 0.005) and MSSA bacteremia	No reduction in LOS. Mortality reduced (15% vs. 6%, P = 0.36). Reduction in ICU costs.	Short ICU stay in Filmarray group may have affected costs

		BCID testing was introduced.			(P < 0.001). Patients with VRE bacteremia received active therapy earlier than historical controls (P = 0.047).	
FIlmarray	Ray et al., 2016	Prospective intervention study, pediatric hospital	Gram positive, negative and Candida	Yes	Antibiotics were changed in 19% episodes and de-escalated/withheld / stopped in 25% episodes	14 bed day stays saved	Small study, no outcomes data

AS – antibiotic stewardship, AS-I – antibiotic stewardship interventions, BC-GP – blood culture Gram positive, BC-GN – blood culture Gram negative, TT-targeted therapy, EAT – effective antibiotic therapy, OAT – optimal antibiotic therapy, AAT – appropriate antibiotic therapy, LOS – length of hospital stay, I – LOS-infection related LOS, DDD – defined daily dose, GPCC – gram-positive cocci in clusters, CPCPC – gram-positive cocci in pairs and chains, MSSA – Methicillin-susceptible *S. aureus*, MRSA – Methicillin-resistant *S. aureus*, CoNS – *Coagulase-negative staphylococci*, VSE – vancomycin sensitive *Enterococcus*, VRE – vancomycin-resistant *Enterococcus*

B. How will education of clinicians occur?

Education in medical schools and residency programs on rapid microbiologic testing is virtually non-existent. Therefore, any new laboratory test introduced into a clinical environment needs to be supplemented with education to clinicians prior to implementation of the assay to ensure that test results are interpreted appropriately.[24] Development and dissemination of algorithms prior to implementation can educate clinicians and result in a more immediate and robust response to the novel assay. Often this needs to be supplemented with direct contact by the ASP as results become available, at least when the test is first introduced.

C. Is a system in place to report results to clinicians?

Results need to be reported in terms understandable to clinicians. Clinicians may not understand the significance of the "mecA" gene or the "bla_{KPC}" gene so results should be presented in more understandable language. For example, "A bla_{CTX-M} gene has been detected. This means your patient may be infected with an extended-spectrum beta-lactamase (ESBL) producing organism. Carbapenems are generally considered the first choice for ESBL-producing organisms." For resistance mechanisms where additional information is needed to guide treatment options, the results can suggest contacting the ASP. The onus of recommending treatment for specific organisms or resistance mechanisms should not be placed on the clinical microbiology laboratory. Additionally, there should be a clear plan of how to handle reporting of resistance markers. "Unidentifiable" organisms also need an action plan. For example, the Verigene GN-BC platform in the US does not report S. maltophilia and calls it unidentifiable. Having a plan to address organisms not detected by the panel, is important.

Immediate reporting enhances the impact of rapid molecular testing results. Texting, paging and phone calls are superior to leaving a note in the EMR.[37] Developing treatment guidelines or algorithms can help with the process. It is clear that leaving providers to their own devices typically results in failure to impact antibiotic utilization and patient care.

D. How will discrepant test results be managed?

The expectations of new rapid diagnostics can be extremely high for many providers and far outweigh what is rational. No test is 100% accurate and discrepancies between the test result and the final culture can lead to loss of confidence in the test by clinicians. Having a system in place to review the discrepancy which could be anything from test performance to human error is just as important as ensuring appropriate turnaround time.

Assays for Pathogen Detection Directly from Blood/Serum

There are three platforms for the diagnosis of sepsis directly on blood samples: one broad-range and two multiplex PCR assays. None of these platforms are cleared for commercial usage in the USA; however, they are licensed for use in Europe. The tests are the LightCycler SeptiFast Test (Roche Molecular Systems, Branchburg, NJ), SepsiTest (Molzym, Bremen, Germany), and Vyoo (SIRS-Lab, Jena, Germany).[64]

SeptiFast is the only multiplex real-time PCR assay available for the diagnosis of sepsis. It is capable of detecting genetic material belonging to several bacterial and fungal pathogens, representing approximately 90% of the species responsible for nosocomial bacteremia.[65] The SeptiFast panel of bacteria and fungi that can be detected is shown in Table 1.[64] The PCR test has a detection limit range from 3 to 30 CFU/ml, and the turnaround time is approximately 6 hours.[65] This test has many studies showing rapid detection of pathogens in blood compared to routine blood cultures.[66–68] In a prospective single-center observational study, all patients with severe sepsis admitted to the intensive care unit had SeptiFast testing.[68] There was a 13-fold higher probability of detecting at least 1 microorganism compared to blood cultures.[68] In a double-blind randomized study in patients with sepsis, Tafelski et al. showed that Septifast testing reduced time to identification by 16 hours when the initial pathogen was identified in septic patients.[69] A meta-analysis of all studies comparing Septifast to blood cultures showed a sensitivity and specificity for SeptiFast compared with blood culture as 68% (95% CI 0.63–0.73) and 86% (95% CI 0.84–0.89), respectively.[70] Future evaluation of this platform should involve the evaluation of stewardship input in impacting clinical outcomes.

For SepsiTest, a broad-range PCR-based assay and Vyoo there are no available clinical data. Both tests require eight hours or more for results. These technologies are expensive to perform- approximately $500 per test.[68] Their role in patient care is yet to be determined.

T2 Magnetic Resonance

The T2Candida Panel (T2 biosystems) is an FDA-cleared rapid diagnostic approach that enables target amplification of the multicopy internal transcribed spacer region 2 (ITS2) region of the *Candida* genome. The resulting amplicons are detected using nanoparticles coated with oligonucleotide capture probes to enable sensitive and specific detection directly from whole blood.[71] Mylonakis et al. performed a clinical study using the T2Candida panel with 1,801 consecutive blood specimens from patients, but over 460 (20%) were excluded due to technical error or indeterminate results.[72] The median time to identification was 4 hours and, based on spiked blood bottles, was 99% specific. There were 31 discordant results; 2 with positive blood cultures and negative T2Candida panel, 29 with positive T2Candida and negative blood cultures.[72] Less than 2% of all tested specimens yielded a positive result. Development of algorithms with the laboratory and ASP are necessary to prevent overtesting and subsequent overtreating before adopting a a costly and poorly understood test.

Future Rapid Technologies

There are several rapid technologies that could emerge over the next few years that will impact both microbiology laboratories and stewardship programs. These rapid phenotypic susceptibility identification systems include digital automated microscopy, next generation sequencing, pathogen-specific bioparticles (GeneWEAVE, Los Gatos, CA), and laser light scattering (BacterioSCAN, St Louis, Mo).

Digital automated microscopy (Accelerate Diagnostics, Tuscon, Az) can give pathogen identification in 1 hour and antibiotic susceptibility results within 5 hours direct from blood culture and other specimens such as sputum, wound, and urine.[73] Currently, there are a few papers on the utility this assay on respiratory specimens, but the technology is novel and integrating these data with the stewardship programs may present a new challenge.[73, 74] The other technologies are currently in early stages of development and clinical data are not yet available.

Procalcitonin

Procalcitonin (PCT) is a 13-kDa peptide precursor of calcitonin. In a healthy population, PCT concentrations are negligible however, when there is a systemic bacterial or fungal infection, plasma concentrations become elevated; concentrations are low in viral infections.[75–77] Compared to the previous methodologies, PCT testing does not need to be performed in the microbiology laboratory. The test is automated on an analyzer (BRAHMS, Biomerieux, Durham, NC) and takes approximately twenty minutes. If the first test is negative, the test should be repeated 6 hours later.[77]

In two meta-analyses, PCT demonstrated superior diagnostic accuracy for severe bacterial infections compared to C-reactive protein.[78, 79] The limitations of PCT are that it can be elevated for a wide range of inflammatory conditions including pancreatitis, traumatic injury, major surgery, burns, and massive stress.[80] Its role in the diagnosis of bacterial sepsis in patients with febrile neutropenia is even less certain.[81, 82] Antibiotic therapy is generally strongly discouraged for PCT levels <0.25 µg/L, discouraged for PCT <0.5 µg/L, encouraged for PCT >0.5 µg/L, and strongly encouraged ≥1 µg/L in the majority of studies. If therapy is withheld PTC levels should generally be repeated 6–24 hours later and if therapy is initiated PCT levels should be repeated every 2–3 days to assist with decisions to discontinue antibiotics. The non-adherence to designated PCT treatment algorithms has been shown to be a limitation in previous studies, suggesting the potential benefit of stewardship interventions to supplement any new diagnostic assay.[24, 83–87]

Several randomized controlled trials have demonstrated that PCT can successfully reduce antibiotic initiation and duration of therapy in acute respiratory tract infections in a variety of settings including primary care clinics, emergency departments, and hospital wards without a negative impact on clinical outcomes.[80, 88–91] Reduction in the duration of antibiotic therapy has also been demonstrated in septic ICU adult and neonatal patients using PCT-guided therapy.[87, 92–98]

There are few published studies that have examined the role of ASP interventions on the utility of PCT-guided therapy. An abstract from a community hospital showed that an ASP with PCT had an almost 1.5 day reduction in antibiotic usage in a retrospective analysis of its usage.[99] Although not formally evaluated, ASPs could improve the use of PCT by developing diagnostic and treatment algorithms for incorporation into clinical practice, particularly for outpatient and emergency department patients presenting with respiratory illnesses.[24]

Conclusion

The collaboration between clinical microbiology laboratories and antibiotic stewardship programs needs to be strong – particularly with the rapid proliferation of new technologies that can identify organisms, resistance mechanisms, and antibiotic susceptibilities faster than with traditional methods. Having a collaborative approach to assessing the validity of these assays, their workflow in the microbiology laboratory, and methods of reporting and applying the results is critical to ensure they enhance patient care.

References

1. Dellit TH, Owens RC, McGowan JE, Jr., Gerding DN, Weinstein RA, Burke JP, et al. Infectious Diseases Society of America and the Society for Healthcare Epidemiology of America guidelines for developing an institutional program to enhance antimicrobial stewardship. *Clin Infect Dis* 2007; 44(2):159–177.

2. Barlam TF, Cosgrove SE, Abbo LM, MacDougall C, Schuetz AN, Septimus EJ, et al. Implementing an antibiotic stewardship program: guidelines by the Infectious Diseases Society of America and

the Society for Healthcare Epidemiology of America. *Clin Infect Dis* 2016; 62(10): e51–77.

3. Procop GW, Winn W, Microbiology Resource Committee CoAP. Outsourcing microbiology and offsite laboratories. Implications on patient care, cost savings, and graduate medical education. *Arch Pathol Lab Med* 2003; 127(5):623–624.

4. Bauer KA, Perez KK, Forrest GN, Goff DA. Review of rapid diagnostic tests used by antimicrobial stewardship programs. *Clin Infect Dis* 2014; 59(Suppl 3):S134–145.

5. Baron EJ, Miller JM, Weinstein MP, Richter SS, Gilligan PH, Thomson RB, Jr., et al. A guide to utilization of the microbiology laboratory for diagnosis of infectious diseases: 2013 recommendations by the Infectious Diseases Society of America (IDSA) and the American Society for Microbiology (ASM). *Clin Infect Dis* 2013; 57(4):e22–e121.

6. Park GE, Kang CI, Wi YM, Ko JH, Lee WJ, Lee JY, et al. Case-control study of the risk factors for acquisition of Pseudomonas and Proteus species during tigecycline therapy. *Antimicrob Agents Chemother* 2015; 59(9):5830–5833.

7. Clinical and Laboratory Standards Institute (CaLSI). Analysis and presentation of cumulative antimicrobial susceptibility test data: approved guideline – 4th edition. CLSI document M39–4A, 2014.

8. Hindler JF, Stelling J. Analysis and presentation of cumulative antibiograms: a new consensus guideline from the Clinical and Laboratory Standards Institute. *Clin Infect Dis* 2007; 44(6):867–873.

9. Magee JT. Effects of duplicate and screening isolates on surveillance of community and hospital antibiotic resistance. *J Antimicrob Chemother* 2004; 54(1):155–162.

10. Shannon KP, French GL. Validation of the NCCLS proposal to use results only from the first isolate of a species per patient in the calculation of susceptibility frequencies. *J Antimicrob Chemother* 2002; 50(6):965–969.

11. Binkley S, Fishman NO, LaRosa LA, Marr AM, Nachamkin I, Wordell D, et al. Comparison of unit-specific and hospital-wide antibiograms: potential implications for selection of empirical antimicrobial therapy. *Infect Control Hosp Epidemiol* 2006; 27(7):682–687.

12. Kaufman D, Haas CE, Edinger R, Hollick G. Antibiotic susceptibility in the surgical intensive care unit compared with the hospital-wide antibiogram. *Arch Surg* 1998; 133(10):1041–1045.

13. Saxena S, Ansari SK, Raza MW, Dutta R. Antibiograms in resource limited settings: are stratified antibiograms better? *Infect Dis (London)* 2015; 48(4):299–302.

14. Zatorski C, Jordan JA, Cosgrove SE, Zocchi M, May L. Comparison of antibiotic susceptibility of Escherichia coli in urinary isolates from an emergency department with other institutional susceptibility data. *Am J Health Syst Pharm* 2015; 72(24):2176–2180.

15. Dahle KW, Korgenski EK, Hersh AL, Srivastava R, Gesteland PH. Clinical value of an ambulatory-based antibiogram for uropathogens in children. *J Pediatric Infect Dis Soc* 2012; 1(4):333–336.

16. McGregor JC, Bearden DT, Townes JM, Sharp SE, Gorman PN, Elman MR, et al. Comparison of antibiograms developed for inpatients and primary care outpatients. *Diagn Microbiol Infect Dis* 2013; 76(1):73–79.

17. Ferrer R, Martin-Loeches I, Phillips G, Osborn TM, Townsend S, Dellinger RP, et al. Empiric antibiotic treatment reduces mortality in severe sepsis and septic shock from the first hour: results from a guideline-based performance improvement program. *Crit Care Med* 2014; 42(8):1749–1755.

18. Christoff J, Tolentino J, Mawdsley E, Matushek S, Pitrak D, Weber SG. Optimizing empirical antimicrobial therapy for infection due to gram-negative pathogens in the intensive care unit: utility of a combination antibiogram. *Infect Control Hosp Epidemiol* 2010; 31(3):256–261.

19. Hsu AJ, Carroll KC, Milstone AM, Avdic E, Cosgrove SE, Vilasoa M, et al. The use of a combination antibiogram to assist with the selection of appropriate antimicrobial therapy for carbapenemase-producing Enterobacteriaceae infections. *Infect Control Hosp Epidemiol* 2015; 36(12):1458–1460.

20. Randhawa V, Sarwar S, Walker S, Elligsen M, Palmay L, Daneman N. Weighted-incidence syndromic combination antibiograms to guide empiric treatment of critical care infections: a retrospective cohort study. *Crit Care* 2014; 18(3):R112.

21. Hebert C, Ridgway J, Vekhter B, Brown EC, Weber SG, Robicsek A. Demonstration of the weighted-incidence syndromic combination antibiogram: an empiric prescribing decision aid. *Infect Control Hosp Epidemiol* 2012; 33(4):381–388.

22. Var SK, Hadi R, Khardori NM. Evaluation of regional antibiograms to monitor antimicrobial resistance in Hampton Roads. *Virginia. Ann Clin Microbiol Antimicrob* 2015; 14:22.

23. Moehring RW, Hazen KC, Hawkins MR, Drew RH, Sexton DJ, Anderson DJ. Challenges in preparation of cumulative antibiogram reports for community hospitals. *J Clin Microbiol* 2015; 53(9):2977–2982.

24. Avdic E, Carroll KC. The role of the microbiology laboratory in antimicrobial stewardship programs. *Infect Dis Clin North Am* 2014; 28(2):215–235.

25. Forrest GN. PNA FISH: present and future impact on patient management. *Expert Rev Mol Diagn* 2007; 7(3):231–236.

26. Forrest GN, Mankes K, Jabra-Rizk MA, Weekes E, Johnson JK, Lincalis DP, et al. Peptide nucleic acid fluorescence in situ hybridization-based identification of Candida albicans and its impact on mortality and antifungal therapy costs. *J Clin Microbiol* 2006; 44(9):3381–3383.

27. Forrest GN, Mehta S, Weekes E, Lincalis DP, Johnson JK, Venezia RA. Impact of rapid in situ hybridization testing on coagulase-negative staphylococci positive blood cultures. *J Antimicrob Chemother* 2006; 58(1):154–158.

28. Forrest GN, Roghmann MC, Toombs LS, Johnson JK, Weekes E, Lincalis DP, et al. Peptide nucleic acid fluorescent in situ hybridization for hospital-acquired enterococcal bacteremia: delivering earlier effective antimicrobial therapy. *Antimicrob Agents Chemother* 2008; 52(10):3558–3563.

29. Jabra-Rizk MA, Johnson JK, Forrest G, Mankes K, Meiller TF, Venezia RA. Prevalence of Candida dubliniensis fungemia at a large teaching hospital. *Clin Infect Dis* 2005; 41(7):1064–1067.

30. Ly T, Gulia J, Pyrgos V, Waga M, Shoham S. Impact upon clinical outcomes of translation of PNA FISH-generated laboratory data from the clinical microbiology bench to bedside in real time. *Ther Clin Risk Manag* 2008; 4(3):637–640.

31. Heil EL, Johnson JK. Impact of CLSI breakpoint changes on microbiology laboratories and antimicrobial stewardship programs. *J Clin Microbiol* 2016; 54(4):840–844.

32. Holtzman C, Whitney D, Barlam T, Miller NS. Assessment of impact of peptide nucleic acid fluorescence in situ hybridization for rapid identification of coagulase-negative staphylococci in the absence of antimicrobial stewardship intervention. *J Clin Microbiol* 2011; 49(4):1581–1582.

33. Wong JR, Bauer KA, Mangino JE, Goff DA. Antimicrobial stewardship pharmacist interventions for coagulase-negative staphylococci positive blood cultures using rapid polymerase chain reaction. *Ann Pharmacother* 2012; 46(11):1484–1490.

34. Carver PL, Lin SW, DePestel DD, Newton DW. Impact of mecA gene testing and intervention by infectious disease clinical pharmacists on time to optimal antimicrobial therapy for *Staphylococcus aureus* bacteremia at a University Hospital. *J Clin Microbiol* 2008; 46(7):2381–2383.

35. Bauer KA, West JE, Balada-Llasat JM, Pancholi P, Stevenson KB, Goff DA. An antimicrobial stewardship program's impact with rapid polymerase chain

reaction methicillin-resistant *Staphylococcus aureus/S. aureus* blood culture test in patients with *S. aureus* bacteremia. *Clin Infect Dis* 2010; 51(9):1074–1080.

36. Nguyen DT, Yeh E, Perry S, Luo RF, Pinsky BA, Lee BP, et al. Real-time PCR testing for mecA reduces vancomycin usage and length of hospitalization for patients infected with methicillin-sensitive staphylococci. *J Clin Microbiol* 2010; 48(3):785–790.

37. Frye AM, Baker CA, Rustvold DL, Heath KA, Hunt J, Leggett JE, et al. Clinical impact of a real-time PCR assay for rapid identification of staphylococcal bacteremia. *J Clin Microbiol* 2012; 50(1):127–133.

38. Sharff KA, Monecke S, Slaughter S, Forrest G, Pfeiffer C, Ehricht R, et al. Genotypic resistance testing creates new treatment challenges: two cases of oxacillin-susceptible methicillin-resistant *Staphylococcus aureus*. *J Clin Microbiol* 2012; 50(12):4151–4153.

39. Sango A, McCarter YS, Johnson D, Ferreira J, Guzman N, Jankowski CA. Stewardship approach for optimizing antimicrobial therapy through use of a rapid microarray assay on blood cultures positive for *Enterococcus* species. *J Clin Microbiol* 2013; 51(12):4008–4011.

40. Box MJ, Sullivan EL, Ortwine KN, Parmenter MA, Quigley MM, Aguilar-Higgins LM, et al. Outcomes of rapid identification for gram-positive bacteremia in combination with antibiotic stewardship at a community-based hospital system. *Pharmacotherapy* 2015; 35(3):269–276.

41. Beal SG, Thomas C, Dhiman N, Nguyen D, Qin H, Hawkins JM, et al. Antibiotic utilization improvement with the Nanosphere Verigene Gram-Positive Blood Culture assay. *Proc (Bayl Univ Med Cent)* 2015; 28(2):139–143.

42. Bork JT, Leekha S, Heil EL, Zhao L, Badamas R, Johnson JK. Rapid testing using the Verigene Gram-negative blood culture nucleic acid test in combination with antimicrobial stewardship intervention against Gram-negative

bacteremia. *Antimicrob Agents Chemother* 2015; 59(3):1588–1595.

43. Suzuki H, Hitomi S, Yaguchi Y, Tamai K, Ueda A, Kamata K, et al. Prospective intervention study with a microarray-based, multiplexed, automated molecular diagnosis instrument (Verigene system) for the rapid diagnosis of bloodstream infections, and its impact on the clinical outcomes. *J Infect Chemother* 2015; 21(12):849–856.

44. Rand KH, Delano JP. Direct identification of bacteria in positive blood cultures: comparison of two rapid methods, FilmArray and mass spectrometry. *Diagn Microbiol Infect Dis* 2014; 79(3):293–297.

45. Rand KH, Tremblay EE, Hoidal M, Fisher LB, Grau KR, Karst SM. Multiplex gastrointestinal pathogen panels: implications for infection control. *Diagn Microbiol Infect Dis* 2015; 82(2):154–157.

46. Rhein J, Bahr NC, Hemmert AC, Cloud JL, Bellamkonda S, Oswald C, et al. Diagnostic performance of a multiplex PCR assay for meningitis in an HIV-infected population in Uganda. *Diagn Microbiol Infect Dis* 2016; 84(3):268–273.

47. Pardo J, Klinker KP, Borgert SJ, Butler BM, Giglio PG, Rand KH. Clinical and economic impact of antimicrobial stewardship interventions with the FilmArray blood culture identification panel. *Diagn Microbiol Infect Dis* 2016; 84(2):159–164.

48. Ray ST, Drew RJ, Hardiman F, Pizer B, Riordan A. Rapid identification of microorganisms by FilmArray(R) blood culture identification panel improves clinical management in children. *Pediatr Infect Dis J* 2016; 35(5):e134–138.

49. Banerjee R, Teng CB, Cunningham SA, Ihde SM, Steckelberg JM, Moriarty JP, et al. Randomized trial of rapid multiplex polymerase chain reaction-based blood culture identification and susceptibility testing. *Clin Infect Dis* 2015; 61(7):1071–1080.

50. Laakso S, Kirveskari J, Tissari P, Maki M. Evaluation of high-throughput PCR and microarray-based assay in conjunction

with automated DNA extraction instruments for diagnosis of sepsis. *PLoS One* 2011; 6(11):e26655.

51. Tang YW, Kilic A, Yang Q, McAllister SK, Li H, Miller RS, et al. StaphPlex system for rapid and simultaneous identification of antibiotic resistance determinants and Panton-Valentine leukocidin detection of staphylococci from positive blood cultures. *J Clin Microbiol* 2007; 45(6):1867–1873.

52. Duncan R, Kourout M, Grigorenko E, Fisher C, Dong M. Advances in multiplex nucleic acid diagnostics for blood-borne pathogens: promises and pitfalls. *Expert Rev Mol Diagn* 2016; 16(1):83–95.

53. Patel R. Matrix-assisted laser desorption ionization-time of flight mass spectrometry in clinical microbiology. *Clin Infect Dis* 2013; 57(4):564–572.

54. Tan KE, Ellis BC, Lee R, Stamper PD, Zhang SX, Carroll KC. Prospective evaluation of a matrix-assisted laser desorption ionization-time of flight mass spectrometry system in a hospital clinical microbiology laboratory for identification of bacteria and yeasts: a bench-by-bench study for assessing the impact on time to identification and cost-effectiveness. *J Clin Microbiol* 2012; 50(10):3301–3308.

55. March-Rossello GA, Munoz-Moreno MF, Garcia-Loygorri-Jordan de Urries MC, Bratos-Perez MA. A differential centrifugation protocol and validation criterion for enhancing mass spectrometry (MALDI-TOF) results in microbial identification using blood culture growth bottles. *Eur J Clin Microbiol Infect Dis* 2013; 32(5):699–704.

56. Prod'hom G, Bizzini A, Durussel C, Bille J, Greub G. Matrix-assisted laser desorption ionization-time of flight mass spectrometry for direct bacterial identification from positive blood culture pellets. *J Clin Microbiol* 2010; 48(4):1481–1483.

57. Clerc O, Prod'hom G, Vogne C, Bizzini A, Calandra T, Greub G. Impact of matrix-assisted laser desorption ionization time-of-flight mass spectrometry on the clinical management of patients with Gram-negative bacteremia: a prospective observational study. *Clin Infect Dis* 2013; 56(8):1101–1107.

58. Perez KK, Olsen RJ, Musick WL, Cernoch PL, Davis JR, Land GA, et al. Integrating rapid pathogen identification and antimicrobial stewardship significantly decreases hospital costs. *Arch Pathol Lab Med* 2013; 137(9):1247–1254.

59. Huang AM, Newton D, Kunapuli A, Gandhi TN, Washer LL, Isip J, et al. Impact of rapid organism identification via matrix-assisted laser desorption/ionization time-of-flight combined with antimicrobial stewardship team intervention in adult patients with bacteremia and candidemia. *Clin Infect Dis* 2013; 57(9):1237–1245.

60. Tamma PD, Tan K, Nussenblatt VR, Turnbull AE, Carroll KC, Cosgrove SE. Can matrix-assisted laser desorption ionization time-of-flight mass spectrometry (MALDI-TOF) enhance antimicrobial stewardship efforts in the acute care setting? *Infect Control Hosp Epidemiol* 2013; 34(9):990–995.

61. Vlek AL, Bonten MJ, Boel CH. Direct matrix-assisted laser desorption ionization time-of-flight mass spectrometry improves appropriateness of antibiotic treatment of bacteremia. *PLoS One* 2012; 7(3):e32589.

62. Wenzler E, Goff DA, Mangino JE, Reed EE, Wehr A, Bauer KA. Impact of rapid identification of *Acinetobacter Baumannii* via matrix-assisted laser desorption ionization time-of-flight mass spectrometry combined with antimicrobial stewardship in patients with pneumonia and/or bacteremia. *Diagn Microbiol Infect Dis* 2016; 84(1):63–68.

63. Timbrook TT, Morton JB, McConeghy KW, Caffrey AR, Mylonakis E, LaPlante KL. The effect of molecular rapid diagnostic testing on clinical outcomes in bloodstream infections: a systematic review and meta-analysis. *Clin Infect Dis* 2017; 64(1):15–23.

64. Mancini N, Carletti S, Ghidoli N, Cichero P, Burioni R, Clementi M. The era of molecular and other non-culture-based

methods in diagnosis of sepsis. *Clin Microbiol Rev* 2010; 23(1):235–251.

65. Lehmann LE, Hunfeld KP, Emrich T, Haberhausen G, Wissing H, Hoeft A, et al. A multiplex real-time PCR assay for rapid detection and differentiation of 25 bacterial and fungal pathogens from whole blood samples. *Med Microbiol Immunol* 2008; 197(3):313–324.

66. Dark P, Wilson C, Blackwood B, McAuley DF, Perkins GD, McMullan R, et al. Accuracy of LightCycler(R) SeptiFast for the detection and identification of pathogens in the blood of patients with suspected sepsis: a systematic review protocol. *BMJ Open* 2012; 2(1): e000392.

67. Mancini N, Sambri V, Corti C, Ghidoli N, Tolomelli G, Paolucci M, et al. Cost-effectiveness of blood culture and a multiplex real-time PCR in hematological patients with suspected sepsis: an observational propensity score-matched study. *Expert Rev Mol Diagn* 2014; 14(5):623–632.

68. Suberviola B, Marquez-Lopez A, Castellanos-Ortega A, Fernandez-Mazarrasa C, Santibanez M, Martinez LM. Microbiological diagnosis of sepsis: polymerase chain reaction system versus blood cultures. *Am J Crit Care* 2016; 25 (1):68–75.

69. Tafelski S, Nachtigall I, Adam T, Bereswill S, Faust J, Tamarkin A, et al. Randomized controlled clinical trial evaluating multiplex polymerase chain reaction for pathogen identification and therapy adaptation in critical care patients with pulmonary or abdominal sepsis. *J Int Med Res* 2015; 43(3):364–377.

70. Dark P, Blackwood B, Gates S, McAuley D, Perkins GD, McMullan R, et al. Accuracy of LightCycler® SeptiFast for the detection and identification of pathogens in the blood of patients with suspected sepsis: a systematic review and meta-analysis. *Intensive Care Med* 2015; 41(1):21–33.

71. Neely LA, Audeh M, Phung NA, Min M, Suchocki A, Plourde D, et al. T2 magnetic resonance enables nanoparticle-mediated rapid detection of candidemia in whole blood. *Sci Transl Med* 2013; 5(182):182ra54.

72. Mylonakis E, Clancy CJ, Ostrosky-Zeichner L, Garey KW, Alangaden GJ, Vazquez JA, et al. T2 magnetic resonance assay for the rapid diagnosis of candidemia in whole blood: a clinical trial. *Clin Infect Dis* 2015; 60(6):892–899.

73. Douglas IS, Price CS, Overdier KH, Wolken RF, Metzger SW, Hance KR, et al. Rapid automated microscopy for microbiological surveillance of ventilator-associated pneumonia. *Am J Respir Crit Care Med* 2015; 191(5):566–573.

74. Metzger S, Frobel RA, Dunne WM, Jr. Rapid simultaneous identification and quantitation of *Staphylococcus aureus* and *Pseudomonas aeruginosa* directly from bronchoalveolar lavage specimens using automated microscopy. *Diagn Microbiol Infect Dis* 2014; 79(2):160–165.

75. Assicot M, Gendrel D, Carsin H, Raymond J, Guilbaud J, Bohuon C. High serum procalcitonin concentrations in patients with sepsis and infection. *Lancet* 1993; 341(8844):515–518.

76. Barassi A, Pallotti F, Melzi d'Eril G. Biological variation of procalcitonin in healthy individuals. *Clin Chem* 2004; 50(10):1878.

77. Cheval C, Timsit JF, Garrouste-Orgeas M, Assicot M, De Jonghe B, Misset B, et al. Procalcitonin (PCT) is useful in predicting the bacterial origin of an acute circulatory failure in critically ill patients. *Intensive Care Med* 2000; 26(Suppl 2):S153–158.

78. Simon L, Gauvin F, Amre DK, Saint-Louis P, Lacroix J. Serum procalcitonin and C-reactive protein levels as markers of bacterial infection: a systematic review and meta-analysis. *Clin Infect Dis* 2004; 39(2):206–217.

79. Uzzan B, Cohen R, Nicolas P, Cucherat M, Perret GY. Procalcitonin as a diagnostic test for sepsis in critically ill adults and after surgery or trauma: a systematic review and meta-analysis. *Crit Care Med* 2006; 34(7):1996–2003.

80. Schuetz P, Christ-Crain M, Thomann R, Falconnier C, Wolbers M, Widmer I, et al.

Effect of procalcitonin-based guidelines vs standard guidelines on antibiotic use in lower respiratory tract infections: the ProHOSP randomized controlled trial. *JAMA* 2009; 302(10):1059–1066.

81. Giamarellou H, Giamarellos-Bourboulis EJ, Repoussis P, Galani L, Anagnostopoulos N, Grecka P, et al. Potential use of procalcitonin as a diagnostic criterion in febrile neutropenia: experience from a multicentre study. *Clin Microbiol Infect* 2004; 10(7):628–633.

82. Robinson JO, Lamoth F, Bally F, Knaup M, Calandra T, Marchetti O. Monitoring procalcitonin in febrile neutropenia: what is its utility for initial diagnosis of infection and reassessment in persistent fever? *PLoS One* 2011; 6(4):e18886.

83. Schuetz P, Albrich W, Christ-Crain M, Chastre J, Mueller B. Procalcitonin for guidance of antibiotic therapy. *Expert Rev Anti Infect Ther* 2010; 8(5):575–587.

84. Schuetz P, Briel M, Christ-Crain M, Stolz D, Bouadma L, Wolff M, et al. Procalcitonin to guide initiation and duration of antibiotic treatment in acute respiratory infections: an individual patient data meta-analysis. *Clin Infect Dis* 2012; 55(5):651–662.

85. Schuetz P, Christ-Crain M, Wolbers M, Schild U, Thomann R, Falconnier C, et al. Procalcitonin guided antibiotic therapy and hospitalization in patients with lower respiratory tract infections: a prospective, multicenter, randomized controlled trial. *BMC Health Serv Res* 2007; 7:102.

86. Schuetz P, Muller B, Christ-Crain M, Stolz D, Tamm M, Bouadma L, et al. Procalcitonin to initiate or discontinue antibiotics in acute respiratory tract infections. *Evid Based Child Health* 2013; 8(4):1297–1371.

87. Shehabi Y, Sterba M, Garrett PM, Rachakonda KS, Stephens D, Harrigan P, et al. Procalcitonin algorithm in critically ill adults with undifferentiated infection or suspected sepsis. A randomized controlled trial. *Am J Respir Crit Care Med* 2014; 190(10):1102–1110.

88. Burkhardt O, Ewig S, Haagen U, Giersdorf S, Hartmann O, Wegscheider K, et al. Procalcitonin guidance and reduction of antibiotic use in acute respiratory tract infection. *Eur Respir J* 2010; 36(3):601–607.

89. Christ-Crain M, Muller B. Procalcitonin in bacterial infections – hype, hope, more or less? *Swiss Med Wkly* 2005; 135(31–32):451–460.

90. Kristoffersen KB, Sogaard OS, Wejse C, Black FT, Greve T, Tarp B, et al. Antibiotic treatment interruption of suspected lower respiratory tract infections based on a single procalcitonin measurement at hospital admission–a randomized trial. *Clin Microbiol Infect* 2009; 15(5):481–487.

91. Stolz D, Christ-Crain M, Bingisser R, Leuppi J, Miedinger D, Muller C, et al. Antibiotic treatment of exacerbations of COPD: a randomized, controlled trial comparing procalcitonin-guidance with standard therapy. *Chest* 2007; 131(1):9–19.

92. Bouadma L, Luyt CE, Tubach F, Cracco C, Alvarez A, Schwebel C, et al. Use of procalcitonin to reduce patients' exposure to antibiotics in intensive care units (PRORATA trial): a multicentre randomised controlled trial. *Lancet* 2010; 375(9713):463–474.

93. Hochreiter M, Kohler T, Schweiger AM, Keck FS, Bein B, von Spiegel T, et al. Procalcitonin to guide duration of antibiotic therapy in intensive care patients: a randomized prospective controlled trial. *Crit Care* 2009; 13(3):R83.

94. Nobre V, Harbarth S, Graf JD, Rohner P, Pugin J. Use of procalcitonin to shorten antibiotic treatment duration in septic patients: a randomized trial. *Am J Respir Crit Care Med* 2008; 177(5):498–505.

95. Oliveira CF, Botoni FA, Oliveira CR, Silva CB, Pereira HA, Serufo JC, et al. Procalcitonin versus C-reactive protein for guiding antibiotic therapy in sepsis: a randomized trial. *Crit Care Med* 2013; 41(10):2336–2343.

96. Rodriguez AH, Aviles-Jurado FX, Diaz E, Schuetz P, Trefler SI, Sole-Violan J, et al. Procalcitonin (PCT) levels for ruling-out bacterial coinfection in ICU patients with influenza: A CHAID decision-tree analysis. *J Infect* 2015.

97. Stocker M, Fontana M, El Helou S, Wegscheider K, Berger TM. Use of procalcitonin-guided decision-making to shorten antibiotic therapy in suspected neonatal early-onset sepsis: prospective randomized intervention trial. *Neonatology* 2010; 97(2):165–174.

98. Wacker C, Prkno A, Brunkhorst FM, Schlattmann P. Procalcitonin as a diagnostic marker for sepsis: a systematic review and meta-analysis. *Lancet Infect Dis* 2013; 13(5):426–435.

99. Newton J, Lim, C., Robinson S, Kuper, K, Garey K.W., Trivedi, K.K. Impact of procalcitonin (PCT) guidance on antimicrobial stewardship in a community hospital. *Open forum Infect Dis* 2015; 2(Suppl 1):217.

Chapter 1

Informatics and Stewardship

Francesca Lee and Kristi M. Kuper

Introduction

Manual review of patient data to improve antibiotic use can be onerous and inefficient. Antibiotic stewardship programs (ASPs) that integrate data and functionality from information technology (IT) resources are able to more quickly and consistently identify opportunities to optimize antibiotic therapy in a large number of patients across the healthcare spectrum. If the IT systems include support for a clinical decision support system (CDSS), data extraction may be further enhanced.

A CDSS, by definition, is an electronic system that matches patient information to a clinical knowledge base and generates patient-specific recommendations to improve patient outcomes.[1] These systems combine individual patient data, population trends, and evidence-based medicine into their informatics infrastructure to produce meaningful, actionable alerts. In addition, they have the ability to collate data on interventions, measure antibiotic use, and quantify cost savings. A CDSS can be integrated within the electronic medical record (EMR) system or can exist as stand-alone systems. CDSS have been shown to reduce the use of broad-spectrum antibiotics, improve antibiotic dosing and selection, reduce antibiotic-associated adverse events, and reduce lengths of stay and mortality.[2, 3]

History

The term "clinical decision support" first appeared in the literature in 1969,[4] well before the modernization and widespread adoption of technology in healthcare. Two decades later, Pestonik and colleagues published a prospective study of outcomes associated with "home-grown" therapeutic antibiotic monitoring alerts (TAMs) that were developed within the integrated hospital informatics system at a 520-bed academic hospital in Salt Lake City, UT.[5] TAMs were based on algorithms that would screen for inconsistencies between in vitro antibiotic-susceptibility test results and patients' antibiotic therapy. TAM alerts were divided into three categories: 1) the organism identified was resistant to current antibiotic therapy; 2) no antibiotic susceptibilities reported for the isolated organism; and 3) a clinical isolate was identified but antibiotics were not given. Approximately one-third of TAMs resulted in a physician adjusting or starting antibiotic therapy. This study demonstrated that computer-based alerts generated from a predefined algorithm led to improved antibiotic prescribing.

A decade later, these same investigators published a landmark trial describing the outcomes associated with a more robust version of the system.[2] In this prospective study, they evaluated outcomes associated with a CDSS that was utilized to manage anti-infectives in a 12-bed intensive care unit (ICU) over a one-year period. During the study period, all

545 patients admitted to the ICU had their antibiotics evaluated by the CDSS. Process measures and clinical outcomes were compared to 1,136 patients admitted to the same unit two years prior to the intervention period. Use of CDSS-based interventions compared to the period prior to CDSS-based interventions led to a significant reduction in medication orders for drugs to which patients were allergic (35 patients vs. 146 patients, $p < 0.01$), supratherapeutic dosing (87 patients vs. 405 patients, $p < 0.01$), and antibiotic-susceptibility mismatches (12 patients vs. 206 patients, $p < 0.01$). In addition, those patients who received an antibiotic regimen that was recommended by the computer program ($n = 203$) had lower antibiotic costs, lower total hospital costs, and a reduction in lengths of stay (all parameters $p < 0.001$) when compared to those in the pre-intervention cohort. Taken together, these findings showed that the use of a modern-day CDSS was able to improve patient care with an added financial benefit.

Types of Clinical Decision Technology

CDSS terminology is not yet standardized. For the purposes of this chapter, we will use the definitions created by Forrest et al. in their 2014 review entitled "Use of electronic health records and clinical decision support systems for antibiotic stewardship."[6] The authors divide CDSS programs into those which are based on electronic medical records (EMRs) and third-party systems which they term "Add-on CDSS."

Add-On CDSS

An add-on CDSS runs in parallel with the EMR, and are dependent on the data which they can extract from the institution's native data sources (EMR, microbiology informatics system, etc.).[6, 7] The general functionality among the add-on systems currently available is similar. They incorporate a minimum number of elements including admission, discharge, transfer data, pharmacy records, and microbiology results. A series of algorithms, written by either the end user or vendor, analyze these data and report intervention targets in the background for integration. Examples of ASP interventions available through add-on CDSS include identification of redundant antibiotic coverage, drug-bug mismatches, pharmacokinetic (PK)/pharmacodynamics (PD) optimization targets, sterile site culture reports, and antibiotic time-out reports. Some add-on CDSS can also create unit-specific antibiograms. While these systems are robust, they are dependent on the quality and accuracy of the data extracted from the EMR. A listing of commercial systems available in the US market can be found in Table 1.

EMR-Based Systems

Electronic Medical Record (EMR) systems are digital versions of a patient's chart.[8] EMR systems should have the capabilities of an EMR, plus the ability to share information with other areas of the healthcare system, and be accessible to all clinicians involved in a patient's care (ideally across multiple healthcare organizations).[9] Although there are hundreds of EMR vendors in the United States alone, 67% of the market share is held by three companies.[10] The adoption of EMRs across the US healthcare system increased significantly due to financial incentives provided through the Center for Medicare and Medicaid's (CMS) Meaningful Use Program for eligible professionals and hospitals to invest in EMRs in order to improve quality, safety, privacy, and patient care.[11]

Table 1 Listing of Select Available Add-On Systems for Antibiotic Stewardship

Product Name	Company (also known as)	City, State, Country
360 Care Insights	Truven	Ann Arbor, MI, USA
ABX Alert	Baxter Healthcare/ICNet	Warrensville, IN, USA
Dynamic Monitoring Suite	Vigilanz	Minneapolis, MN, USA
ILUM Insight	Merck Healthcare Services and Solutions	Kenilworth, NJ, USA
Medici	Asolva Inc	Pasadena, CA, USA
Patient Event Advisor	BD (Care Fusion/Medmined)	Birmingham, AL, USA
QC Pathfinder	Vecna	Cambridge, MA, USA
RL Solutions	RL Solutions	Cambridge, MA, USA
Sentri 7	Wolters Kluwer (Pharmacy One Source)	Bellevue, WA, USA
Teqqa	Teqqa	Philadelphia, PA, USA
Theradoc	Premier	Charlotte, NC, USA

EMR systems were not initially created with the goal of meeting the needs of ASPs, but they have evolved over time. Vendors such as Epic (Verona, WI) and Cerner (Kansas City, MO) embed antibiotic stewardship and infection prevention functionality within their systems. Some components are included in the basic EMR structure, but additional functionality requires additional financial investment. In Epic, for example, basic features include iVents, antibiotic order forms, dose-checking alerts, best practice alerts, 96-hour stop dates for restricted antibiotics, and intravenous to oral interchange.[7] The iVents feature is unique to Epic and allows for retrievable, searchable documentation of pharmacist interventions that are not readily accessible to all clinicians. In Cerner, order sets and proprietary "PowerPlans" can be customized to ensure compliance with ASP recommendations and allow flexibility for prescribing practices.[12]

The advantages of utilizing an EMR vendor system over an add-on CDSS for AS include increased visibility of actionable AS interventions across disciplines (rather than only being visible by ASP teams or personnel with access to the system), expansion to the non-acute care setting, and fewer potential data system-interface data errors. Within the EMR, programmers can design the system such that actionable alerts are visible to any care provider, as long as that person has access to the patient's medical record. Another key distinction between EMR and add-on CDSS is prospective intervention capabilities upon order entry. With CDSS, the alerts are typically generated retrospectively, meaning after the medication has been ordered or the lab result reported. As most EMRs include computerized order entry (CPOE) functionality, the order sets and algorithms that are embedded within the system can be customized to proactively guide the prescriber to select the appropriate antibiotic, thereby reducing the number of required retrospective interventions.

Another function built into some EMRs is a scoring system, which helps to triage patients and prioritize those that would benefit most from an intervention. Rules are built that help to determine the acuity of the patient based on multiple variables. Each service that is needed (e.g., intravenous to oral conversion, PK monitoring, renal dosing) is scored.

The sum of each of the individual element scores produces an acuity score. When the practitioner reviews the list, it is typically sorted with the highest acuity score at the top, indicating that this patient should be the first person reviewed by the pharmacist or treating clinicians.

Most acute care facilities utilize CDSS for the inpatient setting but these systems are slowly being integrated into non-acute areas such as ambulatory clinics. A cluster randomized trial among 33 primary care practices that are members of a larger health system in central Pennsylvania showed that the use of an EMR-based CDSS decreased the percentage of adolescents and adults that were prescribed antibiotics unnecessarily for uncomplicated acute bronchitis.[13] In this study, there were three groups of 11 practices each: a control group, a group that utilized a print-based strategy, and the EMR intervention group. In the print-based strategy group, when the triage nurse entered "cough" as the chief symptom, a best practice alert would prompt the nurse to provide the patient with an educational brochure prior to clinical evaluation. The EMR intervention included a structured template for documenting history and physical exam results and included an embedded algorithm that would categorize the patient's probability of having pneumonia. Groups of electronic order sets streamlined testing and treatment options for those patients likely to have upper respiratory tract infections. As a result, the percentage of patients prescribed antibiotics in the EMR intervention group decreased from 74% to 61% compared to the control group ($p = 0.01$).

Practical Considerations When Selecting a System

General Functionality

Both EMR-based and add-on CDSS require IT support resources, and it can be difficult to determine how extensive those resource needs will be until the user has "hands on" experience work with the system. EHR-based systems typically have a few preprogrammed alert algorithms for common interventions such as drug-bug mismatches or redundant therapy, and more limited reporting capabilities. For example, in an EMR-based system, a drug utilization report may require data download and manipulation in a spreadsheet, whereas it is available on demand from a list of preprogrammed reports in an add-on CDSS. Add-on CDSS typically have a graphic user interface that simplifies the processes for building customized alerts, but require significant effort in validation of the reports generated, and in ensuring correct transfer of data from the original source to the add-on program.[6, 7]

Information exchange can vary depending on the system. In EMR-based systems, the information is self-contained and available for current as well as past admissions. Some add-on CDSS can exchange information between the EMR and/or transitions of care (e.g., ambulatory, acute care, long-term care). Information can also be shared from previous hospital admissions or outpatient treatment records. Patients with a previous history of a multidrug-resistant organism (MDRO) can easily be identified and a history performed with a single search as opposed to having to search individual records from past admissions, assisting with both infection control and empiric treatment guidance.

The user interface screen in most systems will either be a home screen or dashboard. This provides a streamlined view of the actions that need to be taken by the user and helps to prioritize activities. The user view should be customizable. Patient lists should be sortable by patient name, location, intervention type, or service line. Some systems display icons, which, when selected, take the user to the data behind the icon.

The portability of the EHR and add-on systems has increased over time. Earlier generations were loaded directly onto computer desktops and could only be accessed through that specific computer. Current CDSS are now web-based and have applications that can be downloaded to "smart devices." However, because of the extensive amount of information contained in patient records that antibiotic stewards may need to review, the desktop computer with a larger screen or multiple screens is generally more convenient and user-friendly.

Reporting Functionality

There is extensive variability among the various systems in terms of their capacity for tracking metrics and benchmarking. Most systems have the ability to measure antibiotic use by days of therapy (DOT) or defined daily dose (DDD) but only some systems can report denominator data (per 1,000 patient days, 1,000 days present, etc.) Most CDSS, either add-on or EMR-based, lack antibiotic utilization benchmarking capabilities beyond the single institution. Another important differentiator is the ability of the system to report data into CDC's National Healthcare Safety Network (NHSN) Antimicrobial Use and Resistance (AUR)[14] module. Some CDSS have the capacity to report into the AUR module, while others lack this functionality.

Ideally, CDSS should have the ability to track and report workload statistics and system efficiencies. Examples include classifying the type of alerts where interventions are occurring, the frequency in which orders are being acted upon by the pharmacist or physician, the number of dismissed alerts, and alert actions by individual pharmacists. These reports can be helpful to managers and system administrators in evaluating performance improvement. These interventions can also be cross-referenced with auto-populated or customized financial costs to measure cost savings and return on investment.

One of the key reporting features imperative to ASPs is the ability to produce on-demand antibiograms. These may be created for a selected timeframe, a specific unit, or for select organisms. Some add-on systems and EMR-based systems have this capability, but the output quality is variable. Compliance with Clinical Laboratory Standards Institute guidelines [15] such as that only the first non-duplicate isolate for the reporting period is included in the antibiogram, is variable.

Unique Functionality of EMR and Add-On Systems

Of the available systems on the market, some offer unique functionality. Newer add-on CDSS have embedded predictive modeling tools that allow the system to assist with increasing the likelihood for the correct diagnosis. For example, one CDSS has an "intelligent user interface" that allows the user to input relevant information about the patient's background and clinical symptoms, and combines this with relevant information such as vital signs and key laboratory values to produce a list of suggested diagnoses, and possible antibiotic treatment regimens.[16] Another system offers a personalized prediction score for the clinician. A background application within the system combines institutional antibiogram data, current diagnostic information, patient demographics (e.g., age, length of stay, previous admissions) and integrates risk factors from published literature in order to predict, at the individual patient level, the likely organism and predicted susceptibility to key antibiotics.[17]

The EMR-based systems have the advantage of allowing the prescriber to enter an indication for use at the point of CPOE. For example, in Epic, there are abbreviated phrases that when selected, auto-populate certain characteristics of the medication order such as indication for use, making it easier to have this information available to other prescribers and pharmacists upon retrospective review.[7] Cerner also has the ability to capture antibiotic indications.[12] When the prescriber orders an antibiotic, a drop down menu of indications appears, allowing for quick selection and assurance that the indication is recorded before proceeding to the next order entry screen. Researchers at Northwestern Memorial Hospital utilized this functionality to improve compliance with the surgical care improvement project by allowing the ASP to identify problem areas related to appropriate utilization of empiric and prophylactic antibiotics.[18]

Several add-on systems are owned by companies that also have drug information references in their product portfolio. The systems that have embedded links to external drug information resources can offer the clinician immediate access to information on dosing, indications, adverse effects, and drug interactions. This has the potential to improve prescribing appropriateness if the CDSS is available to the prescriber.

Determining the Right Program to Enhance Antibiotic Stewardship Activities

Whether to purchase increased functionality within the existing EMR, maximize existing EMR functionality, or purchase an add-on system is a challenging decision. Identifying a group of key stakeholders is crucial before evaluating which type of CDSS is best to meet institutional needs. Suggested members of the team include clinical champions (e.g., infectious diseases physicians – or physicians with an interest in AS if infectious diseases physicians are not available), epidemiologists, pharmacists, infection preventionists, IT personnel, a sub-group of end users, and an executive sponsor. A financial analyst is helpful, as systems can be quite costly.[7]

These stakeholders can map out the needs for each department. For example, members of the pharmacy team should determine if they want a system that can identify intervention opportunities related to both antibiotics and other medication classes (e.g., anticoagulation). Most, but not all, commercially available systems now have alerts that are generated for all categories of drugs (Table 2). Other pharmacy-related needs may include the ability

Table 2 Examples of Electronic Alerts

Antibiotic Alerts [22]	Non-Antibiotic Alerts
• Drug Interactions • De-escalation • Duplicate antibiotic therapy • Supratherapeutic vancomycin level • Supratherapeutic aminoglycoside level • Consideration for intravenous to oral switch • Renal dosing adjustment needed • Positive culture but no antibiotic • Positive culture but incorrect antibiotic	• Heparin and platelet decrease • High international normalized ratio and receiving warfarin • Receiving granulocyte colony stimulating factor and high white blood cell count • Rising serum creatinine in presence of angiotensin converting enzyme inhibitors • Hypoglycemia with active order for insulin • Active anticoagulant and low hemoglobin

to identify situations where an adverse drug reaction has occurred, an active list of patients receiving certain medications, or using the system for medication reconciliation.

IT personnel should analyze how many data feeds will be required, which can increase both the time to implementation and the cost of the system. The amount of oversight or interaction required to maintain data flow to keep the system functional is an important consideration as many hospital IT systems are already overburdened and have to prioritize limited resources. An inventory of hardware required for the system is also advisable; additional investments in monitors and servers may also increase the cost. A clinician or pharmacist viewing the alerts on a computer desktop may need a large computer screen, or two screens, to make the alerts easily visible; this viewing flexibility may not be available at all institutions, and may be difficult for some to implement. The location of the server (on or off site) may also influence the decision. Some hospitals prefer to maintain control of their data and will not allow it to be stored outside of their firewall. However, newer systems utilizing the "cloud" based format may eventually make servers and server location an obsolete issue. Most importantly, IT will want to conduct a review of the CDSS company's compliance with HIPAA regulations and the Health Information Technology for Economic and Clinical Health Act (HI-TECH) requirements. Additional oversight may be required if the CDSS has a mobile interface, as this may create possible risk exposure should the mobile device be involved in a security breach.

Another important consideration is how to validate data provided by a third party CDSS. However, the completeness of this data can only be verified if compared to a source of truth, using an alternate reporting system (**Box 1**). There can be problems in the interface between the Healthcare Information Management (HIM) system and the CDSS, leading to incomplete data. Complicating this, many clinical laboratories use a laboratory informatics system which is separate from the HIM.

The general functionality of an add-on CDSS versus using the EMR needs to be investigated. Add-on system alerts or reports are generally only accessible from within that system, meaning that the user needs to have both this program, and the EMR, opened simultaneously. Also, although the CDSS may provide real-time alerts, these must be reviewed by an ASP, which will then need to communicate with the clinician to implement a change. This approach does not allow for interventions at the time an order is placed, so the EMR will need to remain an integral part of any AS efforts. Conversely, while EMR-based alerts may be configured to trigger at the time of order entry, these could conceivably lead to alert fatigue and provider frustration.

Box 1   Real-World Examples to Support Need for Data Validation

- Institutional practice changed from testing *Clostridium difficile* by toxin to polymerase chain reaction (PCR). The test name was changed to reflect this. However, the code that the third-party CDSS recognized for *Clostridium difficile* was not updated, leading to a sudden drop in *C. difficile* infections noted by the infection preventionists. A code update by the IT analysts was required to allow the CDSS to recognize the organism name so that new cases could be properly identified.

- Reports for restricted antibiotics are printed daily. Many of the positive results were for patients who had been on a restricted agent during previous admissions, but were not receiving the antibiotics during the current admission. After months of investigation, an error was identified in the interface between the EMR and the CDSS resulting in past orders being classified as active during the current admission.

Consideration of these factors should help stakeholders as they determine the necessary components to establish "system readiness" so that when the CDSS is active, it is functional and provides useful alerts. For some systems, this may be as early as 60–90 days after integration, but they may provide less functionality. Other systems may offer very robust alert capabilities and reporting but require a year or more to refine and finalize rules. In a study by Hermsen and colleagues,[19] up to five hours was spent daily on reviewing alerts produced by a CDSS, which included up to 70% of non-actionable alerts. Institutions may need to allow additional, dedicated personnel not only at the time of implementation, but on an ongoing basis, to increase the robustness of the system, to help build and refine alerts, and to validate data. Table 3 includes a checklist that may help guide stakeholders reviewing the systems and lists key points to consider throughout the CDSS assessment process.

Table 3 Checklist for Assessing CDSS Functionality

Functionality/Need	EHR Vendor	Add-On CDSS	Notes
Antibiotic Stewardship Specific Needs			
Method of tracking antibiotic use? Examples include: • DOT per 1,000 patient days • DDD per 1,000 patient days • DOT per 1,000 days present			
Ability to track intervention and acceptance rates?			
Average number of alerts fired per day?			
Is there the ability to customize the antibiotic list for monitoring?			
Identifies duplicate (redundant) antibiotic therapy? Examples include • Duplicate anti-anaerobic therapy (except if patient has *Clostridium difficile*) • Double beta-lactam therapy			
Identifies patients on treatment at specific intervals? (e.g., 48–72 hours) without supporting cultures identified? • Probing question – is this time frame customizable			
Opportunities for IV to PO conversion identified? • Is this rule customizable or based on certain fixed criteria?			
Outpatient functionality described?			
Dashboard present?			
Infection Prevention Needs			
Can the systems identify NHSN healthcare associated infection, multidrug-resistant organisms, and *Clostridium difficile* cases?			
Can it create specific lists or generate specific queries such as isolation lists?			
Does it export directly to NHSN?			
Can the system identify clusters of infections?			

Table 3 *(cont.)*

Functionality/Need	EHR Vendor	Add-On CDSS	Notes
Does the system have the ability to identify organisms with unusual resistance patterns?			
Pharmacy Needs- Non-Antibiotic Stewardship			
Can the system do the following?			
Anticoagulation/antiplatelet monitoring?			
Drug related laboratory abnormalities?			
Adverse drug reactions			
Target medication monitoring			
Support Risk Evaluation and Mitigation Strategy (REMS)			
Perform key word searches in radiology and surgery reports?			
General Functionality			
Does the system interface with the EHR? (Add-on CDSS only)	Not applicable		
Can reports run at specific times?			
Are data or alerts available on mobile devices?			
Describe security protocols			
Where are data stored? • Cloud • Off-site server • On-site server			
Ability to send interventions directly to prescriber through application?			
What training is available for IT to support the project?			
What interfaces are required?			
Can the program go through a test drive prior to purchase?			
Ease of use – how many clicks /actions does it take to respond to high use alerts?			
Provide links to literature references to support recommendations?			
Can you customize alerts at each campus [for multi- hospital systems]			
Financial			
Ability to quantify savings from interventions?			
Cost of system before upgrades?			
Additional charge for supplemental data feeds? NHSN? Other?			
Are cost-savings estimates customizable?			

Putting Clinical Decision Support Technology to Work

Due to financial incentives from the federal government, the majority of acute care hospitals in the US have moved or will be moving to some type of computerized data management system, which may be a limited EMR system or a full-fledged EMR product. Availability in other settings of care such as skilled nursing facilities, long-term care, and in ambulatory care clinics will vary. The robustness of system will determine the types of data that are available for the ASP, which will guide the decisions on the types of interventions to be pursued.

ASPs early in their development or programs with limited CDSS resources can still use technology to assist with their daily antibiotic stewardship activities. Even the most basic EHRs and add-on systems allow for the creation of lists. A good place to start is to generate lists of patients on targeted antibiotics or antibiotic classes such as broad-spectrum agents (e.g., carbapenems, flouroquinolones). After targeted antibiotic lists, a next step would be to generate daily reports of culture results from normally sterile sites. These can be created either from the EMR/add-on CDSS or through the laboratory information system. Other lists that may be helpful include lists of patients on three or more antibiotics, those who have been receiving intravenous antibiotics for oral equivalents are available (to identify IV to oral conversion opportunities), or lists of patients receiving antibiotics for a specific duration (e.g., 48 hours) to identify opportunity for an antibiotic "time out." Finally, disease-state specific interventions can be designed and tracked with daily or real-time lists of patients with specific diagnoses on their problem list (for example, "pneumonia" or "*Clostridium difficile*"). Alternately, unit or service-line specific interventions could be targeted with a daily report showing patients on antibiotics for a given unit. These are all reasonably straightforward requests for most IT Departments.

For both add-on and EMR-based CDSS, generating rules based on microbiology results can be very effective in reducing inappropriate antibiotic use and improving quality of care (**Box 2**). Antworth and colleagues [20] developed a rule in their add-on CDSS that would send an alert to the ASP team when a patient had a positive blood culture for any species of *Candida*. Once the AS team received the alert, they would not only review therapy appropriateness based on culture and susceptibility results, but expand their review to include assessment of intravascular catheter needs, repeat blood culture obtainment every 48 hours, appropriate duration, and ophthalmologic examination to evaluate *Candida* endophthalmitis [collectively referred to as a *Candida* bundle]. Compared to a historical group, the patients in the bundle group had significant improvements in ophthalmologic

---

Box 2 Case Study Demonstrating a Positive Outcome from the Use of a CDSS

The ASP at a 576-bed healthcare system noted that many of the prescriptions for carbapenems were being written for extended-spectrum beta lactamase (ESBL) positive *Escherichia coli* urinary isolates. Upon review, a number of these cases were clinically identified as asymptomatic bacteriuria. Of the documented clinical infections, the majority were diagnosed as cystitis, allowing treatment with alternate, oral agents. By using the CDSS, a customized alert was created to identify patients with ESBL-positive *E. coli* and *Klebsiella* spp. in the urine who were treated with a carbapenem. When the alert was generated, the ASP reviewed the susceptibility report and contacted the clinician whom ordered the carbapenem and recommended fosfomycin. This alert has led to a significant reduction in the use of carbapenems for the treatment of ESBL-positive urinary isolates.

examination rates, appropriateness of therapy selection, and fewer excess total DOT beyond the recommended duration (5 vs. 83 total antifungal days).

Advanced programs with robust add-on CDSS or EMRs allow for manipulation of patient lists in more complex ways using underlying algorithms to generate actionable interventions. For example, a successful penicillin allergy assessment program was undertaken by Chen et al.[21] with initial patient identification starting in the EMR. Any inpatient with a documented penicillin allergy was cross-referenced to remove patients actively receiving antihistamines (which would impact allergy testing). Patients with active discharge orders were also filtered out. The remaining patients were then reviewed for consideration for penicillin allergy testing. Of 228 patients who ultimately underwent testing, 223 (98%) had the penicillin allergy flag removed.

Data Aggregation and Analysis

A strength of any CDSS is the ability to generate reports that can be used to identify opportunities or drive change in practice or process. Each alert, intervention, or action can be measured and then a query generated to produce aggregate reports. Aggregate data can be used to measure quality, medication use opportunities, cost savings, and safety. Quality metrics assessed may include readmissions due to infectious diseases complications, adherence to evidence based guidelines, and appropriateness of initial antibiotic therapy. Medication use opportunities can become apparent through measurement of antibiotic utilization (e.g., DOT or DDD per patient census metric such as per 1,000 patient days). Reports generated can track drug utilization by individual antibiotic, area of the hospital (**Figure 1**), or prescriber (**Figure 2**). Reports in both systems can measure hard and soft costs in an aggregate fashion. An example of "hard costs" is measuring the difference in

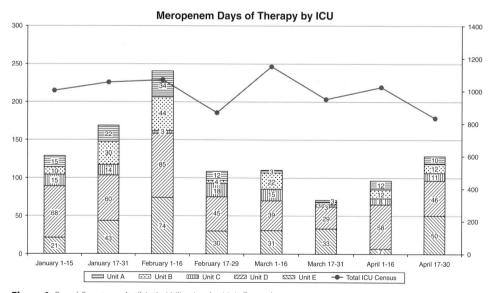

Figure 1 Broad-Spectrum Antibiotic Utilization by Unit Example
In this figure, meropenem utilization data from Electronic Health Record-based reports is downloaded and cross-plotted against total ICU days to monitor trends and to identify which unit of the hospital has the highest prescribing rates of meropenem.

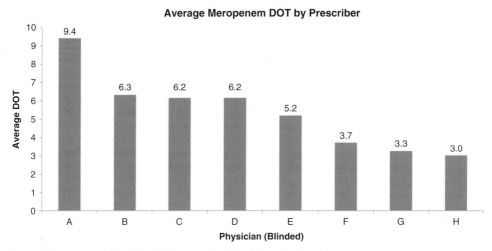

Figure 2 Meropenem Utilization in DOT Per 1,000 Patient Days by Prescriber
In this figure, total DOT and total number of patients by individual prescriber are downloaded from the EMR-based reports and then transposed for graphic output. Physician names are intentionally blinded.

costs for IV vs. oral therapy by drug as part of an IV to oral conversion program or costs savings associated with a measured reduction in antibiotic utilization. "Soft costs," or costs that do not impact the budgetary bottom line, might include total number of PK levels reviewed each month or process measures such as redundant therapy events.

Lessons Learned

Integrating clinical decision support into a new ASP can be overwhelming upon initial start. There can be anywhere from 10 to 100 actionable alerts preprogrammed in the system, and it is very difficult to manage all of them. One approach is to query the CDSS end users and/ or ASP subject matter experts to identify the target areas where the system may be helpful in driving or sustaining change. Once these target areas are identified, the initiatives should be categorized into high, medium, and low priority. One suggestion is to cross plot each of the initiatives on a scatter diagram so that the x axis represents priority and the y axis represents degree of difficulty. The high priority items should be manageable (i.e., no more than 5) and obtainable without significant investment in time or programming resources. Once these are on track or completed, then the ASP team can work numerically through the list, implementing medium and low priority alerts based on resource requirements to operationalize. In addition, if the alerts built into a system are standardized across multiple hospitals, a committee or streamlined alert approval process should be developed to allow for efficient approval and implementation of new alerts or changes to existing alerts.

One of the most significant challenges that accompany implementing a CDSS is managing the impact on workflow. This analysis should not be rushed during the implementation phase as it can impact productivity, system adoption, and patient safety. The analysis should answer the questions of who will receive the alerts (e.g., by practitioner type, location of the hospital, or shift) and how the alert view should be customized such that it only displays information needed to allow efficient and accurate review of the intervention opportunity. Post-implementation, ongoing analysis must be performed to review the differences between actionable alerts and real interventions in order to measure system efficiency. The goal is to have the number of actionable alerts be as close to the number of interventions as possible. The narrower the gap, the more relevant the rules.

Workload analysis for the system administrators should also be considered due to the need for continued maintenance of alerts to ensure accuracy and to maximize return on time investment. In one study of a 793-bed academic medical center, 399,979 individual alerts were triggered over a single year, with an average of one alert firing every 80 seconds.[22] The system managers were able to suppress 325 of the 417 master alerts. This reduced alert fatigue and allowed the pharmacists to focus on alerts that had a high likelihood of resulting in an intervention. The method in which information is shared from shift to shift should also be determined. For example, pending trough levels in a patient receiving vancomycin may not be finalized until the next shift. Therefore, having an area to document notes for information transfer during handoffs in care is important to ensure consistency.

Regardless of whether an add-on or EMR-based system is used, there should be a clear method for documenting and tracking interventions. First, all stakeholders should agree about whether or not interventions will be consistently documented as part of the medical record, or only visible to members of the ASP or pharmacy. Second, there should be a consistent manner of documentation with standardized terminology, that is quantifiable and able to be monitored. The ability to display the data gathered and the interventions that have been successful are crucial to demonstrating the impact of the ASP.

Conclusion

CDSS, either commercially available or EMR-based, should be considered key components of any ASP. The technology can efficiently identify patients who are candidates for antibiotic de-escalation, escalation, renal dosing, and intravenous to oral conversion, and may be customizable to include other actionable alerts. These systems provide useful reports on frequency of therapeutic interventions, staff performance, and financial cost savings. They can rapidly accelerate the development of antibiograms through on-demand reporting. Finally, some systems can provide predictive diagnostic capabilities to help improve the accuracy of diagnosis and treatment outcomes based on individual and aggregate data. The challenge is to determine which type of CDSS will best fulfill the needs of an institution in a cost-efficient, and workflow efficient manner.

References

1. Eicher J, Das M. Challenges and barriers to clinical decision support (CDS) design and implementation experienced in the agency for healthcare research and quality cds demonstrations. Prepared for the AHRQ National Resource Center for Health Information Technology under Contract No. 290–04–0016.). AHRQ Publication No. 10–0064-EF. Rockville, MD: Agency for Healthcare Research and Quality, 2010.

2. Evans RS, Pestonik SL, Classen DC, et al. A computer-assisted management program for antibiotics and other antiinfective agents. N Engl J Med 1998; 338(4):232–8.

3. Pestonik SL, Classen DC, Evans RS, Burke JP. Implementing antibiotic practice guidelines through computer-assisted decision support: clinical and financial outcomes. Ann Intern Med 1996; 124 (10):884–90.

4. Goertzel G. Clinical decision support system. Ann N Y Acad Sci 1969; 161(2):689–693.

5. Pestonik SL, Evans RS, Burke JP, Gardner RM, Classen DC. Therapeutic antibiotic monitoring: surveillance using a

computerized expert system. *Am J Med* 1990; 88(1):43–48.

6. Forrest GN, VanSchooneveld TC, Kullar R, Schulz LT, Duong P, Postelnick M. Use of electronic health records and clinical decision support systems for antimicrobial stewardship. *Clin Infect Dis* 2014; 59(Suppl 3):S122–133.

7. Kullar R, Goff DA, Schulz LT, Fox BC, Rose WE. The "epic" challenge of optimizing antimicrobial stewardship: the role of electronic medical records and technology. *Clin Infect Dis* 2013; 57 (7):1005–1013.

8. Electronic Medical Record Systems. Health Information Technology. (Accessed May 1, 2017, at https://healthit.ahrq.gov/ key-topics/electronic-medical-record-systems.)

9. Garrett PAS, Seidman J. EMR vs EHR – what is the difference. HealthITBuzz 2011. (Accessed May 1, 2017 at www.healthit.gov/buzz-blog/electronic-health-and-medical-records/emr-vs-ehr-difference/.)

10. Vaidya A. Epic, Cerner hold 50% of hospital EHR market share: 8 things to know. *Health Information Technology* 2017. (Accessed May 1, 2017 at www.beckershospitalreview.com/ healthcare-information-technology/epic-cerner-hold-50-of-hospital-ehr-market-share-8-things-to-know.html.)

11. Center for Medicare and Medicaid Services, Electronic health records (EHR) incentive programs. 2017. (Accessed at www.cms.gov/Regulations-and-Guidance/ Legislation/EHRIncentivePrograms/.)

12. Pogue JM, Potoski BA, Prostelnik M, et al. Bringing the "power" to Cerner's PowerChart for antimicrobial stewardship. *Clin Infect Dis* 2014; 59(3):416–424.

13. Gonzales R, Anderer T, McCulloch CE, et al. A cluster randomized trial of decision support strategies for reducing antibiotic use in acute bronchitis. *JAMA Intern Med* 2013; 173(4):267–273.

14. Centers for Disease Control. NHSN antimicrobial use and resistance module. (Accessed May 2, 2017, at www.cdc.gov/ nhsn/pdfs/pscmanual/ 11pscaurcurrent.pdf.)

15. Clinical and Laboratory Standards Institute, Analysis and presentation of cumulative antimicrobial susceptibility test data; approved guideline. 4th ed. CLSI document M39-A4. 2014.

16. Treat systems antimicrobial stewardship. (Accessed May 2, 2016, at www.treatsystems.com/.)

17. Teqqa antimicrobial stewardship. (Accessed May 2, 2017, at www.teqqa.com/ stewardship/.)

18. Patel JA, Esterly JS, Scheetz MH, Postelmick MJ. An analysis of the accuracy of physician-entered indications on computerized antimicrobial orders. *Infect Control Hosp Epidemiol* 2012; 33 (10):1066–1067.

19. Hermsen ED, Vanschooneveld TC, Sayles H, Rupp ME. Implementation of a clinical decision support system for antimicrobial stewardship. *Infect Control Hosp Epidemiol* 2012; 33(4):412–415.

20. Antworth A, Collins CD, Kunapuli A, et al. Impact of an antimicrobial stewardship program comprehensive care bundle on management of candidemia. *Pharmacotherapy* 2013; 33(2):137–143.

21. Chen JR, Tarver SA, Alvarez KS, Tran T, Khan DA. A proactive approach to penicillin allergy testing in hospitalized patients. *J Allergy Clin Immunology Pract* 2017; 5(3):686–693.

22. Hohlfelder B, Stashek C, Anger KE, Szumita PM. Utilization of a pharmacy clinical surveillance system for pharmacist alerting and communication at a tertiary academic medical center. *J Med Syst* 2016; 40(1):24.

Antibiotic Allergies and Antibiotic Stewardship

Keith W. Hamilton and Holly D. Maples

Background

Allergies to antibiotics are frequently reported in medical practice. Penicillin is the most commonly reported antibiotic allergy, described in 5%–15% of all patients, followed by sulfa antibiotics (Table 1).[1–4] Risk factors for drug allergies include female gender and a prior history of allergies to other medications.[5–7] Overall, 15.3% of patients report an allergy to at least one antibiotic class, 2.5% to 2 classes, and 0.8% to 3 or more classes.[7] The types of reactions reported by patients with multiple drug allergies are variable, and some likely represent non-immunologic reactions. The mechanisms behind these risk factors are not well understood. Although not an independent risk factor for development of antibiotic allergies, history of asthma or other allergic conditions increase the risk of *severe* drug reactions such as anaphylaxis.

Uncertainty can exist among healthcare providers and patients on the appropriate classification of and approach to antibiotic allergies, leading to inappropriate treatment and adverse outcomes. Better understanding of antibiotic allergies and potential interventions to improve antibiotic prescribing related to antibiotic allergies are essential for a robust antibiotic stewardship program (ASP). Even if ASPs do not undertake formal interventions to address antibiotic allergies, being versed in the appropriate evaluation and classification of antibiotic allergies is essential to making appropriate antibiotic recommendations. This chapter will review important characteristics and outcomes of patients with antibiotic allergies as well as how ASPs can leverage this information to promote more appropriate antibiotic prescribing.

Classification of Adverse Events Related to Antibiotics

Ultimately, the decision to prescribe an antibiotic in the setting of a prior adverse reaction must be made by carefully assessing the risks and benefits of an antibiotic in a given clinical context. This risk assessment can be facilitated by systematically categorizing adverse reactions. There are two main categories of adverse reactions to antibiotics: type A and type B reactions (Figure 1). Both types of reactions are clinically relevant, but the implications and approach to these reactions often differ.

Type A reactions, which make up at least 85% of all adverse reactions to drugs, are largely dose-dependent, related to the known pharmacologic properties of the drug, and usually reversible. They can be further characterized by severity with mild reactions including diarrhea, nausea, and vomiting as well as severe reactions including QT prolongation, nephrotoxicity, and hepatitis. Patients at increased risk for these reactions include those with drug-drug interactions and underlying organ dysfunction. Of type

Table 1 Incidence of Reported Antibiotic Allergies

Antibiotic	Percentage of Patients Reporting Allergies
Penicillin	5–15
Sulfonamide	7–10
Erythromycin	2
Cephalosporin	1.7
Fluoroquinolone	1.2
Tetracycline	1
Vancomycin	0.7
Clindamycin	0.4
Gentamicin	0.3
Clarithromycin	0.3
Nitrofurantoin	0.2
Metronidazole	0.2

Adapted from CE Lee, TR Zembower, MA Fotis, et al. The incidence of antimicrobial allergies in hospitalized patients: implications regarding prescribing patterns and emerging bacterial resistance. *Arch Intern Med* 2000; 160:2819–2822.

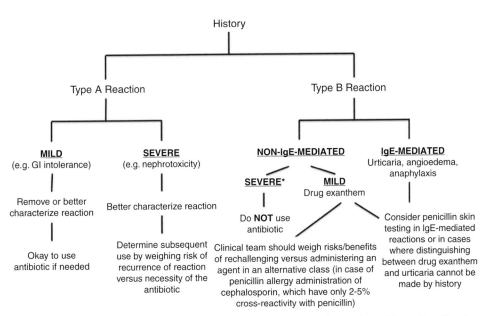

Figure 1 Suggested Approach to Classification and Decision-Making Related to Antibiotic Adverse Drug Reactions
*Severe non-IgE-mediated reactions include reactions such as Stevens-Johnson syndrome, toxic epidermal necrolysis, hemolytic anemia, granulocytopenia, thrombocytopenia, serum sickness, cutaneous or visceral vasculitis, drug reaction with associated eosinophilia and systemic symptoms (DRESS), pneumonitis, hepatitis, and drug-induced systemic lupus erythematosis.

A reactions, gastrointestinal symptoms are the most common. Diarrhea occurs in 5%–10% of patients taking ampicillin, 10%–25% of patients taking amoxicillin-clavulanate, 15%–20% of patients taking cefixime, and 2%–5% of patients receiving other classes of antibiotics including macrolides, fluoroquinolones, and tetracyclines.[8, 9] Patient tolerance and preference should be considered when prescribing any antibiotic, but antibiotics causing mild type A reactions should still be considered if needed with minimal long-term risk to patients. Severe type A reactions are often predictable based on dose and underlying patient risk factors so the decision to prescribe an antibiotic in this setting should be made by considering the severity of the reaction as well as the likelihood of the reaction being reproduced. For instance, in a patient who had QT prolongation in the setting of fluoroquinolone use in the past, future risk may be considered less likely if the patient was previously on other drugs that cause QT prolongation, but is no longer on those drugs, especially if other antibiotic options are deemed less ideal. Nonetheless, close monitoring should be performed in any setting in which there is the potential for a severe reaction.

Most type B reactions are immune-mediated and idiosyncratic. Immune-mediated type B reactions are best classified by their pathophysiology.[10] There are four types of immune-mediated, or hypersensitivity, reactions: type I (immunoglobulin E, or IgE, mediated), type II (cytotoxic), type III (immune complex), and type IV (cellular mediated) (Table 2). Type I reactions are mediated by IgE and symptoms are related to activation of mast cells and basophils after drug exposure. In many cases, patients who develop type I reactions have had prior drug exposure, or sensitization, but lack of prior drug exposure does not preclude presence of type I reaction. Symptoms of type I reaction occur along the spectrum of urticaria, angioedema, and anaphylaxis. Urticaria, the most common and least severe symptom of type I reaction, is characterized by a wheal and flare reaction, or the rapid development of irregular, pruritic, blanched papules on erythematous bases. Wheals can range from pinpoint to several centimeters in diameter and can have an appearance similar to that of mosquito or insect bites. Angioedema is characterized by swelling of the face, extremities, and airways that may lead to respiratory compromise by bronchospasm or asphyxia. Anaphylaxis, the most serious type I reaction, is characterized by the rapid onset over minutes to hours of symptoms that may include urticaria, but also includes life-threatening symptoms such as respiratory compromise and hypotension. Type I reactions typically occur within minutes to hours of exposure to the drug. A reaction that occurs greater than 72 hours after drug exposure can still be mediated by IgE, but the more delayed a reaction is, the less likely it is to be type I.[11]

Type II reactions occur as a result of cytotoxic response to antibodies, typically immunoglobulin G (IgG). Some examples include drug-induced hemolytic anemia, granulocytopenia, and thrombocytopenia. Type III reactions occur as a result of deposition of antigen–antibody complexes and activation of complement. Examples include serum sickness and drug-induced vasculitis. Type IV reactions result from the activation of T cells (type IVc) and occasionally other white blood cells such as macrophages (type IVa), eosinophils (type IVb), and neutrophils (type IVd).[12] Type IV reactions range from mild reactions that may resolve with continued exposure to the drug to severe, life-threatening reactions. More mild reactions include contact dermatitis, morbilliform drug exanthem, and drug fever. Severe reactions include acute generalized exanthematous pustulosis (AGEP), Stevens-Johnson Syndrome (SJS), toxic

Table 2 Classification of Immune-Mediated Type B Drug Reactions

Classification	Pathophysiology	Examples	Characteristics
Type I	IgE activation of mast cells and basophils	Urticaria (hives)	Irregular, pruritic, blanched papules on erythematous base pinpoint to several centimeters in diameter
		Angioedema	Rapid accumulation of edema in the dermis, subcutaneous tissues, and mucosal tissues often of the face and hands
		Bronchospasm	Sudden constriction of bronchiolar muscles causing shortness of breath and wheezing
		Anaphylaxis	Systemic reaction that occurs when previously sensitized patient is re-exposed to a drug with findings that may include pruritic rash, angioedema, and hypotension, or shock occurring minutes to hours after drug exposure
Type II (Cytotoxic)	Antibody (usually IgG) destruction of cells	Hemolytic anemia	Shortness of breath, fatigue, jaundice, dark urine
		Granulocytopenia	Fever, stomatitis, severe infection
		Thrombocytopenia	Bleeding, petechiae
Type III	IgG-immune complex deposition and activation of complement	Vasculitis	Palpable purpura, fever, urticaria, joint pain, lymphadenopathy
		Serum sickness	Fever, purpuric, or urticarial rash, joint pain, lymphadenopathy
Type IV	T-cell mediated reaction	Drug exanthem	Maculopapular rash
		Contact dermatitis	Local erythema with vesicles or bullae and swelling
		Drug fever	Fever is sole symptom of drug reaction
		Stevens-Johnson Syndrome	Blistering of epidermis involving <10% of skin
		Toxic Epidermal Necrolysis	Blistering of epidermis involving >30% of skin
		Drug rash with eosinophilia and systemic symptoms	Rash, fever, eosinophilia, organ involvement (kidney, liver, heart, lungs)
		Acute generalized exanthematous pustulosis	Diffuse cutaneous pustules

epidermal necrolysis (TEN), and drug reaction with eosinophilia and systemic symptoms (DRESS).

Drug exanthems are the most common kind of type B reactions.[11] In many cases of reported allergy, clinicians have to distinguish between drug exanthems and urticarial; this distinction is important because rechallenging a patient with history of urticaria has a risk of precipitating anaphylaxis. Unlike urticaria, drug exanthems are delayed in onset and typically manifest during the second week of initial drug exposure. However, when the same medication is used again, drug exanthems can have a more rapid and widespread onset. Although the rash may have varying appearances, it normally is morbilliform, or consists of erythematous macules or papules that first appear on the face and torso but then may become more generalized. It is generally safe to rechallenge patients who have had drug exanthems to medications. In fact, many cases in which a patient develops a drug exanthem, the rash resolves with continued use of the drug due to the development of tolerance.[11] If the rash does not resolve, antihistamines or topical corticosteroids can be used to control symptoms if the drug is preferred to alternative options.

SJS and TEN are blistering skin reactions to medications that involve mucous membranes as well as skin. The spectrum includes SJS involving less than 10% of the skin area and TEN involving greater than 30%, with intermediate form involving 10%–30% of skin area referred to SJS/TEN. Initial appearance of rash is typically that of red or dusky macules that may become necrotic and eventually blister. These reactions are life threatening and often lead to substantial morbidity. As with other type IV hypersensitivity reactions, they typically occur during the second week of exposure, but may occur more rapidly with reexposure to a drug.[13]

DRESS is a severe drug reaction that involves fever, eosinophilia, diffuse maculopapular rash, and organ involvement. Lymphadenopathy can be found in 30%–60% of cases.[14] Organs involved include the liver (80%), kidneys (40%), and to a lesser extent other organs (38%) including the lungs, heart, pancreas, thyroid, and brain.[11] Some symptoms can occur several weeks after stopping the offending agent.

AGEP is an uncommon reaction that is also associated with fever and rash. The rash is characterized by the formation of pustular lesions on a base of an erythematous coalescent rash.[8] AGEP can also involve mucous membranes and cause swelling of the hands and face. Unlike DRESS, however, internal organ involvement is rare.

In addition, an immune-mediated reaction may occur in response to an antibiotic that is related to administration during concurrent Epstein-Barr virus (EBV) infection. A rash typically occurs in EBV infection with administration of amoxicillin or ampicillin, but has also been described with other antibiotics as well.[15] The mechanisms of these reactions are not completely understood. Although these reactions are immune-mediated, they often do not represent reproducible reactions to the antibiotics themselves so may be mistaken for an antibiotic allergy.

Differentiating between type A and B reactions and within type B reactions among type I, II, III, and IV reactions can help clinicians and ASPs accurately record the nature of drug reactions as well as take informative allergy histories to help guide antibiotic prescribing. A proposed algorithm for approaching antibiotic reactions is depicted in Figure 1. Using a systematic approach, clinicians and ASPs can also make more accurate risk assessments when deciding whether or not to use a particular antibiotic. Accurate assessment of antibiotic reactions is crucial, as antibiotic allergies have significant implications for clinical outcomes.

Cross-Reactivity between Antibiotics and Implications for Antibiotic Stewardship

Because antibiotics within the same class are related to each other as well as to antibiotics in some other classes, a reaction to one antibiotic may have implications for other antibiotics as well. Understanding the cross-reactivity among different antibiotics is crucial for stewardship personnel. The most frequently encountered consideration is the cross-reactivity among beta-lactam antibiotics, including penicillins, cephalosporins, carbapenems, and monobactams because first-line treatment recommendations for most infectious conditions generally fall into one of these classes. Therefore, a reaction to an antibiotic in any of these classes has significant implications on optimal treatment regimens and often forces clinicians to choose less ideal antibiotics. This section focuses on the cross-reactivity among beta-lactam antibiotics because of their importance to clinical practice and because concerns of cross-reactivity among these antibiotics often motivate providers to select less optimal antibiotics.

Penicillin Cross-Reactivity Penicillin and aminopenicillins such as amoxicillin and ampicillin are structurally similar and have high rates of cross-reactivity with 94% of patients with allergic reaction to ampicillin cross-reacting with penicillin determinants.[16] Penicillins and cephalosporins are also structurally similar with both having a beta-lactam ring and sulfur-containing ring.[17] Many also contain similar side chains (Table 3). These similarities would suggest a high rate of cross-reactivity between penicillins and cephalosporins. Initial estimates of cross-reactivity placed estimates of cross-reactivity at least as high as 15% based on clinical and immunologic analysis.[18] However, the degradation products of penicillins and cephalosporins, the molecules that trigger allergic reactions, are significantly different. [19] Later studies suggest that of patients with penicillin allergy, only 5% will have an allergic reaction to first-generation cephalosporins and only 2% will have an allergic reaction to third or fourth-generation cephalosporins.[20] This difference in estimates has been suggested to be due to factors such as the contamination of cephalosporins with penicillin during the manufacturing process and increased similarity in early cephalosporin drugs compared to newer drugs.[18, 20, 21] Older 1st-generation cephalosporins such as cephaloridine and cephalothin have identical side chains to penicillin, whereas newer 1st-generation cephalosporins such as cefadroxil and cephalexin are less related to penicillin.[22] Third and 4th-generation cephalosporins are even more structurally different from penicillin. In assessing the side chains of the beta-lactam rings, it is important to note that penicillins have only one side chain (R1) while cephalosporins have two side chains (R1 and R2), but both could have the same R1 side chain, which explains why some penicillins and cephalosporins have higher cross-reactivity than others.[23, 24]

Carbapenems also have similar structures to penicillins. The original study examining the cross-reactivity between penicillin and imipenem estimated the rate at 47%; however, this study was limited by a small size. More recent studies estimate rate of cross-reactivity at less than 10% but caution should still be practiced in patients with history of severe reactions to penicillin.[25–27] Aztreonam, a monobactam, has been shown to lack cross-reactivity in penicillin allergic patients.[28] Immunogenicity studies have demonstrated that antibodies involved in allergic reactions to aztreonam are directed to the side chain instead of the β-lactam ring.[29]

Cephalosporin Cross-Reactivity Cephalosporin allergies are reported in less than 2% of all patients, but these allergies still have considerable consequences for the treatment of many conditions.[4] For patients with cephalosporin allergies, cross-reactivity does not

Table 3 β-Lactams with Cross-Sensitivity Due to Common Side Chain

Penicillins	Cephalosporins	Monobactams

β-Lactams with Common R1 Side Chains (each column indicates a common side chain)

Amoxicillin	Ampicillin	Benzyl penicillin	Ceftriaxone	Ceftazidime
Cefadroxil	Cephalexin	Cephalothin	Cefuroxime	Aztreonam
Cefatrizine	Cefaclor		Cefotaxime	
Cefprozil	Cephradine		Cefepime	
	Cephaloglycin			
	Loracarbef			

β-Lactams with Common R2 Side Chains (each column indicates a common side chain)

Cephalexin	Cefotaxime	Cefuroxime	Cefotetan	Cefaclor	Cefibuten
Cefadroxil	Cephalothin	Cefoxitin	Cefamandole	Loracarbef	Ceftizoxime
Cephradine	Cephaloglycin		Cefmetazole		
			Cefpiramide		

Adapted from J Trubiano and E Phillips. Antimicrobial stewardship's new weapon? A review of antibiotic allergy and pathways to "de-labeling." *Curr Opin Infect Dis* 2013; 26:526–537.

appear to be class-wide. Studies have shown that patients with cephalosporin allergies can receive a cephalosporin containing a different side chain without adverse reactions.[30, 31] Side chain similarity appears to correlate with likelihood of cross-reactivity among cephalosporins, but this comparison is not entirely predictive (Table 3).[23, 32] However, if the reaction to a cephalosporin is a mild non-IgE-mediated reaction, other cephalosporins, especially those with different side chains may be used. If a patient has an allergic reaction to a cephalosporin, the likelihood that patient will have a reaction to penicillin derivative is unclear; however, this rate is likely small so penicillins should be used in patients with mild non-IgE-mediated reactions if they are deemed the best agents for treatment.[23, 32] In patients with IgE-mediated reactions to cephalosporins, penicillin skin testing, which is discussed later, can be used to determine the safety of using penicillins. The risk of cross-reactivity between cephalosporins and carbapenems is likely minimal with only 1% of patients skin test positive to both cephalosporins and carbapenems.[32] Although there is no cross-reactivity between penicillin and aztreonam, aztreonam does share a side chain with ceftazidime and cross-reactivity between the two agents has been reported clinically.[30, 33, 34]

Carbapenem Cross-Reactivity The current incidence of hypersensitivity to carbapenems is estimated to be less than 11%.[35] Minimal data exist assessing allergic reactions within the carbapenem class. However, one case report cites a patient who developed an allergic reaction to imipenem-cilastatin, but tolerated meropenem.[35] Animal models have also shown this weaker cross-reactivity between meropenem and imipenem-cilastatin.[36] While data support the potential that a different carbapenem could be utilized following an allergic reaction to another carbapenem, caution should be given, and use of another carbapenem should definitely be avoided in cases of severe immune-mediated or IgE-mediated reaction.

Beta-lactams are often preferred treatment options based upon efficacy and tolerability. Because the rates of cross-reactivity between penicillin and other beta-lactams is low, clinicians can consider prescribing beta-lactams to patients who had a penicillin allergy classified as mild type A or a drug exanthem. However, these agents should be avoided in cases where the reaction was a type I reaction or another severe non-type I reaction. Ultimately, the decision to prescribe an antibiotic should consider the following: 1) the certainty with which a prior allergy occurred, 2) the risk of severe reaction upon rechallenge, 3) cross-reactivity between the agent being prescribed and the agent that elicited the previous reaction, and 4) the necessity of giving a particular agent relative to other available options. In some clinical situations, the benefit of using an agent with a low likelihood of cross-reactivity may outweigh the risks.

Implications of Antibiotic Allergies

When patients report an antibiotic allergy, it alters a prescriber's choice of antibiotic approximately 30% of the time.[3] When treated for infections, patients with reported antibiotic allergies often receive broader spectrum, suboptimal, and more toxic therapy than patients without penicillin allergies.[3] Reported antibiotic allergy, especially penicillin allergy, has been associated with increased antibiotic resistance, cost, length of hospital stay, and mortality.[3, 4, 37] Patients with reported penicillin allergy receive significantly more fluoroquinolones, clindamycin, and vancomycin compared with patients who do not report such allergies.[3, 4, 37] Patients with reported antibiotic allergies are approximately 40% more likely to be admitted to an intensive care unit and 60% more likely to experience in-hospital mortality.[2] Reported allergy has also been associated with decreased adherence to guidelines and greater risk of readmission for infection in certain populations.[38] Because of these consequences, clarification of allergies by clinicians and the ASP has the potential to improve patient outcomes.

Clarification of Reported Allergy through History

Although the incidence of reported penicillin allergy ranges from 5% to 10%, the incidence of life-threatening reaction ranges from only 0.004% to 0.015%.[4] Even though the rates of severe allergy are low, they should be taken seriously in all situations in which a patient may be at risk. However, appropriate history can better classify most of these reactions. Patients with an antibiotic allergy recorded in their medical records often have not had appropriate investigation into the nature of the reaction. Mild type A reactions, such as gastrointestinal intolerance, are often recorded as an allergy, inappropriately classified, and perpetuated in the medical record as "true" allergic reactions. In fact, up to 68% of allergies in the medical record lack documentation as to the nature and severity of the reaction, and 22% have major discrepancies from verbal history provided by the patient.[39, 40] Electronic medical records allow many different types of medical providers to enter allergy information, making quality assurance of allergy information challenging. De-labeling inappropriate allergies in these settings has the potential to improve patient outcomes and stewardship efforts by decreasing broad-spectrum antibiotic use and increasing appropriate therapy.

There are several components of an effective history that can help to characterize antibiotic reactions (Table 4). An initial objective of the history is to classify the reaction as a type A reaction such as diarrhea or nephrotoxicity or a type B such as rash or anaphylaxis. If the antibiotic caused a rash, inquiring about the nature of the rash is important. Key queries about a rash include *location* classified as local or generalized; *extent* classified as estimate of proportion of body surface area and involving or not involving mucous membranes; and *description* classified as raised, flat, blistering, or pustular and pruritic or non-pruritic. Inquiry should also evaluate the presence of systemic symptoms including fever, respiratory symptoms, edema particularly of the hands and face, and organ involvement. Other questions should focus on the severity of the reaction, specifically whether it led to hospitalization or ICU admission.

Characteristics that would suggest a type I or IgE-mediated reaction, include the presence of a pruritic, raised rash that may appear similar to mosquito bites, swelling of the hands and face, hypotension or shock, and shortness of breath. Urticaria is incredibly pruritic so if a rash is not pruritic, it almost certainly is *not* urticaria. Qualities that would suggest a drug exanthem, or mild type IV reaction, include morbilliform rash and *lack* of all of the following symptoms: fever, respiratory symptoms, edema of the hands and face, involvement of mucous membranes, and hospital admission. The presence of any of these findings indicates a more severe reaction and suggests that the reported allergy was unlikely a mild drug exanthem. Even after a systematic evaluation, some patients still may not be able to recall the nature of the reaction so the reaction has to be classified as unknown.

Another important question when evaluating a type I reaction is time since reaction. Up to 80% of patients with true IgE-mediated reactions lose anti-penicillin IgE antibodies after 10 years, and many patients who skin test positive for penicillin allergy will revert to negative over time (Figure 2).[41, 42] In addition, older patients are less likely to have a positive skin test to penicillin than younger patients (Figure 3).[41, 42]

Table 4 Type B Adverse Drug Reactions and Associated Symptoms

Clinical Manifestation	Type I	Type II	Type III		Type IV			
	Hives Angioedema Anaphylaxis	Hemolytic anemia Thrombocytopenia Agranulocytosis	Vasculitis	Serum sickness	Drug Exanthem	TEN/ SJS	DRESS	AGEP
Rash								
Hives	✓	–	✓	✓	–	–	–	–
Morbilliform	–	–	–	✓	✓	–	✓	–
Blisters	–	–	–	–	–	✓	–	–
Pustules	–	–	–	–	–	–	–	✓
Palpable purpura	–	✓	✓	✓	–	–	–	–
Mucosal involvement	✓	–	✓	–	–	✓	✓	–
Typical Onset	Minutes to hours	1–3 weeks	1–3 weeks	1–3 weeks	1–3 weeks	1–3 weeks	1–3 weeks	<48 hours
Systemic Symptoms								
Fever	–	–	✓	✓	–	✓	✓	✓
Respiratory symptoms	✓	–	–	–	–	–	✓	–
Edema	✓	–	✓	✓	–	–	✓	✓
Lymphadenopathy	–	–	✓	✓	–	–	✓	–
Hepatitis	–	–	–	–	–	–	✓	✓
Leukocytosis	–	–	–	✓	–	–	✓	✓
Eosinophilia	–	–	–	–	–	–	✓	✓
Hospital/ICU Admission	✓	–	✓	✓	–	✓	✓	✓

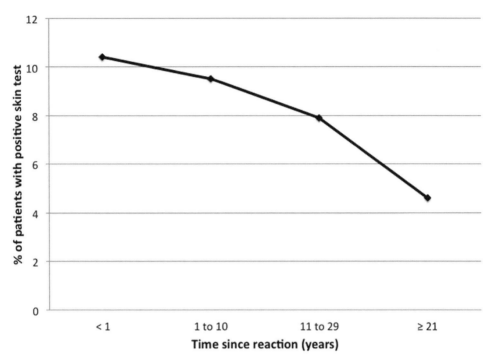

Figure 2 Correlation of the Proportion of Positive Skin Tests with Time Since Reaction
Adapted from TJ Sullivan, HJ Wedner, GS Shatz, et al. Skin testing to detect penicillin allergy. *J Allergy Clin Immunol* 1981; 68:171–180.

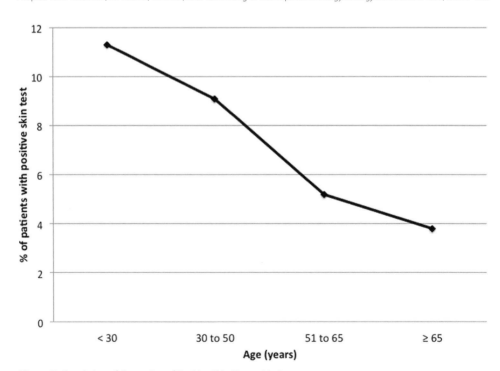

Figure 3 Correlation of Proportion of Positive Skin Tests with Age
Adapted from TJ Sullivan, HJ Wedner, GS Shatz, et al. Skin testing to detect penicillin allergy. *J Allergy Clin Immunol* 1981; 68:171–180.

Inquiring whether a patient has received and tolerated another antibiotic in the same or similar class subsequent to the reaction can also be informative. In the case of penicillin allergy, if a patient has received an antibiotic such as an aminopenicillin, cephalosporin, or carbapenem after the reported penicillin allergy occurred, these agents could be administered safely without additional testing. Reviewing the patient's medical record for historical information can also be helpful, especially for prior antibiotic exposure. In many cases, a patient may not recall the receipt of certain antibiotics, but the ASP team may find that these antibiotics were administered safely in the past by another prescriber and thus can be given again.

Reported allergies have a significant effect on antibiotic prescribing decisions. However, records of these allergies are fraught with inaccuracies. Education of prescribers as well as centralized efforts by stewardship personnel to clarify reported allergies offers a promising strategy to improve antibiotic prescribing.

The Role of Skin Testing to Clarify Allergy

Skin testing can be used as a supplement to historical evaluation of allergy because it can be used to determine the likelihood of type I reactions (Figure 1). Penicillin is the only drug with a commercially available skin test in the United States.

Type I reactions to penicillin occur following a process of degradation and haptenation. After the drug is administered, penicillin breaks down to smaller molecules. However, these molecules are too small to elicit an allergic response but can be bound by proteins called haptens, a process called haptenation. The complex of penicillin intermediate and hapten can trigger a reaction in the sensitized patient.[3] The reactive intermediates of penicillin are referred to as major determinants and minor determinants, with the major determinant benzylpenicilloyl polylysine representing 85% to 90% of all intermediates while the minor determinants comprise the remaining 10%–15%.[3]

The penicillin skin testing procedure should utilize both major and minor determinants of penicillin because using benzylpenicilloyl polylysine alone can miss up to 30% of type I penicillin allergies (Table 5).[3] If both major and minor determinants are used, penicillin skin testing has a 97%–99% negative predictive value and a 50% positive predictive value.[3] The skin test should also utilize positive (histamine) and negative (normal saline) controls. Because only the major determinant benzylpenicilloyl polylysine is available in the United States, diluted penicillin G should be used as a substitute for the minor determinants. The process of skin testing begins with introducing the reagents via a skin prick, and, if the test is negative, these same reagents are introduced via intradermal injection. If either of these steps elicits a reaction to one of the penicillin determinants and the normal saline control is negative, the test is considered positive. If the positive control is negative or the negative control is positive, the test is considered indeterminate. If skin testing is negative, a single dose of a beta-lactam such as amoxicillin or penicillin V potassium can be administered or a graded challenge with escalating doses of the desired antibiotic can be performed subsequently to confirm drug tolerability. If a patient has a positive skin test, penicillin and related drugs should be avoided, but desensitization can be performed if use of a beta-lactam is necessary.

Because skin testing evaluates only the possibility of a type I reaction, it cannot exclude the presence of another type of reaction.[7, 43, 44] However, if a provider needs to distinguish between a type I and a type IV drug exanthem and cannot do so by history

Table 5 Procedure for Performing Penicillin Skin Testing

Step	Components
Preparation	Label sections on each arm with a pen to make areas for each reagent: (1) benzylpenicilloyl polylysine (major determinant) (6.0×10^{-5} mol/L), (2) penicillin G (minor determinant) (10,000 units/mL), (3) histamine (positive control) (1 mg/mL), and (4) normal saline (negative control) (0.9%). Use alcohol-based disinfectant on the arm prior to performing the test. Ensure epinephrine, steroids, and diphenhydramine are available in case of severe IgE-mediated reaction.
Skin prick test	Place 1–2 drops of each reagent in the area of the corresponding label. Puncture the skin at the site of the drop with a sterile 22--28-guage or bifurcating needle using twisting motion. Use a new needle for each reagent. Observe for 15 minutes for any reaction. • **Positive**: wheal with zone or erythema ≥3 mm in diameter compared to negative control. • **Indeterminate**: absence of positive control reaction or wheal from positive control similar in size to that of negative control. • **Negative**: absence of wheal or diameter <3 mm in diameter compared to negative control.
Intradermal test	If the skin prick test is negative, inject 0.02 mL of each reagent intradermally using 26- to 30-gauage, short-bevel needle. Observe for 15 minutes. Results are interpreted similar to skin prick test.
Penicillin challenge	If the intradermal test is negative, patients should receive a challenge with either 500 mg of oral penicillin V potassium or amoxicillin. Observe for 60 minutes. Another option is the graded challenge, which may be performed by starting at 1/100 to 1/10 of the planned starting dose and escalate the dose in a graded fashion every 30–60 minutes as tolerated.

Consultation with a clinician experienced in performing penicillin skin testing should be performed prior to implementing penicillin skin testing. Testing should be performed only by a provider who has been trained to place and interpret the skin test. Adapted from NR Unger, TP Gauthier, LW Cheung. Penicillin skin testing: potential implications for antimicrobial stewardship. *Pharmacotherapy* 2013; 33:856–867.

alone, evaluation of the possibility of a type I reaction is still helpful. In addition, if the nature of a penicillin allergy remains unknown despite focused history, penicillin skin testing can help to exclude type I reaction. Based on the given clinical situation, exclusion of type I reaction may be sufficient to administer a beta-lactam antibiotic following a dose or graded challenge. Penicillin skin testing should not be performed to evaluate patients with severe non-IgE-mediated reactions such as TEN and Stevens-Johnson syndrome. The skin test cannot predict recurrence of these reactions, and therefore the antibiotic suspected to have caused these reactions should be avoided outright, and healthcare providers should counsel patients to permanently avoid these medications as well as other structurally related drugs.

Skin testing is a limited resource and may not be convenient in certain settings because the process takes several hours. Therefore, certain patient populations or infection types must be prioritized for effective utilization of skin testing. Clinical pathways, developed in collaboration with allergists, can be developed by the ASP to guide appropriate testing. Infections that can be prioritized are those in which penicillin or beta-lactam antibiotics offer a clear treatment advantage over other classes of antibiotics or in infections in which a broader spectrum or more expensive antibiotic would otherwise be used.[45] Patient populations that can be prioritized are those in settings in which skin testing would be practical or those in which antibiotics are likely to be administered. One such setting in which skin testing has been effective is in preoperative evaluation, as these patients will certainly receive antibiotics in the perioperative setting.

Penicillin skin testing does have limitations. As previously noted, it can evaluate for only type I reactions. Therefore, it is arguably most useful in cases where a strong suspicion for prior type I reaction exists based on history or in cases where differentiating between drug exanthem and urticaria is difficult by history alone. Interpreting skin tests in certain patient populations can also be challenging because many patients in the inpatient and ambulatory settings have received antihistamines, steroids, and other immunosuppressive medications, which may interfere with test performance. If possible, medications that could affect the performance of the skin test should be held for at least 72 hours prior to skin testing. However, the test does include a positive histamine control, allowing clinicians interpreting the test to classify a test as invalid, or indeterminate, if a patient does not react to the histamine. In addition, many hospitalized patients, especially in the ICU, have anasarca or diffuse edema, which makes interpretation of the test challenging. Some studies have reported an indeterminate skin testing rate of 10%–20% in the ICU.[46] Although the negative predictive value of penicillin skin testing is quite high, there are rare instances where the antibiotic challenges precipitate potentially severe reactions so testing should be performed in the appropriate setting with trained personnel. These limitations are not reasons to avoid penicillin skin testing, but should be taken into account when interpreting and performing the test. Allergists have expertise in interpretation of skin testing in complicated situations. Because of the complexity of interpretation, consultation with an allergist experienced in performing and interpreting penicillin skin testing should be undertaken before implementing this strategy of antibiotic stewardship. Determination of which providers should perform and interpret the skin testing should be made in the context of the patient population, provider expertise, and available personnel.

Use of Allergy De-Labeling to Enhance Antibiotic Stewardship

Because reported antibiotic allergies are associated with worse clinical outcomes, implementation of strategies to de-label penicillin allergies when they are inaccurate or inactive has the potential to improve clinical care. Several retrospective case-control studies in the inpatient setting demonstrate that patients who have had a negative penicillin skin test are less likely to receive alternative therapy. Medications such as vancomycin, aminoglycosides, fluoroquinolones, clindamycin, and broad-spectrum cephalosporins were stopped in 52%–73% of patients after a negative skin test in acute care hospitals.[3, 46–48] Rates of positive penicillin skin testing in this setting were low, ranging from 10% to 12%, and there were no adverse events reported in the cases that received skin testing. Use of de-labeling interventions in the ICU setting has also been shown to be feasible with 82% of patients who tested negative changed to a beta-lactam antibiotic.[46] No adverse events were found in this study either, but there was a relatively high rate of indeterminate testing of 10%, likely due to factors more common among ICU patients such as presence of anasarca and use of antihistamines and immunosuppressive medications. In the emergency department, use of penicillin skin testing was also demonstrated to be feasible and if used to direct antibiotic prescribing would have improved cost savings and increased guideline adherence.[49] De-labeling has also been shown to be both feasible and effective in certain specialized populations with high rates of antibiotic exposure. In the perioperative setting, same-day skin testing has been performed in preoperative clinics.[50] Up to 95% of patients had a negative skin test and patients with negative skin tests had lower use rates of vancomycin and other alternative antibiotics with no adverse events.

Several studies have demonstrated minimum to moderate cost savings when penicillin skin testing is used. However, there are limitations to some of these studies because they do not consider at least one of several key cost elements including skin test reagent(s), personnel cost to place and interpret test, cost of allergy specialist consultation, and clinical outcomes.[45, 51] Although the economic impact of skin testing is unclear, it is very likely at the least a cost neutral method of decreasing the use of broad-spectrum antibiotics. Because skin testing is a limited resource, various testing algorithms have been proposed, but design of these programs should be based on local resources and should focus on highest yield patient populations and settings.[45]

Different methods of identifying patients for antibiotic de-labeling include diagnosis-based identification (e.g., bacteremia, endocarditis, meningitis), condition-based identification (e.g., hematologic malignancy, preoperative), and antibiotic-based identification (e.g., patients receiving aminoglycoside, clindamycin, fluoroquinolone). Collaboration between ASPs and allergy specialists has the potential for identification and de-labeling of patients who have high likelihood of receiving an antibiotic, are receiving less optimal antibiotics, or are undergoing treatment for conditions in which beta-lactam antibiotics are clearly preferred.

Conclusion

In light of suboptimal antibiotic choices, inferior clinical outcomes, and increased antibiotic resistance observed in patients who report antibiotic allergies, ASPs should at least be competent in the evaluation and characterization of antibiotic allergies in order to make sound recommendations to prescribers. For those programs with the available resources, programs designed to de-label antibiotic allergies including those incorporating penicillin skin testing offers an innovative, cost-effective, and safe strategy to enhance antibiotic stewardship programs in a variety of healthcare settings.

References

1. Macy E, Contreras R. Health care use and serious infection prevalence associated with penicillin "allergy" in hospitalized patients: a cohort study. *J Allergy Clin Immunol* 2014; 133:790–796.

2. Charneski L, Deshpande G, Smith SW. Impact of an antimicrobial allergy label in the medical record on clinical outcomes in hospitalized patients. *Pharmacotherapy* 2011; 31:742–747.

3. Unger NR, Gauthier TP, Cheung LW. Penicillin skin testing: potential implications for antimicrobial stewardship. *Pharmacotherapy* 2013; 33:856–867.

4. Lee CE, Zembower TR, Fotis MA, et al. The incidence of antimicrobial allergies in hospitalized patients: implications regarding prescribing patterns and emerging bacterial resistance. *Arch Intern Med* 2000; 160:2819–2822.

5. Park MA1, Matesic D, Markus PJ, Li JT. Female sex as a risk factor for penicillin allergy. *Ann Allergy Asthma Immunol* 2007; 99:54–58.

6. Moseley EK, Sullivan TJ. Allergic reactions to antimicrobial drugs in patients with a

history of prior drug allergy. *J Allergy Clin Immunol* 1991; 87:226.

7. Macy E, Poon K-Y. Self-reported antibiotic allergy incidence and prevalence: age and sex effects. *Am J Med* 2009; 122:778.

8. Bartlett JG. Antibiotic-associated diarrhea. *Clin Infect Dis* 1992;15:573–581.

9. Gilbert DN. Aspects of the safety profile of oral antimicrobial agents. *Infect Dis Clin Pract* 1995; 4(Suppl 2):S103–S112.

10. Solensky R, Khan DA. Evaluation of antibiotic allergy: the role of skin tests and drug challenges. *Curr Allergy Asthma Rep* 2014; 14:459.

11. Rive CM, Bourke J, Phillips EJ. Testing for drug hypersensitivity syndromes. *Clin Biochem Rev* 2013; 34:15–38.

12. Pichler WJ. Delayed drug hypersensitivity reactions. *Ann Intern Med* 2003; 139:683–693.

13. Bastuji-Garin S, Rzany B, Stern RS, et al. Clinical classification of cases of toxic epidermal necrolysis, Stevens-Johnson syndrome, and erythema multiforme. *Arch Dermatol* 1993; 129:92.

14. Cacoub P, Musette P, Descamps V, et al. The DRESS syndrome: a literature review. *Am J Med.* 2011; 124:588.

15. McCloskey GL, Massa MC. Cephalexin rash in infectious mononucleosis. *Cutis* 1997; 59:251–254.

16. Romano A, Torres MJ, Fernandez J, et al. Allergic reactions to ampicillin: studies on the specificity and selectivity in subjects with immediate reactions. *Clin Exp Allergy* 1997; 27:1425–1431.

17. Petz LD. Immunologic cross-reactivity between penicillins and cephalosporins: a review. *J Infect Dis* 1978. 137 (Suppl):S74–79.

18. Newton GG, Hamilton-Miller JMT. Cephaloridine: chemical and biochemical aspects. *Postgrad Med* 1967; 43:10–13.

19. Park MA, Li JT. Diagnosis and management of penicillin allergy. *Mayo Clin Proc* 2005; 80:405–410.

20. Anne S, Reisman RE. Risk of administering cephalosporin antibiotics to patients with histories of penicillin allergy. *Ann Allergy Asthma Immunol* 1995; 74:167–170.

21. Joint Task Force on Practice Parameters, American Academy of Allergy, Asthma and Immunology; American College of Allergy, Asthma and Immunology; Joint Council of Allergy, Asthma and Immunology. Drug allergy: an updated practice parameter. *Ann Allergy Asthma Immunol* 2010; 105:259–273.

22. Trubiano J, Phillips E. Antimicrobial stewardship's new weapon? A review of antibiotic allergy and pathways to "de-labeling." *Curr Opin Infect Dis* 2013; 26:526–537.

23. Antunez C, Blanca-Lopez N, Torres MJ. Immediate allergic reactions to cephalosporins: evaluation of cross-reactivity with a panel of penicillins and cephalosporins. *J Allergy Clin Immunol* 2006; 117:404–410.

24. Miranda A, Blanca M, Vega JM, et al. Cross-reactivity between a penicillin and a cephalosporin with the same side chain. *J Allergy Clin Immunol* 1996; 98:671–677.

25. Romano A, Viola M, Guéant-Rodriguez RM, et al. Imipenem in patients with immediate hypersensitivity to penicillins. *N Engl J Med* 2006; 354:2835–2837.

26. Saxon A, Adelman DC, Patel A, et al. Imipenem cross-reactivity with penicillin in humans. *J Allergy Clin Immunol* 1988; 82:213–217.

27. Prescott WA Jr., Kusmierski KA. Clinical importance of carbapenem hypersensitivity in patients with self-reported and documented penicillin allergy. *Pharmacotherapy* 2007; 27:137–142.

28. Gaeta F, Valluzzi RL, Alonzi C, et al. Tolerability of aztreonam and carbapenems in patients with IgE-mediated hypersensitivity to penicillins. *J Allergy Clin Immunol* 2015; 135:972–976.

29. Adkinson NF, Swabb EA, Sugerman AA. Immunology of the monobactam aztreonam. *Antimicrob Agents Chemother* 1984; 25:93–97.

30. Romano A, Gaeta F, Valluzzi RL, et al. IgE-mediated hypersensitivity to cephalosporins: cross-reactivity and

tolerability of penicillins, monobactams, and carbapenems. *J Allergy Clin Immunol* 2010; 126:994–999.

31. Romano A, Gaeta F, Valluzzi RL, et al. IgE-mediated hypersensitivity to cephalosporins: cross-reactivity and tolerability of alternative cephalosporins. *J Allergy Clin Immunol* 2015; 136:685–691.

32. Romano A, Gaeta F, Valluzzi RL, et al. IgE-mediated hypersensitivity to cephalosporins: cross-reactivity and tolerability of penicillins, monobactams, and carbapenems. *J Allergy Clin Immunol* 2010; 126:994–999.

33. Pérez Pimiento A, Gómez Martínez M, Mínguez Mena A, et al. Aztreonam and ceftazidime: evidence of in vivo cross allergenicity. *Allergy* 1998; 53:624–625.

34. Frumin J, Gallagher JC. Allergic cross-sensitivity between penicillin, carbapenem, and monobactam antibiotics: what are the chances? *Ann Pharmacother* 2009; 43:304–315.

35. Bauer SL, Wall GC, Skoglund K, Peters LK. Lack of cross-reactivity to meropenem in a patient with an allergy to imipenem-cilastatin. *J Allergy Clin Immunol* 2004; 113:173–175.

36. Nakanishi T, Kohda A, Kato T, et al. Antigenicity tests of meropenem. *Chemotherapy* (Tokyo) 1992; 40:251–257.

37. Neuman MI, Kelley M, Harper MB, et al. Factors associated with antimicrobial resistance and mortality in pneumococcal bacteremia. *J Emerg Med* 2007; 23:349–357.

38. Trubiano JA, Leung VK, Chu MY, et al. The impact of antimicrobial allergy labels on antimicrobial usage in cancer patients. *Antimicrob Resist Infect Control* 2015; 4:23.

39. Weingart SN, Toth M, Sands DZ, et al. Physicians' decisions to override computerized drug alerts in primary care. *Arch Intern Med* 2003; 163:2625–2631.

40. Lutomski DM, LaFollette JA, Biaglow MA, Haglund LA. Antibiotic allergies in the medical record: effect on drug selection and assessment of validity. *Pharmacotherapy* 2008; 28:1348–1353.

41. Fernandez T, Torres MJ, R-Pena R, et al. Decrease of selective immunoglobulin E response to amoxicillin despite repeated administration of benzylpenicillin and penicillin V. *Clin Exp Allergy* 2005; 35:1645–1650.

42. Sullivan TJ, Wedner HJ, Shatz GS, et al. Skin testing to detect penicillin allergy. *J Allergy Clin Immunol* 1981; 68:171–180.

43. Macy E, Ho NJ. Adverse reactions associated with therapeutic antibiotic use after penicillin skin testing. *Perm J* 2011; 15:31–37.

44. Macy E, Ho NJ. Multiple drug intolerance syndrome: prevalence, clinical characteristics, and management. *Ann Allergy Asthma Immunol* 2012; 108:88–93.

45. Forrest DM, Schellenberg R, Thien VV, et al. Introduction of a practice guideline for penicillin skin testing improves the appropriateness of antibiotic therapy. *Clin Infect Dis* 2001; 32:1685–1690.

46. Arroliga ME, Radojicic C, Gordon SM, et al. A prospective observational study of the effect of penicillin skin testing on antibiotic use in the intensive care unit. *Infect Control Hosp Epidemiol* 2003; 24:347–350.

47. Park MA, McClimon BJ, Ferguson B, et al. Collaboration between allergists and pharmacists increases β-lactam antibiotic prescriptions in patients with a history of penicillin allergy. *Int Arch Allergy Immunol* 2011; 154:57–62.

48. del Real GA, Rose ME, Ramirez-Atamoros MT, et al. Penicillin skin testing in patients with a history of beta-lactam allergy. *Ann Allergy Immunol* 2007; 98:355–359.

49. Raja AS, Lindsell CJ, Bernstein JA, et al. use of penicillin skin testing to assess the prevalence of penicillin allergy in an emergency department setting. *Ann Emerg Med* 2009; 54:72–77.

50. Park M, Markus P, Matesic D, Li JT. Safety and effectiveness of a preoperative allergy clinic in decreasing vancomycin use in patients with a history of penicillin allergy. *Ann Allergy Asthma Immunol* 2006; 97:681–687.

51. Rimawi RH, Cook PP, Gooch M, et al. The impact of penicillin skin testing on clinical practice and antimicrobial stewardship. *J Hosp Med* 2013; 8:341–345.

Chapter 12

Antibiotic Stewardship in Post-Acute Care Facilities

Anurag N. Malani and Christopher J. Crnich

Introduction

Utilization of post-acute care services has escalated sharply over the past decade.[1] Nursing homes (NHs), the majority of which are dually certified to provide skilled post-acute and long-term residential care services, are occupied by 1.4 million persons on any given day [2] and nearly 3.2 million persons will reside in one of the 15,700 US nursing home facilities at some point in any given year.[3] Nursing homes increasingly provide a wide variety of skilled care services, including intensive rehabilitation, basic wound care, and administration of parenteral medications. Nevertheless, there are an increasing number of hospitalized patients who require continued complex care and acute medical needs including mechanical ventilator dependence, administration of intravenous antibiotics, and complex wound care, precluding their discharge to a NH. For these patients, long-term acute care hospitals (LTACHs), which are defined by the Centers for Medicare & Medicaid Services (CMS) as hospitals with a mean length of stay equal or greater to 25 days, are an increasingly common destination on the path to recovery.[4] There are over 500 LTACHs across the United States, primarily of two types: free-standing LTACHs (located on their own property) and hospital-within-the-hospital LTACHs (located in an acute care hospital).[4, 5]

Nursing home residents and LTACH patients are highly susceptible to infection.[6–8] Age-related frailty and comorbidities are ubiquitous among individuals in these settings as are chronic wounds [9, 10] and exposure to invasive medical devices.[8, 11, 12] These patients have increased risk of acquiring multidrug-resistant organisms (MDROs). Nearly 50% of NH residents are colonized with one or more species of antibiotic-resistant bacteria, including methicillin-resistant *Staphylococcus aureus* (MRSA) and resistant gram-negative bacteria.[6, 13] The situation in LTACHs may be even more dire; a majority of *S. aureus* isolates recovered from clinical cultures in LTACHs are resistant to methicillin and multiply drug-resistant gram-negative bacteria can be recovered from a large number of patients hospitalized in these facilities.[8, 14–16] While a substantial number of individuals are colonized with MDROs at admission to a NH or LTACH,[17, 18] intra-facility cross-transmission of MDROs is common in these facilities.[19–22] The concentration and amplification of MDROs in these facilities coupled with the large number of resident/patient transitions that occur from NHs and LTACHs to hospitals [23, 24] are important drivers of antibiotic resistance in communities.[25, 26]

While resident/patient characteristics and infection control practices are important factors in the observed burden of antibiotic resistance and *Clostridium difficile* (CDI) in NHs and LTACHs, antibiotic use in these facilities is an equally, if not more, important determinant. While daily antibiotic utilization in NHs is lower than in hospitals and LTACHs,[27–30] the extended lengths of stay in these facilities means that up to 75% of residents who stay in a NH for six months or longer will receive at least one course of antibiotics.[31] Over half of the antibiotic courses initiated in NHs are unnecessary [32–38] and, even when necessary, the antibiotics prescribed are often excessively broad spectrum [34, 36] or administered for a duration longer than necessary for treatment of the underlying infection.[29] Antibiotic utilization in LTACHs is comparable to that observed in hospitals, likely as a result of the more complicated respiratory and skin and soft tissue infections encountered in these facilities.[4] When benchmarked against antibiotic use in medical intensive care units (MICUs) that submitted data to the Centers for Disease Control and Prevention (CDC) previous infection control and antibiotic use surveillance system called the National Nosocomial Infection Surveillance system, utilization of fluoroquinolone antibiotics in LTACHs approached the 90th percentile while utilization of vancomycin and carbapenem antibiotics ranged between the 50th and 75th percentiles compared to use observed in MICUs.[14] To our knowledge, there are no studies that have quantified the frequency of inappropriate antibiotic use in LTACHs. Nevertheless, if patterns mirror those observed in hospitals,[39] it is reasonable to assume that up to 50% of the antibiotic prescribing in LTACHs is inappropriate.[40]

Increasing concerns about a future devoid of effective antibiotic therapies [41–43] has prompted calls for widespread implementation of antibiotic stewardship programs (ASPs). [44, 45] Initial antibiotic stewardship policy efforts have appropriately centered on recommendations for implementation of ASPs in hospitals.[46, 47] Many of these existing policy initiatives affect LTACHs, which are regulated in many states similarly to acute care hospitals. Proposed modifications to the CMS Conditions for Participation would require that acute care hospitals and LTACHs have ASPs in order to qualify for payment.[48] Policy initiatives addressing antibiotic stewardship in NHs have recently been released. The CDC has published guidance detailing the core elements of antibiotic stewardship in NHs,[49] and CMS will require NHs participating in the federal payment system implement ASPs by 2018.[50] While these policy initiatives create much needed external pressure for change, implementation of ASPs in post-acute and long-term care facilities is not without its challenges. In this chapter, we will attempt to describe the major barriers to stewardship in NHs and LTACHs, the types of successes that have been achieved with stewardship interventions in both settings, and an approach for starting and expanding an ASP in these facilities.

Challenges to Antibiotic Stewardship in Post-Acute Care Facilities

Antibiotic stewardship programs were initially developed in tertiary care hospitals with ample access to infectious disease (ID) sub-specialists, pharmacists, and laboratory and informatics resources.[51, 52] These programs are becoming more common in non-tertiary care hospitals. Nevertheless, implementing ASPs in more resource-limited settings like NHs and LTACHs faces a number of challenges (Table 1).[53–59]

Barriers in Nursing Homes

Clinician contact with residents who experience a change-in-condition potentially caused by an infection is less frequent than in other healthcare settings.[29, 33, 60] Consequently, most antibiotic decisions in NHs are made remotely during brief telephone interactions with facility nursing staff.[61, 62] The knowledge and skill of nursing staff responsible for

Table 1 Comparison of Resources for ASPs in Facilities

	Nursing Homes (NHs)	Long-Term Acute Care Hospitals (LTACHs)
Located within an acute care hospital	Uncommon	++
Member of large system group	+	++
On-site diagnostic testing	Uncommon	++
Reporting to National Healthcare Safety Network	+	++
Informatics infrastructure	+	++
Use of electronic medical record	Uncommon	+
Electronic record analytic tools		
Ability to measure antibiotic costs	Uncommon	++
Ability to measure antibiotic use	Uncommon	+
Clinical staffing resources	+	++
Daily on-site physician or nurse practitioner presence	+	++
Daily pharmacist presence		
Availability of stewardship expertise:	Uncommon	+
ID physician	Uncommon	+
Pharmacy specialists		
Quality improvement infrastructure	Uncommon	+

+ = little availability/presence; ++ = readily available/present

the primary assessment of residents experiencing a change-in-condition and the quality of communication with providers vary widely.[63, 64] Similarly, the ability of clinicians in NHs to recognize and treat commonly encountered infections can vary considerably across settings [65] and access to providers and pharmacists with ID training is largely non-existent in these facilities.[66] While most NHs possess the capacity to perform basic laboratory and imaging tests, the turnaround time and/or quality of the results are often sub-optimal.[67, 68] Finally, while electronic medical records (EMRs) are becoming more common in NHs, a majority of the records employed in resident care, including laboratory and microbiology reports, remain paper-based.[69] Taken together, these barriers suggest that the structure and process of antibiotic stewardship in NHs differ substantially from that observed in hospitals.

Barriers in LTACHs

While many LTACHs have a primary relationship with a single host acute care facility, >50% of admissions often come from facilities outside these referral networks. Consequently, access to pertinent documentation, laboratory results (i.e., cultures), and antibiotic administration records is problematic. Lack of complete and timely information is compounded by the high prevalence of MDROs and device utilization in these facilities,[8, 14–16, 25, 70, 71] which creates a strong pressure to prescribe broad-spectrum antibiotic therapy.

Prospective audit and feedback is a strategy that many hospitals use to control the use of broad-spectrum antibiotic regimens. However, the effectiveness of this strategy is reliant on robust informatics systems that facilitate the identification of specific antibiotic agents and combinations. While most LTACHs have systems to track costs of antibiotic agents, their ability to track use and appropriateness of specific antibiotic agents in real-time is more limited.

Strategies to Improve Antibiotic Stewardship in Post-Acute Care Facilities

Antibiotic stewardship is accomplished through centralized and/or decentralized processes. Centralized processes include formulary restriction and pre-authorization as well as prospective audit and feedback. These approaches typically rely on individuals with specific training and expertise in the diagnosis and management of infectious diseases.[72] Non-centralized antibiotic stewardship interventions, which seek to positively impact antibiotic prescribing quality through education and during frontline staff-driven post-prescriptive review, are alternative approaches that have been promulgated in settings with more limited access to individuals with ID and/or antibiotic stewardship expertise.[73, 74] Examples of both types of approaches have been studied in NHs and LTACHs.

Centralized Antibiotic Stewardship Interventions

There have been three studies that have examined the impact of a centralized antibiotic stewardship approach in NHs (Table 2). Implementation of an ID consultative service in a Veterans Affairs (VA) Community Living Center, the VA equivalent of a NH, was associated with significant improvements in antibiotic utilization.[75] The ID service performed in-person consultation on residents with active antibiotic orders once-weekly and was available for remote consultations the remainder of the week, completed 291 consults on 250 study facility residents during the 15-month intervention period (~7 patient visits and 5–10 calls per week). Ninety-five percent of the consultative team recommendations were accepted. Compared to a three-year baseline period, total antibiotic use in the study facility decreased by 30% (175–122 days of therapy [DOT] per 1,000 resident days, P-value < 0.01) with statistically significant reductions in the use of fluoroquinolones, sulfamethoxazole/trimethoprim, β-lactam/β-lactamase inhibitors, clindamycin, and tetracycline antibiotics. Rates of hospitalization during the intervention period did not change; however, rates of *C. difficile* infection declined significantly relative to the baseline period.

While current levels of pharmacist involvement in stewardship activities in most NHs are limited,[76] pharmacist-driven interventions have been shown to positively impact the quality of antibiotic prescribing in this setting.[38, 77] A pharmacist-led prospective audit and feedback intervention focused on antibiotics initiated for treatment of culture-positive infections was associated with a 50% reduction in inappropriate antibiotic therapy in a single hospital-affiliated NH.[77] More recently, prospective audit and feedback intervention of antibiotics initiated for treatment of UTIs in three California nursing homes were associated with a significant reduction in UTI-specific and all-cause antibiotic starts.[38] The intervention in this study involved once-weekly site visits by an ID-trained pharmacist who performed chart reviews, discussed the cases with an off-site ID physician, and communicated recommendations to facility prescribers. Due to limited available contact

Centralized Stewardship Interventions in NHs

Reference	Study characteristics	Interventions	Outcomes
Jump et al. [75]	Design: Before/after single-center study Focus: all infections Randomization: N/A	Weekly ID consultant review of residents receiving antibiotics with feedback of recommendations to providers 24/7 telephone ID consultative services made available to prescribing providers	Total antibiotic DOT decreased from 175.1 to 122.3 days per 1,000 resident days (IRR = 0.60; $p < 0.001$) Oral antibiotic DOT decreased from 136.1 to 93.1 days per 1,000 resident days (IRR = 0.59; $p < 0.001$) Intravenous antibiotic DOT decreased from 39.0 to 29.3 days per 1,000 resident days (IRR = 0.75; $p = 0.01$)
Gugkaeva et al. [77]	Design: Before/after single-center study Focus: urinary tract infections Randomization: N/A	Pharmacist-led prospective audit and feedback of suspected urinary tract infections in which urine cultures were obtained	Percentage of inappropriate antibiotic courses decreased from 40% to 21% (RR = 0.50, $p = 0.11$)
Doernberg et al. [38]	Design: Before/after multi-center study ($n = 3$) Focus: urinary tract infections Randomization: N/A	ID physician and pharmacist-led prospective audit and feedback of all orders for antibiotics to treat urinary tract infection	Antibiotic starts for urinary tract infection declined 6% (IRR = 0.94, 95% CI = 0.92 – 0.97, $p < 0.001$) Antibiotic starts for all indications declined 5% (IRR = 0.95, 95% CI = 0.92 – 0.98, $p = 0.001$)

Centralized Stewardship Interventions in Long-Term Acute Care Hospitals

Reference	Study characteristics	Interventions	Outcomes
Kravitz et al. [56]	Design: before/after single-center study Focus: all infections Randomization: N/A	ID physician and pharmacist-led prospective audit and feedback of targeted antibiotic orders	Antibiotic utilization in defined daily doses per 1,000 patient days decreased 43% Antibiotic costs decreased 42% ($17.31–$10.05 per patient day)

Table 2 (cont.)

Centralized Stewardship Interventions in Long-Term Acute Care Hospitals

Reference	Study characteristics	Interventions	Outcomes
Pate et al. [57]	Design: before/after single-center study Focus: all infections Randomization: N/A	Non-ID-trained pharmacist devoted 5 hours per week reviewing and preparing charts ID physician and pharmacist reviewed charts for one hour per week Non-binding recommendations communicated to providers	Antibiotic utilization decreased from 914 to 712 defined daily doses per 1,000 patient days (IRR = 0.79; $p = 0.007$) Antibiotic costs decreased from $26.9 to $18.2 per patient day (RR = 0.68; $p = 0.001$)
Benson [58]	Design: before/after single-center study Focus: all infections Randomization: N/A	Pharmacy students performed structured review of charts of patients with active antibiotic orders Cases discussed with ID and clinical pharmacist(s) and recommendations made to providers ID physician available for questions	Antibiotic costs decreased from $75.4 to $64.1 per patient day (RR = 0.85; $p = 0.022$)
Beaulac et al. [59]	Design: before/after single-center study Focus: all infections Randomization: N/A	Off-site ID pharmacists and ID physicians remotely reviewed the records of patients who were receiving target antibiotics for at least 7 days. Recommendations sent to LTACH providers by email.	Antibiotic utilization declined 6.6 defined daily doses per 1,000 patient days per month ($P = 0.01$) C. difficile infection rates dropped 43% (IRR = 0.57, 95% CI = 0.35–0.92, $p = 0.02$)

Non-Centralized Stewardship Interventions in NHs

Reference	Study characteristics	Interventions	Outcomes
Naughton et al. [90]	Design: cluster-randomized study in 10 NHs Focus: nursing home-acquired	Prescriber-only facilities	Guideline adherence of IV antibiotics increased from 62.2% to 73.4% ($p < 0.02$)

Study	Design / Methods	Intervention	Outcomes
	Randomization: 5 NHs allocated to an educational intervention targeted at prescribers-only (5 NHs) and 5 NHs allocated to an educational intervention targeted at prescribers and nursing staff	Small group sessions in which guidelines were modified based on prescriber feedback • Small group sessions in which guidelines were modified based on prescriber feedback • Laminated pocket cards summarizing treatment of pneumonia Prescriber and nursing staff facilities: • Small group sessions for providers and nursing staff • Laminated pocket cards summarizing treatment of pneumonia • Laminated posters placed near facility telephones used to contact prescribing providers	
Loeb et al. [79]	Design: cluster-randomized study in 24 NHs Focus: urinary tract infection Randomization: 12 NHs allocated to a multifaceted intervention and 12 NHs allocated to usual care	Diagnostic and treatment algorithm for UTI Education of nursing staff (small group) and prescribers (individual) Pocket cards and posters with algorithms	Antibiotic starts for suspected urinary tract infection was significantly lower in intervention facilities (1.17 per 1,000 resident days) versus control facilities (1.59 per 1,000 resident days). Antibiotic utilization for treatment of urinary tract infection was lower in intervention facilities (6.9 defined daily doses [DDD] per 1,000

Table 2 *(cont.)*

Non-Centralized Stewardship Interventions in NHs			
Reference	**Study characteristics**	**Interventions**	**Outcomes**
			resident days) versus control facilities (10.9 DDD per 1,000 resident days) Total antibiotic utilization did not differ between intervention and control facilities
Schwartz et al. [87]	Design: before/after single-center study Focus: all infections Randomization: N/A	Locally developed prescribing guideline Audit of baseline rates of antibiotic resistance in the study facility Four small group sessions demonstrating case-based application of guidelines and review of resistance audit Pocket booklet of prescribing guideline	Charted diagnostic accuracy improved from 38% to 62% ($p = 0.006$) Treatment courses that were guideline concordant increased from 11% to 39% ($p < 0.001$) Antibiotic starts declined 5.9% ($p = 0.06$) Antibiotic DOT declined 29.7% ($p < 0.001$)
Monette et al. [88]	Design: cluster-randomized study in 8 NHs Focus: all infections Randomization: 4 NHs allocated to multifaceted intervention and 4 NHs allocated to usual care	Antibiotic guide mailed to prescribers; initial mailing followed by 2nd mailing 4 months later Individual profile of prescribing patterns (guideline adherence) over previous 3 months mailed to providers; initial mailing followed by a 2nd mailing 4 months later	Likelihood of guideline non-adherence in intervention arm • After 1st mailing: 0.47 (95% CI 0.21–1.05) • After 2nd mailing: 0.36 (95% CI 0.18–0.73) • 6-month follow-up: 0.48 (95% CI 0.23–1.02)

| Zabarsky et al. [81] | Design: before/after single-center study
Focus: urinary tract infections
Randomization: N/A | Baseline and semi-annual education of nursing staff focused on indications for testing resident urine samples.

Baseline and semi-annual education of primary care staff focused on diagnosis of UTI and avoiding treatment of ASB

Pocket reference cards tailored by nursing and primary care staff role

Posters displayed at computer stations used by nursing and primary care staff

Audit and feedback to nursing and primary care staff when inappropriate testing and treatment of ASB identified | Urine culture rate (pre/post): 3.7 to 1.5 cultures per 1,000 resident days (IRR = 0.41; 95% CI: 0.27–0.64; $p < 0.001$)

ASB treatment rate (pre/post): 1.7 to 0.6 events per 1,000 resident days (IRR = 0.37; 95% CI: 0.19–0.72; $p = 0.002$)

Antibiotic days of treatment (pre/post): 167.1–117.4 antibiotic days per 1,000 resident days ($p<0.001$) |
| Pettersson et al. [89] | Design: cluster-randomized study in 58 NHs
Focus: all infections (guideline intervention primarily focused on management of UTI in women)
Randomization: 29 NHs allocated to multifaceted intervention (26 included in final analyses) and 29 NHs allocated to usual care (20 included in final analyses)
Outcome data collected by participants rather than investigators. | Regionally developed antibiotic prescribing guideline

Audit of baseline prescribing patterns and local antibiotic resistance patterns

Two educational sessions delivered to nursing staff and prescribing providers that focused on: | Primary outcome |

Table 2 (cont.)

Non-Centralized Stewardship Interventions in NHs

Reference	Study characteristics	Interventions	Outcomes
		• Content of prescribing guideline • Review of facility-specific prescribing patterns and local antibiotic resistance patterns • Identification of barriers to change Printed educational materials focused on hygiene and prescribing guideline disseminated	• Change in % of female residents receiving a fluoroquinolone antibiotic for treatment of UTI: −0.196 in intervention NHs versus -0.224 in control NHs (diff-in-diff: 0.028; 95% CI: −0.193, 0.249 Secondary outcomes • Change in % of residents receiving an antibiotic for treatment of any infection (pre/post): −0.076 in intervention NHs and 0.048 in control NHs (diff-in-diff: −0.124; 95% CI: −0.228, −0.019) • Change in % of residents managed with "wait and see" approach (pre/post): 0.093 in intervention NHs versus -0.051 in control NHs (diff-in-diff: 0.143; 95% CI: 0.047, 0.240) • Change in % of residents receiving an antibiotic for UTI (pre/post): −0.031 in intervention NHs versus -0.070 in control NHs (diff-in-diff: 0.038; 95% CI: −0.013, 0.089)

Linnebur et al. [121]	Design: Quasi-experimental study in 16 NHs Focus: nursing home-acquired pneumonia Randomization: 8 NHs in Colorado non-randomly allocated to a multifaceted intervention and 8 NHs in Kansas and Missouri served as controls	Change tools • Evidence-based pneumonia care pathway developed • Standardized order forms Implementation strategies • A brief educational session focused on guidelines and pneumonia pathway delivered to prescribing providers at baseline • Reinforcement phone calls 3 months after baseline education and in year 2 of study • Paid a nurse liaison in study NHs to champion use of pneumonia pathway and collect study data	Change in guideline adherence (pre/post): +6% in intervention NHs versus +7% in control NHs ($p = 0.3$) Change in delivery of antibiotic within 4 hours (pre/post): +18% in intervention NHs versus −7% ($p < 0.001$)
Frentzel et al. [85]	Design: Quasi-experimental study in 12 NHs Focus: urinary tract infections Randomization: 4 NHs allocated to the standardized form intervention using a high-intensity implementation plan, 4 NHs were allocated to the standardized form intervention using a low-intensity implementation plan and 4 NHs were allocate to usual care	Change tools • Standardized form designed to structure documentation of resident signs/symptoms and facilitate decision-making around treatment of UTI Implementation strategies	Change in treatment of ASB • High fidelity NHs (n = 4; pre/post): 73.2%–49.4% (regression adjusted OR = 0.35; 95% CI: 0.16–0.76) • Low fidelity and control NHs (n = 8; pre/post): 69.6%–68.8% (regression adjusted OR = 1.93; 95% CI 1.05–3.56)

Table 2 (cont.)

Non-Centralized Stewardship Interventions in NHs

Reference	Study characteristics	Interventions	Outcomes
		• Letter describing purpose of form sent out to providers • In-person training of nursing staff (1 session in low-intensity and 2 sessions in high-intensity) • Technical support to intervention nursing homes (passive in low-intensity NHs and active in high-intensity NHs)	All antibiotic starts per 1,000 resident days (pre/post): −3.65 in intervention NHs and −0.90 in control NHs (diff-in-diff −2.75; regression adjusted IRR = 0.86; 95% CI = 0.79–0.95) Antibiotic starts for respiratory tract infection: IRR = 0.71 (95% CI = 0.56–0.90) Antibiotic starts for UTI: IRR = 0.84 (95% CI = 0.66–1.05) Antibiotic starts for skin and soft tissue infection: IRR = 0.89 (95% CI = 0.62–1.28)
Zimmerman et al. [86]	Design: Quasi-experimental study in 12 NHs Focus: respiratory and urinary tract infections Randomization: 6 NHs in one geographic region allocated to multifaceted intervention and 6 NHs in another geographic region assigned to usual care	Standardization of inter-professional communication through medical care referral form (MCRF) Nurse in-services focused on use of MCRF as well as identification and testing of residents with suspected infection Prescriber education focused on purpose of MCRF as well as diagnosis and treatment of common infections Pocket cards summarizing content of educational sessions Resident/family informational pamphlet focused on benefits and risks of antibiotic therapy Facility-level review of adherence to treatment recommendations	

| Furuno et al. [117] | Design: Before/after single-center study
Focus: culture-confirmed infections
Randomization: N/A | Facility-specific antibiograms (frequency tables summarizing rates of resistance to selected antibiotics among different types of bacteria) were developed

Results of antibiograms were presented at in-services with advice on how to use these data when selecting antibiotic therapy | Culture-concordant antibiotic therapy increased from 32% to 45% ($p = 0.32$) |
| Fleet et al. [92] | Design: Cluster-randomized study in 30 NHs
Focus: all infections
Randomization: 15 NHs allocated to a prescribing care bundle intervention and 15 NHs allocated to usual care | "Initiation of Treatment" form focused on the following process elements
• Documentation of resident signs/symptoms
• Documentation of diagnosis
• Obtaining tests before starting antibiotic
• Timing and appropriateness of antibiotic

"Review of Treatment" form focused on the following process elements
• Review of resident progress
• Review of test results
• Stop date and outcomes of treatment documented | Antibiotic starts per 100 residents (pre/post): +0.06 ($p = 0.94$) in intervention NHs versus +0.56 ($p = 0.4$) in control NHs

Antibiotic consumption (defined daily doses) per 1,000 resident days (pre/post): −3.25 ($p = 0.02$) in intervention NHs versus +2.24 ($p = 0.04$) in control NHs |

Table 2 (cont.)

Non-Centralized Stewardship Interventions in NHs

Reference	Study characteristics	Interventions	Outcomes

Doron et al. [83]	Design: Before/after study in 17 NHs
	Focus: urinary tract infections
	Randomization: N/A
		Change tools
		• UTI protocol to guide decisions about testing and treatment
		  • Clinician educational curriculum focused on appropriate urine testing and avoidance of treating ASB
		  • Resident/family member educational curriculum about UTI and risks and benefits of antibiotics
		  • Posters and handouts summarizing important aspects of educational curriculum
		e. Data collection instrument and instructional materials
		Implementation strategies
		• 2 full-day workshops focused on rationale for and use of change tools
		• Regular webinars focused on implementing change tools
		• Collaborative conference calls
		• One-on-one coaching
			Urine culture rate:
			IRR = 0.73 (95% CI = 0.66–0.79)
			UTI treatment rate: IRR = 0.67 (95% CI = 0.59–0.76)
			Clostridium difficile rate: IRR = −.55 (95% CI = 0.39–0.78)

Trautner et al. [122]	Design: Before/after study with contemporary control group Focus: urinary tract infections Randomization: N/A	Algorithm created to make CAUTI and ASB guidelines applicable at point of care Use of algorithm taught through case-based audit and feedback during in-services	Number of urine cultures ordered (acute and long-term care) decreased from 41.2 to 23.3 per 1000 bed-days during the intervention year ($p < 0.0001$) and decreased further during the maintenance year to 12.0 per 1,000 bed-days ($p < 0.0001$) Treatment of ASB decreased from 52% to 10% ($p = 0.001$) in long-term care intervention units

ASB = asymptomatic bacteriuria, CI = confidence interval, IRR = incidence rate ratio, MCRF = medical care referral form, N/A = not applicable, NH = nursing home, UTI = urinary tract infection, ns = not significant in the study facilities, the ID pharmacist was only able to review 104 of the 183 UTI treatment events during the intervention phase and left specific modification recommendations for 40 of these cases, 10 of which were accepted by providers (25%). The investigators hypothesized that notifying providers of the intent of the study – to improve the quality of antibiotic prescribing – created an unexpected normative influence that may have led to reductions in antibiotic utilization independent of those driven by pharmacist recommendations.

The evidence supporting the benefit of centralized antibiotic stewardship interventions in LTACHs is more robust (Table 2) with several studies demonstrating reductions in antibiotic costs and utilization as well as improvements in facility rates of CDI and antibiotic susceptibility patterns. During a 12-month study at a 140-bed LTACH in Minnesota, Kravitz et al. performed twice-weekly audit and feedback to prescribers.[56] The ASP team was composed of one clinical pharmacist and one ID physician. Compared to a six-month baseline period, overall antibiotic use, as measured by defined daily doses (DDD) per 1,000 patient days, declined by 43%; antibiotic cost per patient day decreased by 42% from $17.31 to $10.05; and antibiotic acquisitions costs decreased by 44%, resulting in a savings of about $306,000 per year. Reductions in use of cephalopsorins, fluoroquinolones, carbapenems, linezolid, metronidazole, piperacillin/tazobactam, and vancomycin were observed over the study period.

An ID physician and a clinical pharmacist without specialized ID training formed a two-member antibiotic stewardship team in a 60-bed LTACH in Texas.[57] They performed once-weekly audit and feedback of all patients receiving systemic antibiotics and provided prescribers with feedback on how to optimize existing antibiotic therapy. Compared to the baseline period, overall antibiotic use decreased by 21% during the intervention period and anti-infective cost per patient day decreased by 28% for an estimated cost savings of nearly $160,000 during the 15-month intervention period. Statistically significant reductions in use of fluoroquinolone antibiotics, linezolid, metronidazole, and antifungal agents were also observed.

At a 41-bed LTACH in Utah, a six-week elective ID experience was developed for rotating pharmacy students.[58] The primary role of the pharmacy students was to become integral members of the facility's existing ASP, which included an ID physician and ID pharmacist. Prior to the pharmacy students' rotation, the facility ASP lacked time to perform prospective review and feedback activities. Duties on the elective included monitoring all infection-related patient problems, meeting daily with the ID pharmacist and clinical pharmacist to develop recommendations for optimizing antibiotic use, communicating regularly with the ID physician, and providing real-time feedback to prescribers. The study reported a 15% decrease in the antibiotic costs per patient day over a two-year intervention period with an estimated cost savings of nearly $260,000. The pharmacy students consistently reported positive feedback and improved their ability to treat infections.

Recently, antibiotic stewardship using telemedicine via remote electronic medical record review has been described.[59] The ASP consisted of university-based ID physicians and ID pharmacists who spent one to two hours per week reviewing cases and providing recommendations remotely, primarily through daily emails to LTACH providers. The ASP had full access to the electronic medical record at the LTACH and antibiotic review activities specifically focused on patients who received at least seven days of targeted antibiotics. When compared to the one-year pre-implementation period, antibacterial utilization

(-6.6 DDD/1,000 patient days per month, 95% CI -11.5 to -1.7, P-value $= 0.01$) and CDI rates (IRR $= 0.57$, 95% CI 0.35–0.92, P-value $= 0.02$) were significantly lower in the post-implementation period. Statistically significant reductions in the utilization of anti-MRSA and anti-CDI antibiotic agents were also observed.

Non-Centralized Antibiotic Stewardship Interventions

Given existing limitations in access to clinicians with ID expertise, current efforts to influence antibiotic prescribing behaviors in NHs have predominantly focused on non-centralized interventions based on education, practice guidelines, and decision-support tools.[53–55, 78] A large number of the interventions described in published studies (Table 2) have targeted the decision to initiate antibiotic therapy in the NH resident with suspected urinary tract infection (UTI). A cluster-randomized trial in 24 US and Canadian nursing homes found that implementation of UTI testing and treatment pathways was associated with a short-term reduction in antibiotic treatment for UTIs.[79] Treatment effects waned over time and the intervention did not have a significant impact on urine culture utilization, suggesting some issues with intervention sustainability and fidelity.[80] In contrast, a subsequent study in a single VA long-term care facility using the same testing and treatment pathways demonstrated an impressive reduction in urine culture utilization, overtreatment of asymptomatic bacteriuria, and overall DOTs per 1,000 patient days when comparing the three-month pre-intervention phase, the six-month post-intervention phase, and the subsequent two years.[81] While these two studies addressed both testing and treatment decision-making, other studies have shown that interventions focusing on testing decision-making can positively impact antibiotic prescribing in NHs. Implementation of a testing decision-support pathway in 10 acute and long-term care units at a VA medical center was associated with a significant reduction in urine culture utilization and over-treatment of asymptomatic bacteriuria.[82] Similarly, there was a significant decrease in utilization of urine cultures and antibiotic therapy for UTIs following introduction of a UTI diagnostic pathway in 17 Massachusetts nursing homes.[83]

There is substantial evidence that sub-optimal assessment of NH residents experiencing a change-in-condition coupled with poor interdisciplinary communication has an unto-ward influence on antibiotic decision-making by off-site providers.[32, 33, 84] Not surprisingly, interventions focused on improving nursing assessments of residents and standardizing the content of communication with prescribers have been associated with reductions in antibiotic use in NHs.[85, 86] A quality improvement intervention focused on education of NH staff and families and implementation of tools to improve nurse-provider communication led to a 14% reduction in antibiotic utilization in six North Carolina nursing homes relative to control NHs in the same region that did not participate in the quality improvement intervention.[86] Similarly, antibiotic prescribing in Texas nursing homes was 33% lower in facilities that implemented a standardized communication and UTI decision-support form with high fidelity compared to control facilities that imple-mented the form with low fidelity.[85]

Efforts to improve the spectrum and duration of antibiotic therapy through educational interventions have had modest success in NHs. Case-based educational sessions on inter-vention units in a Chicago long-term care facility were associated with a 28% improvement in the frequency of guideline-concordant treatment courses and a 30% reduction in the days of antibiotic therapy. No changes were noted on care units that did not receive the educational intervention.[87] The impact of education-based interventions on a larger scale has been less impressive. A controlled, cluster-randomized study was performed in 8 Canadian nursing homes in which providers in intervention NHs were mailed an antibiotic guide describing treatment of common infections (UTI, lower respiratory tract infection, skin and soft tissue infection) as well as a report of their personal prescribing patterns over the previous three months.[88] While initial guideline-adherent prescribing improved in intervention NHs, adherence rates were no better when compared to control NHs at the conclusion of the study.[88] Similarly, a cluster-randomized study in Swedish nursing homes in which printed educational materials and in-person small group educational sessions were delivered to staff and providers in intervention facilities did not demonstrate a significant impact on the targeted prescribing behavior (reduction in use of fluoroquinolone antibiotics) but was associated with a modest reduction in the numbers of residents treated with antibiotics.[89] Interestingly, the effectiveness of educational interventions may rely on the simultaneous delivery of content to facility nursing staff and prescribing providers. A cluster-randomized trial of an educational intervention to improve antibiotic prescribing for pneumonia in New York nursing homes demonstrated significant improvement in adherence to prescribing guidelines (from 50% to 82%) in facilities where education was targeted at both types of clinical staff.[90] In contrast, guideline adherence remained essentially unchanged in NHs where education was targeted solely at prescribing providers (from 65% to 69%).[90].

While a majority of the stewardship interventions studied in NHs have focused on reducing unnecessary antibiotic use, there is ample evidence that the quality of antibiotic prescribing in NHs could be improved through efforts to reduce the length of treatment courses [29, 91] and decreasing use of broad-spectrum agents.[36] These two goals have been successfully achieved through a centralized prospective audit and feedback approach as detailed above but the scalability of this approach in NHs remains uncertain. Self-directed post-prescriptive review, which has been shown to be modestly effective in the hospital setting,[73, 74] has been studied on a limited basis in NHs. A cluster-randomized study of a multi-component intervention that included protocol-guided post-prescription review of antibiotic courses initiated in 30 NHs in London demonstrated a 5% reduction in antibiotic consumption in intervention facilities compared to control facilities despite only a 26% adherence to the post-prescription review protocol.[92]

Implementation of Antibiotic Stewardship Programs in Post-Acute Care Facilities

The studies described in the preceding section generally centered on interventions rather than programs. Notably, many of the interventions described above, while often exhibiting a positive initial impact, did not have a sustained impact on antibiotic prescribing patterns. This speaks to a critical need for structured ASPs that can proactively: 1) identify local antibiotic prescribing patterns most in need of improvement; 2) determine the best strategies to affect change in these patterns for implementation; and 3) maintain improvement efforts over time. Current guidelines recommend implementation of ASPs in post-acute care facilities although these guidelines are notably silent on how these programs should be structured and the types of actions that should be pursued by them, particularly in the NH setting.[93] The CDC has identified the core elements of ASPs in both hospitals and NHs.[46, 49] Both documents follow a similar structure (Table 3) although it is

Component [46, 49]	Description	Comments
Leadership Commitment	Dedicate support and commitment to safe and appropriate antibiotic use in the facility	Medical director, Chief Nursing Official and Director of Pharmacy should be visible and vocal champions for the facility's ASP
		Structure, roles and responsibilities of facility ASP should be detailed in a policy that is reviewed and approved by the facility leadership (the Quality Assurance/Performance Improvement [QAPI] committee in NHs and the Medical Executive Committee in LTACHs
		Other policies and guidelines developed by the facility ASP should be reviewed and approved through these same committees
		The facility ASP program should periodically report to these committees
Accountability	Identify which members of the facility will be part of the stewardship team and clearly delineate their role and responsibilities	Antibiotic stewardship is a team-based process that requires involvement and collaboration between leadership, providers, nursing staff, and pharmacy
	Assign administrative leadership of the stewardship team to a single individual	While responsibility for completing the various stewardship-related tasks (e.g. policy/guideline development, staff education/training, process/outcome tracking and reporting, stewardship intervention development and implementation) may be delegated to different members of the team, administrative oversight should be assigned to a single individual
		The stewardship team leader should have a clinical background plus a demonstrated

Table 3 *(cont.)*

Component [46, 49]	Description	Comments
		capacity to work and communicate well with stakeholders in other disciplines who operate in the facility: • In nursing homes, the Director of Nursing, Infection Preventionist, Nurse Educator, or facility pharmacist are appropriate for this position • In LTACHs, the Director of Pharmacy or another facility pharmacist are preferred. However, one of the facility ID sub-specialists, a hospitalist or the Director of Quality, if they are available and have a clinical background, could serve in this role
Drug Expertise	Ensure access to individuals with experience and/or training in antibiotic stewardship	Ideally, the individual selected to lead the facility stewardship team will have prior training/expertise in ID and/or antibiotic stewardship but this will be unusual in most NHs and many LTACHs In the absence of local expertise, the facility should: • Provide support for the stewardship team to attend stewardship training opportunities and pursue formal certification, if available • Identify and collaborate with experts in the region (e.g., referring acute care hospital) who can help develop facility policies/guidelines and provide input on selection and implementation of different stewardship interventions

Action

Implement at least one policy or practice to improve antibiotic use in the facility

Specific strategies should be chosen based on facility resources and needs identified through tracking measures

In NHs, strategies that focus on reducing unnecessary testing of urine samples and treatment of asymptomatic bacteriuria appear to have the greatest potential for immediate impact (see text)

In LTACHs, prospective audit and feedback appears to have the greatest potential for impact (see text) although formulary restriction is another strategy that may be equally effective in this setting [123]

Tracking

Monitor at least one *antibiotic utilization outcome* and one *clinical outcome* measure of antibiotic use in the facility

In NHs:

- At a minimum, track facility-initiated antibiotic starts on a monthly basis (ideally, denominate by resident days)
- Other utilization measures to consider include, proportion of antibiotic starts prescribed for >7 days [106] and proportion of antibiotic starts that meet appropriateness criteria[105]
- Clinical outcomes that should be considered include the monthly number of residents colonized or infected with different multidrug-resistant organisms (e.g., methicillin-resistant *Staphylococcus aureus* and *Clostridium difficile*) and the facility antibiogram[117]

Table 3 (cont.)

Component [46, 49]	Description	Comments
		In LTACHs:
		• At a minimum, facilities should track days of antibiotic therapy per 1,000 patient days or 1,000 days present. DDD per 1,000 patient days is a less preferable alternative for measurement of antibiotic use
		• Utilization rates of high-risk antibiotics for the development of CDI and/or serious adverse effects; and or broad-spectrum antibiotics are other utilization measures that facilities should consider tracking
		• Facilities should update their antibiogram annually
		• Rates of *C. difficile* infections and infections caused by selected multidrug-resistant bacteria are other clinical outcomes that should be considered
Reporting	Provide regular feedback of antibiotic use and antibiotic resistance to staff and providers in the facility	In NHs:
		• Antibiotic utilization and clinical outcomes data should be presented at least quarterly at the facility QAPI meeting
		• Providing individual feedback to providers on their prescribing patterns relative to their peers may have a beneficial normative influence on outliers [109, 124]

In LTACHs:

- Antibiotic utilization and clinical outcomes data should be presented at least quarterly at the facility Infection Control Committee meeting, Pharmacy and Therapeutics meeting, and Medical Executive Committee meeting
- Facilities should consider participating in the Centers for Disease Control and Prevention National Healthcare Safety Network's Antimicrobial Use and Antimicrobial Resistance Module

Education

Provide resources to staff, providers, and patients/residents about the risks of antibiotics and opportunities for improving antibiotic use

Education on the importance of antibiotic stewardship and the strategies the facility is using to promote better antibiotic stewardship should be delivered at hire and periodically thereafter

In nursing homes, education should target both nursing staff and prescribers [125, 126]

expected that facilities will tailor implementation of the core elements based on existing organizational structure and resource availability. Importantly, healthcare facilities are encouraged to develop their ASP in a step-wise fashion, starting with one or two activities and gradually adding new strategies over time. Below we describe key aspects of a post-acute facility ASP and highlight some of the key differences between NHs and LTACHs that should be considered when approaching programmatic development in these facilities. As a first step, we recommend that facilities looking to implement or scale up an existing ASP employ one of the checklists developed by the CDC.[94, 95] Use of these tools will help facilities identify and prioritize resource needs and also develop a roadmap for implementation of the various policies and procedures that can be used to improve antibiotic prescribing practices. While ASP development in LTACHs is not explicitly addressed, the hospital-based materials and checklists developed by the CDC are most applicable.

Leadership Commitment

There is little doubt that hospitals and post-acute care facilities will face increasing external pressures to demonstrate action focused around judicious use of antibiotics. For example, CMS has released proposed draft regulations that require NHs and hospitals to have an ASP in order to participate in Medicare and Medicaid programs.[48, 50]

Although external pressures such as those from CMS provide a needed initial impetus for change, it is critical that commitment for developing ASPs be internally motivated. Failure to proactively identify local needs, opportunities and resources for improvement will likely result in a stewardship program that reacts only in response to regulatory actions (i.e., the state survey) and is unlikely to improve the outcomes of patients and residents. Studies in a related field – infection control – have shown that leadership commitment is a critical element of high-performing infection prevention programs.[96] Consequently, one of the first steps on the journey to developing a facility ASP requires commitment and support from facility leadership, including the chief executive officer (CEO), medical director, director of nursing (DON), director of pharmacy, and the quality officer or lead. Discussions that leadership often find persuasive include: 1) need to satisfy regulatory requirements focused on appropriate use of medications; 2) federal mandates to demonstrate meaningful organizational quality assurance and performance improvement (QAPI); [97] 3) emerging federal policies to promote and ultimately require antibiotic stewardship activities across all healthcare settings;[45] 4) organizational costs of treating antibiotic-resistant and *C. difficile* infections;[98, 99] and 5) how antibiotic stewardship interventions, particularly those focused around enhancing interdisciplinary communication, can generate corollary benefits in other processes and outcomes (e.g., enhanced management of resident change-in-condition). While the day-to-day involvement of these individuals in running the ASP may be minimal, leadership is responsible for making stewardship an organizational priority and communicating this to providers and staff, identifying the key stakeholders responsible for implementing the facility ASP, and providing the necessary resources and support needed for these stakeholders to be successful.

Programmatic Structure (Accountability and Expertise)

The background and training of the individuals responsible for implementation of an ASP in the post-acute care setting may differ substantially from those responsible for stewardship in well-resourced hospitals. Ideally, the individual or individuals responsible for developing the facility ASP will possess ID expertise and/or specific training in antibiotic stewardship operations. While it is unrealistic to assume that individuals with these particular skills will be available in many post-acute care contexts, individuals with other operational skills can usually be identified. Ideally, these local stewards will: 1) have general clinical expertise as well as an ability to meaningfully engage nursing staff and providers; 2) understand facility pharmacy operations and how medication administration data are structured and stored; 3) understand facility laboratory services and how results are structured and stored; and 4) be able to interact with other key operational staff (e.g., the infection preventionist as well as pharmacy, laboratory, and information technology staff) to identify opportunities to standardize and automate methods for tracking and reporting important process and outcome measures (see below).

ASP Structure in NHs While there have been a number of antibiotic stewardship interventions studied in the NH setting, there are few examples of how to structure an ASP program in this setting. In general, these facilities have limited access to providers with appropriate expertise and information system resources enjoyed by hospitals and LTACHs. It is, therefore, unrealistic to assume that NHs will be able to employ or even contract with individuals who have specific antibiotic stewardship expertise although this may change in the future. Nevertheless, it is important that NHs, at a minimum, identify a local steward to develop and implement the facility's ASP. While a pharmacist may be the individual best positioned to fill this role, most NHs do not employ pharmacists directly. A majority of pharmacists who work in NHs are contracted by the facilities to provide core services (e.g., monthly medication reconciliation) and these individuals often play a limited role in the facility's day-to-day operations [76] The infection preventionist or DON, who often performs double-duty as the facility infection preventionist, are often the individuals most actively engaged in quality improvement in the NH and, after the pharmacist, may be the individuals best positioned to assume leadership responsibilities for the facility's ASP. When available, the NH should attempt to cultivate collaborative or even formal consultative relationships with ID and antibiotic stewardship experts in referring hospitals. These individuals can be particularly helpful in the development and delivery of educational content for nursing staff and providers, development of guidelines for the treatment of commonly encountered infections, and development of effective antibiotic utilization tracking and reporting systems. The medical director and DON, even if they are not the designated ASP leaders, can play a critical role in growing the facility ASP by publicly affirming its importance and supporting improvement efforts. For example, NHs often have limited organizational influence over providers and the medical director can exert important social influence on his/her peers to adhere to ASP policies and practices. A recent report from a Wisconsin nursing home described case studies of antibiotic stewardship programs in different healthcare settings and identified medical director support and involvement as a key facilitator in the implementation of a facility ASP.[100] High levels of frontline staff turnover is a continuing problem in many NHs [101] and the DON plays an important role in onboarding of new staff and continuing education of existing staff as well as reinforcing expectations of staff responsible for assessment and communication of resident change-in-condition, both of which factor into provider decisions regarding initiation of antibiotics.[32, 33, 84]

ASP Structure in LTACHs LTACHs generally have ample access to individuals with general clinical (i.e., hospitalists) and pharmacy expertise and usually have some level of access to ID specialists, these resources are more readily available at "hospital-within-the-hospital" LTACHs than free-standing hospitals. Nevertheless, many LTACHs do not possess the resources to employ an individual with formal antibiotic stewardship expertise. In this situation, contracting with expert antibiotic stewards at referring hospitals is often a viable option. However, even in those situations where the LTACH has contracted with an outside ASP for specific services, it is still important to identify a local steward – hospitalist, infection preventionist, and/or pharmacist – who can engage frontline staff and providers and work with other employed or contracted operational partners to develop tracking and reporting systems and function as a liaison between the consultant antibiotic steward and facility leadership. The medical director, DON, and director of pharmacy play an important support role, regardless of the existing ASP structure, through endorsement of policies and practices, facilitating buy-in from prescribing providers and nursing staff, reviewing process and outcome measures and identifying opportunities and resources for further programmatic growth.

Tracking and Reporting Antibiotic Utilization and Related Outcomes

A capability to track and report process and outcomes is a fundamental characteristic of successful quality improvement.[102] The infection preventionist in NHs and LTACHs are already engaged in tracking infections [7, 103] and adapting this process to track antibiotic utilization and related outcomes (*C. difficile* and multidrug-resistant organisms) should be feasible in most post-acute care facilities.

Most LTACHs employ an electronic medical record (EMR) that should allow these facilities to more easily track antibiotic and laboratory data. Use of an EMR is likely more available and common across LTACHs than other long-term care facilities. EMR penetration in NHs is more limited, however, tracking methods to identify residents experiencing a change-in-condition, including those residents who are currently receiving antibiotics, is a common practice in these facilities.[104] Consequently, information on antibiotic starts is readily available and can be tracked at predefined time periods by the individual responsible for infection surveillance in the facility. At a minimum, post-acute care facilities should periodically assess antibiotic utilization in the facility using a cross-sectional approach (e.g., the number of residents on antibiotics during a given day, week, or month). However, cross-sectional assessments are not as sensitive to change as measures that are tracked more regularly. In order to monitor the effects of improvement interventions and detect aberrant prescribing patterns, post-acute care facilities should ideally track antibiotic starts and/or antibiotic DOT prospectively. While tracking counts may be reasonable in settings where monthly census patterns are stable, tracking antibiotic utilization using incidence density measures (e.g., antibiotic starts or DOT per 1,000 resident days) is more appropriate in settings where there is variation in monthly census data. Stratifying tracking measures by indication (e.g., UTI) and antibiotic class (e.g., fluoroquinolones) can help facilities better ascertain conditions in need of focused attention and follow the effects of condition-specific interventions. Supplementing utilization measures with assessments of appropriateness (e.g., proportion of monthly antibiotic courses meeting explicit criteria [103, 105] or proportion of monthly antibiotic courses exceeding 7 days [106]) can provide additional insights into opportunities for improvement.

Educational Activities

Education is a foundational activity of the ASP. Educational content should cover the importance of antibiotic stewardship, plans for implementation of specific ASP activities, and the responsibilities of clinical staff in achieving ASP goals. Education should be targeted and tailored to nursing assistants, nursing staff, providers, residents, and families. While not focused on antibiotic prescribing practices, a recently published study performed in 12 Michigan NHs demonstrated that a multi-modal educational intervention focused on common infection prevention practices and care processes associated with indwelling urinary catheters and feeding tubes was associated with a 22% decrease in rates of MRSA acquisition and 31% decreased in catheter-associated UTIs.[107] Resident and family education, when combined with staff and provider education as well as interventions to enhance interdisciplinary communication, has also been shown to be associated with reductions in antibiotic use in NHs.[86] Studies such as these demonstrate that educational interventions can be powerful tools for changing behaviors but likely need to target multiple individuals [90] and be delivered via a number of modalities – including in-service training sessions, newsletters, pocket-guides, posters, and brochures – in order to be maximally effective.

Giving providers feedback on their antibiotic prescribing patterns and engaging in interactive academic detailing are strategies that have been used to improve antibiotic prescribing in hospitals and outpatient settings [108, 109] but has not been well studied in the post-acute care setting. An educational intervention in which the aggregate prescribing practices of providers in a Chicago nursing home were compared to existing guideline recommendations was associated with a significant reduction in antibiotic utilization and improvement in adherence to prescribing guidelines.[87] However, giving providers a summary of the quality of their antibiotic prescribing did not have a sustained impact on antibiotic utilization in a cluster-randomized trial in French NHs.[88]

Starting an ASP

There are a large number of ASP activities from which post-acute care facilities can choose to implement. In general, these strategies map to one of four categories: 1) antibiotic prescribing policies/guidelines; 2) broad interventions; 3) pharmacy-driven interventions; and 4) syndrome-specific interventions. Facilities should select their strategies based on need and degree of match with existing resources. When first implementing a facility ASP, it is easy to get overwhelmed with the time and resources needed simply to establish the organizational and tracking/reporting infrastructure. Consequently, it is recommended that facilities implement stewardship activities in a step-wise fashion rather than attempt to make numerous changes simultaneously.[46, 49]

Antibiotic prescribing policies Post-acute facilities should have policies stipulating that antibiotic orders include clear documentation of the drug, dose, duration and indication for treatment (e.g., UTI).[49] Many hospitals employ standardized antibiotic order forms to ensure that this information is captured reliably.[110] Use of standardized order forms can help the local ASP leader track antibiotic use more effectively and, when adapted to include decision-support content (e.g., preferred agents, dosage adjustments for renal function and appropriateness criteria),[105] these tools can be a mechanism for educating facility providers. Unnecessary laboratory testing is a driver of antibiotic overuse.[111] There is considerable evidence that positive urine culture results exert an undue influence on prescriber decisions to initiate antibiotics, particularly in the post-acute care setting.[112–114] Accordingly, policies focused on reducing utilization of urine cultures should be assigned a high priority. Policies should specifically address testing urine samples with reagent strips (i.e., the dipstick) [115, 116] and performing urine cultures to confirm test-of-cure both of which are unnecessary and likely promote antibiotic overuse in nursing homes.[113] Other policy topics that facilities should consider include appropriate testing for C. *difficile*, prioritizing narrow-spectrum over broad-spectrum agents, in particular the fluoroquinolones which have been increasingly linked to C. *difficile* and antibiotic resistance in the post-acute care setting,[117, 118] and guidelines on how to treat infections commonly encountered in the post-acute care setting, including agent selection and duration of therapy. However, drafting effective treatment guidelines may require input from individuals with ID expertise who may not be easily available.[87]

Broad Interventions Two resource intensive ASP interventions commonly employed in hospitals include: 1) formulary restrictions with prior authorization and 2) expert-led prospective audit and feedback to frontline providers.[119] Almost 50% of LTACHs are facilities within a few large networks (i.e., Select Medical, Kindred Healthcare, Vibra) and likely have an established antibiotic formulary.[5] Moreover, many LTACHs have ready access to consultants with ID expertise suggesting that both of these recommended antibiotic stewardship activities can be implemented in LTACHs (and can be effective as described above). Nevertheless, it is unlikely that most NHs will have the resources to implement either of these intensive ASP activities successfully. Strategies focused on promotion of self-directed stewardship, in which prescribers are trained and/or prompted to engage in review of empirically initiated antibiotics and modify the therapeutic dose, spectrum and/or duration when appropriate ("antibiotic timeout"), has been implemented successfully in a hospital setting with limited access to individuals with stewardship expertise.[73] Implementation of a checklist tool to foster self-directed stewardship activities in a cluster-randomized trial in 30 United Kingdom NHs was associated with a 5% reduction in systemic antibiotic use in intervention facilities versus a 5% increase in antibiotic use in control facilities.[92] Another broad strategy that should be feasible in the NH setting is the introduction of training and tools focused on improving resident assessments and interdisciplinary communication of resident change-in-condition.[120] As noted above, the introduction of standardized communication forms as part of multi-component interventions has been associated with significant reductions in antibiotic utilization in North Carolina and Texas NHs.[85, 86] While the CDC's Core Elements for Antibiotic Stewardship Programs in Nursing Homes advocates for the use of antibiograms, both as a tool to help guide empiric prescribing in the facility and a mechanism by which to raise provider awareness of the consequences of antibiotic prescribing, there is limited evidence of the beneficial impact of antibiograms on antibiotic prescribing patterns in the NH setting.[117] Furthermore, survey studies suggest that many NHs struggle with obtaining antibiotic susceptibility data needed to develop these tools from contracted laboratories.[76]

Pharmacy-Driven Interventions Examples of pharmacy interventions include automatic changes from intravenous to oral antibiotic therapy for highly bioavailable antibiotics (i.e., ciprofloxacin, levofloxacin, trimethoprim-sulfamethoxazole, linezolid, etc.), which reduces the need for intravenous access and improves patient safety and satisfaction. Pharmacists can perform automatic renal dose adjustments and dose optimization based on therapeutic drug monitoring (i.e., vancomycin, aminoglycosides). While post-prescription review and feedback appears to be most effective with models that pair pharmacists with ID specialists, pharmacist-only programs have been effective in the NH [77] and LTACH settings.[58] Pharmacists engaged in post-prescription review and

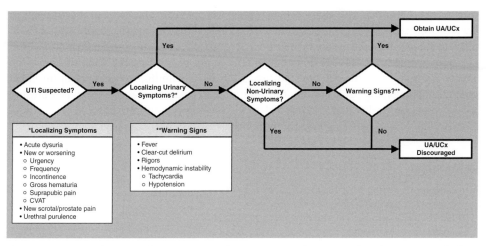

Figure 1 Decision pathway to reduce unnecessary diagnostic testing of urine samples in long-term care facilities (adapted from [113]). (Abbreviations: UTI = urinary tract infection; UA = urinalysis; UCx = urine culture; CVAT = costovertebral angle tenderness)

feedback activities in both cited examples had received specialized training and/or oversight from pharmacists with antibiotic stewardship expertise. Unfortunately, pharmacists with this advanced antibiotic stewardship training are not typically available in most post-acute care facilities currently.[76]

Syndrome-Specific Interventions A number of practices that promote the overuse of antibiotics are common in many post-acute care facilities, specifically NHs. Prescribing prophylactic antibiotics to prevent recurrent UTIs, sending urine cultures to confirm test-of-cure and culturing open wounds are just some examples of questionable practices still encountered in NHs. However, treatment of asymptomatic bacteriuria is probably the most prevalent problem encountered in most NHs.[113, 114] Implementation of protocols that restrict urine testing to residents with a high probability of having a UTI (Figure 1) [83] and similarly designed protocols to limit antibiotic therapy in residents without clear signs and symptoms of UTI [79, 81] have been associated with significant reductions in antibiotic utilization in NHs. These protocols should be operationalized not only through education of providers but, given their influence on provider decision-making,[60, 84] also through engagement of nursing staff who should be empowered to discourage providers from ordering diagnostic tests of the urine in the absence of specific, evidence-based criteria. Tracking the frequency of urine cultures and number of treated UTI events that do not satisfy surveillance definitions [103] provide targets that a facility can follow in order to assess impact of the ASP intervention.

Conclusion

The emerging crisis in antibiotic resistance will require a concerted effort to improve antibiotic stewardship across all healthcare settings.[45] Considerable progress has been made in our understanding of the extent and determinants of inappropriate antibiotic use in post-acute care facilities. While there is accumulating evidence that interventions focused on processes (e.g., urine testing) associated with the initial antibiotic decision can reduce unnecessary antibiotic use, there remains a critical need to identify the effectiveness of interventions that target post-prescribing decision-making (e.g., review and de-escalation) and how these interventions can be delivered in a cost-effective manner. There is also a need for more research on how to implement both types of stewardship interventions with fidelity and sustain them over time, particularly in NHs with limited quality improvement resources. Finally, there is a need for studies that evaluate the effects of stewardship interventions on facility and resident outcomes, including healthcare costs as well as rates of infections caused by *C. difficile* and multidrug-resistant bacteria.

References

1. Chandra A, Dalton MA, Holmes J. Large increases in spending on postacute care in Medicare point to the potential for cost savings in these settings. *Health Aff (Millwood)* 2013; 32:864–872.

2. Harris-Kojetin LD, Sengupta M, Park-Lee E, Valverde E. *Long-term care services in the United States: 2013 Overview. National health care statistics report; no. 1.* Hyattsville, MD: National Center for Health Statistics, 2013.

3. Centers for Medicare and Medicaid Services (CMS). Nursing Home Data Compendium, 2009. 7th ed. 2009. (Accessed April 12, 2016, at www.cms.gov/ Research-Statistics-Data-and-Systems/ Statistics-Trends-and-Reports/ DataCompendium/15_2009_Data_ Compendium.html.)

4. Munoz-Price LS. Long-term acute care hospitals. *Clin Infect Dis* 2009; 49:438–443.

5. Chopra T, Goldstein EJC. *Clostridium difficile* infection in long-term care facilities: a call to action for antimicrobial stewardship. *Clin Infect Dis* 2015; 60(Suppl 2):S72–76.

6. Strausbaugh LJ, Joseph CL. The burden of infection in long-term care. *Infect Control Hosp Epidemiol* 2000; 21:674–679.

7. Smith P, Bennett G, Bradley S, et al. SHEA/ APIC guideline: infection prevention and control in the long-term care facility. *Infect Control Hosp Epidemiol* 2008; 29:785–814.

8. Chitnis AS, Edwards JR, Ricks PM, Sievert DM, Fridkin SK, Gould CV. Device-associated infection rates, device utilization, and antimicrobial resistance in long-term acute care hospitals reporting to the national healthcare safety network, 2010. *Infect Control Hosp Epidemiol* 2012; 33:993–1000.

9. Park-Lee E, Caffrey C. Pressure ulcers among nursing home residents: United States, 2004. National Center for Health Statistics Data Brief 2009:1–8.

10. Milne CT, Trigilia D, Houle TL, Delong S, Rosenblum D. Reducing pressure ulcer prevalence rates in the long-term acute care setting. *Ostomy Wound Manage* 2009; 55:50–59.

11. Mody L, Maheshwari S, Galecki A, Kauffman CA, Bradley SF. Indwelling device use and antibiotic resistance in nursing homes: identifying a high-risk group. *J Am Geriatr Soc* 2007; 55:1921–1926.

12. Crnich CJ, Drinka P. Medical device-associated infections in the long-term care setting. *Infect Dis Clin North Am* 2012; 26:143–164.

13. Bonomo R. Multiple antibiotic-resistant bacteria in long-term-care facilities: an emerging problem in the practice of infectious diseases. *Clin Infect Dis* 2000; 31:1414–1422.

14. Gould C, Rothenberg R, Steinberg J. Antibiotic resistance in long-term acute care hospitals: the perfect storm. *Infect Control Hosp Epidemiol* 2006; 27:920–925.

15. Munoz-Price LS, Stemer A. Four years of surveillance cultures at a long-term acute care hospital. *Infect Control Hosp Epidemiol* 2010; 31:59–63.

16. Marchaim D, Chopra T, Bogan C, et al. The burden of multidrug-resistant organisms on tertiary hospitals posed by patients with recent stays in long-term acute care

facilities. *Am J Infect Control* 2012; 40:760–765.

17. Crnich CJ, Safdar N, Robinson J, Zimmerman D. Longitudinal trends in antibiotic resistance in US nursing homes, 2000–2004. *Infect Control Hosp Epidemiol* 2007; 28:1006–1008.

18. Murphy CR, Quan V, Kim D, et al. Nursing home characteristics associated with methicillin-resistant *Staphylococcus aureus* (MRSA) burden and transmission. *BMC Infect Dis* 2012; 12:269.

19. Furuno JP, Shurland SM, Zhan M, et al. Comparison of the methicillin-resistant *Staphylococcus aureus* acquisition among rehabilitation and nursing home residents. *Infect Control Hosp Epidemiol* 2011; 32:244–249.

20. Fisch J, Lansing B, Wang L, et al. New acquisition of antibiotic-resistant organisms in skilled nursing facilities. *J Clin Microbiol* 2012; 50:1698–1703.

21. Stone ND, Lewis DR, Johnson TM, et al. Methicillin-resistant *Staphylococcus aureus* (MRSA) nasal carriage in residents of Veterans Affairs long-term care facilities: role of antimicrobial exposure and MRSA acquisition. *Infect Control Hosp Epidemiol* 2012; 33:551–557.

22. Haverkate MR, Bootsma MCJ, Weiner S, et al. Modeling spread of KPC-producing bacteria in long-term acute care hospitals in the Chicago region, USA. *Infect Control Hosp Epidemiol* 2015; 36:1148–1154.

23. Mor V, Intrator O, Feng Z, Grabowski DC. The revolving door of rehospitalization from skilled nursing facilities. *Health Aff (Millwood)* 2010; 29:57–64.

24. Kahn JM, Benson NM, Appleby D, Carson SS, Iwashyna TJ. Long-term acute care hospital utilization after critical illness. *JAMA* 2010; 303:2253–2259.

25. Won SY, Munoz-Price LS, Lolans K, et al. Emergence and rapid regional spread of Klebsiella pneumoniae Carbapenemase-producing Enterobacteriaceae. *Clin Infect Dis* 2011; 53:532–540.

26. Lee BY, Song Y, Bartsch SM, et al. Long-term care facilities: important participants of the acute care facility social network? *PLoS ONE* 2011; 6:e29342.

27. Polk RE, Fox C, Mahoney A, Letcavage J, MacDougall C. Measurement of adult antibacterial drug use in 130 US hospitals: comparison of defined daily dose and days of therapy. *Clin Infect Dis* 2007; 44:664–670.

28. Benoit S, Nsa W, Richards C, et al. Factors associated with antimicrobial use in nursing homes: a multilevel model. *J Am Geriatr Soc* 2008; 56:2039–2044.

29. Daneman N, Gruneir A, Newman A, et al. Antibiotic use in long-term care facilities. *J Antimicrob Chemother* 2011; 66:2856–2863.

30. McClean P, Hughes C, Tunney M, Goossens H, Jans B, European Surveillance of Antimicrobial Consumption (ESAC) Nursing Home Project Group. Antimicrobial prescribing in European nursing homes. *J Antimicrob Chemother* 2011; 66:1609–1616.

31. van Buul LW, van der Steen JT, Veenhuizen RB, et al. Antibiotic use and resistance in long term care facilities. *J Am Med Dir Assoc* 2012; 13:568.e1–13.

32. Zimmer JG, Bentley DW, Valenti WM, Watson NM. Systemic antibiotic use in nursing homes: a quality assessment. *J Am Geriatr Soc* 1986; 34:703–710.

33. Warren JW, Palumbo FB, Fitterman L, Speedie SM. Incidence and characteristics of antibiotic use in aged nursing home patients. *J Am Geriatr Soc* 1991; 39:963–972.

34. Pickering T, Gurwitz J, Zaleznik D, Noonan J, Avorn J. The appropriateness of oral fluoroquinolone-prescribing in the long-term care setting. *J Am Geriatr Soc* 1994; 42:28–32.

35. Loeb M, Simor AE, Landry L, et al. Antibiotic use in Ontario facilities that provide chronic care. *J Gen Intern Med* 2001; 16:376–383.

36. Rotjanapan P, Dosa D, Thomas KS. Potentially inappropriate treatment of urinary tract infections in two Rhode Island nursing homes. *Arch Intern Med* 2011; 171:438–443.

37. Vergidis P, Hamer DH, Meydani SN, Dallal GE, Barlam TF. Patterns of antimicrobial use for respiratory tract infections in older residents of long-term care facilities. *J Am Geriatr Soc* 2011; 59:1093–1098.

38. Doernberg SB, Dudas V, Trivedi KK. Implementation of an antimicrobial stewardship program targeting residents with urinary tract infections in three community long-term care facilities: a quasi-experimental study using time-series analysis. *Antimicrob Resist Infect Control* 2015; 4:54.

39. Davey P, Brown E, Fenelon L, et al. Systematic review of antimicrobial drug prescribing in hospitals. *Emerging Infect Dis* 2006; 12:211–216.

40. Dellit TH, Owens RC, McGowan JE, et al. Infectious Diseases Society of America and the Society for Healthcare Epidemiology of America guidelines for developing an institutional program to enhance antimicrobial stewardship. *Clin Infect Dis* 2007; 44:159–177.

41. World Health Organization. *The Evolving Threat of Antimicrobial Resistance: Options for Action.* Geneva, Switzerland: World Health Organization, 2012.

42. Centers for Disease Control and Prevention. *Antibiotic Resistance Threats in the United States, 2013.* Atlanta, GA: US Department of Health and Human Services, Centers for Disease Control and Prevention, 2013.

43. O'Neill J. Antimicrobial resistance: tackling a crisis for the health and wealth of nations. the review on antimicrobial resistance. 2014. (Accessed April 12, 2016, at http://amr-review.org/sites/default/files/AMR%20Review%20Paper%20-%20Tackling%20a%20crisis%20for%20the%20health%20and%20wealth%200f%20nations_1.pdf.)

44. Interagency Taskforce on Antimicrobial Resistance (ITFAR). A Public Health Action Plan to Combat Antimicrobial Resistance. 2012. (Accessed April 12, 2016, at www.cdc.gov/drugresistance/pdf/action-plan-2012.pdf.)

45. The White House. National Strategy for Combatting Antibiotic Resistant Bacteria. 2014. (Accessed April 12, 2016, at www.whitehouse.gov/sites/default/files/docs/carb_national_strategy.pdf.)

46. Pollack LA, Srinivasan A. Core elements of hospital antibiotic stewardship programs from the Centers for Disease Control and Prevention. *Clin Infect Dis* 2014; 59(Suppl 3):S97–100.

47. Department of Veterans Affairs, Veterans Health Administration. VHA directive 1031: antimicrobial stewardship programs (ASP). 2014.

48. CMS. Hospital and Critical Access Hospital (CAH) changes to promote innovation, flexibility, and improvement in patient care (proposed rule). 2016: 1–128. (Accessed April 12, 2016, at https://s3.amazonaws.com/public-inspection.federalregister.gov/2016–13925.pdf.)

49. Centers for Disease Control and Prevention. The core elements of antibiotic stewardship for nursing homes. Atlanta, GA: US Department of Health and Human Services, CDC, 2015: 1–21.

50. Department of Health and Human Services, CMS. Medicare and Medicaid Programs: reform of requirements for long-term care facilities. *Federal Register* 2016; 81:68688–68872.

51. Fishman N. Antimicrobial stewardship. *Am J Med* 2006; 119:S53–61; discussion S62–70.

52. Tamma PD, Cosgrove SE. Antimicrobial stewardship. *Infect Dis Clin North Am* 2011; 25:245–260.

53. Rhee SM, Stone ND. Antimicrobial stewardship in long-term care facilities. *Infect Dis Clin North Am* 2014; 28:237–246.

54. Nicolle LE. Antimicrobial stewardship in long term care facilities: what is effective? *Antimicrob Resist Infect Control* 2014; 3:6.

55. Crnich CJ, Jump R, Trautner B, Sloane PD, Mody L. Optimizing antibiotic stewardship in nursing homes: a narrative review and recommendations for improvement. *Drugs and Aging* 2015; 32:699–716.

56. Kravitz GR, Glynn PF, Bornstein PF, Eirtz JJ, Krason DA, Kahn MA. Implementation

of an antibiotic stewardship program (ASP) at a long-term acute care hospital (LTACH): fertile ground. Nineteenth Annual Scientific Meeting of the Society for Healthcare Epidemiology of America. San Diego, CA: March 18–22, 2009. Abstract 72.

57. Pate PG, Storey DF, Baum DL. Implementation of an antimicrobial stewardship program at a 60-bed long-term acute care hospital. *Infect Control Hosp Epidemiol* 2012; 33:405–408.

58. Benson JM. Incorporating pharmacy student activities into an antimicrobial stewardship program in a long-term acute care hospital. *Am J Health Syst Pharm* 2014; 71:227–230.

59. Beaulac K, Corcione S, Epstein L, Davidson LE, Doron S. Antimicrobial stewardship in a long-term acute care hospital using offsite electronic medical record Audit. *Infect Control Hosp Epidemiol* 2016; 37:1–7.

60. Schweizer AK, Hughes CM, Macauley DC, O'Neill C. Managing urinary tract infections in nursing homes: a qualitative assessment. *Pharm World Sci* 2005; 27:159–165.

61. Katz P, Beam T, Brand F, Boyce K. Antibiotic use in the nursing home. Physician practice patterns. *Arch Intern Med* 1990; 150:1465–1468.

62. Richards CL, Darradji M, Weinberg A, Ouslander JG. Antimicrobial use in post-acute care: a retrospective descriptive analysis in seven long-term care facilities in Georgia. *J Am Med Dir Assoc* 2005; 6:109–112.

63. Longo DR, Young J, Mehr D, Lindbloom E, Salerno LD. Barriers to timely care of acute infections in nursing homes: a preliminary qualitative study. *J Am Med Dir Assoc* 2002; 3:360–365.

64. Kim H, Harrington C, Greene WH. Registered nurse staffing mix and quality of care in nursing homes: a longitudinal analysis. *Gerontologist* 2009; 49:81–90.

65. Fleming A, Bradley C, Cullinan S, Byrne S. Antibiotic prescribing in long-term care facilities: a meta-synthesis of qualitative research. *Drugs and Aging* 2015; 32:295–303.

66. Morrill HJ, Caffrey AR, Jump RLP, Dosa D, LaPlante KL. Antimicrobial Stewardship in Long-Term Care Facilities: A Call to Action. *J Am Med Dir Assoc* 2016; 17:183. e1–183.e16.

67. Loeb MB, Carusone SBC, Marrie TJ, et al. Interobserver reliability of radiologists' interpretations of mobile chest radiographs for nursing home-acquired pneumonia. *J Am Med Dir Assoc* 2006; 7:416–419.

68. Shirts BH, Perera S, Hanlon JT, et al. Provider management of and satisfaction with laboratory testing in the nursing home setting: results of a national internet-based survey. *J Am Med Dir Assoc* 2009; 10:161–166.e3.

69. Rantz MJ, Hicks L, Petroski GF, et al. Cost, staffing and quality impact of bedside electronic medical record (EMR) in nursing homes. *J Am Med Dir Assoc* 2010; 11:485–493.

70. Furuno JP, Hebden JN, Standiford HC, et al. Prevalence of methicillin-resistant *Staphylococcus aureus* and *Acinetobacter baumannii* in a long-term acute care facility. *Am J Infect Control* 2008; 36:468–471.

71. Chitnis AS, Caruthers PS, Rao AK, et al. Outbreak of carbapenem-resistant enterobacteriaceae at a long-term acute care hospital: sustained reductions in transmission through active surveillance and targeted interventions. *Infect Control Hosp Epidemiol* 2012; 33:984–992.

72. Gross R, Morgan AS, Kinky DE, Weiner M, Gibson GA, Fishman NO. Impact of a hospital-based antimicrobial management program on clinical and economic outcomes. *Clin Infect Dis* 2001; 33:289–295.

73. Lee TC, Frenette C, Jayaraman D, Green L, Pilote L. Antibiotic self-stewardship: trainee-led structured antibiotic time-outs to improve antimicrobial use. *Ann Intern Med* 2014; 161:S53–58.

74. Hamilton KW, Gerber JS, Moehring R, et al. Point-of-prescription interventions to improve antimicrobial stewardship. *Clin Infect Dis* 2015; 60:1252–1258.

75. Jump RLP, Olds DM, Seifi N, et al. Effective antimicrobial stewardship in a long-term

care facility through an infectious disease consultation service: keeping a lid on antibiotic use. *Infect Control Hosp Epidemiol* 2012; 33:1185–1192.

76. Taylor L, Adibhatla S, Nace DA, Crnich CJ. Antibiotic stewardship structure and process in Wisconsin nursing homes: a follow-up telephone survey. IDWeek: A Joint Scientific Meeting of the Infectious Disease Society of America, Society for Healthcare Epidemiology of America, HIV Medical Association, and Pediatric Infectious Disease Society, New Orleans, LA. 2016.

77. Gugkaeva Z, Franson M. Pharmacist-led model of antibiotic stewardship in a long-term care facility. *Ann Long Term Care* 2012; 20:22–26.

78. Dyar OJ, Pagani L, Pulcini C. Strategies and challenges of antimicrobial stewardship in long-term care facilities. *Clin Microbiol Infect* 2015; 21:10–19.

79. Loeb M, Brazil K, Lohfeld L, et al. Effect of a multifaceted intervention on number of antimicrobial prescriptions for suspected urinary tract infections in residents of nursing homes: cluster randomised controlled trial. *BMJ* 2005; 331:669.

80. Lohfeld L, Loeb M, Brazil K. Evidence-based clinical pathways to manage urinary tract infections in long-term care facilities: a qualitative case study describing administrator and nursing staff views. *J Am Med Dir Assoc* 2007; 8:477–484.

81. Zabarsky TF, Sethi AK, Donskey CJ. Sustained reduction in inappropriate treatment of asymptomatic bacteriuria in a long-term care facility through an educational intervention. *Am J Infect Control* 2008; 36:476–480.

82. Trautner BW, Grigoryan L, Petersen NJ, et al. Effectiveness of an antimicrobial stewardship approach for urinary catheter-associated asymptomatic bacteriuria. *JAMA Intern Med* 2015; 175:1120–1127.

83. Doron S, McElroy N, Salem-Schatz S, et al. Improved practice and decreased antibiotic utilization for urinary indications in long term care facilities after an educational intervention. Poster presentation at IDWeek, Philadelphia, PA. 2014.

84. Walker S, McGeer A, Simor AE, Armstrong-Evans M, Loeb M. Why are antibiotics prescribed for asymptomatic bacteriuria in institutionalized elderly people? A qualitative study of physicians' and nurses' perceptions. *CMAJ* 2000; 163:273–277.

85. Frentzel E, Moudouni DKM, Garfinkel S, Phillips C, Zhao H, Fuchs S. Standardizing Antibiotic Use in Long-Term Care Settings (SAUL study): final report. Agency for Healthcare Research and Quality Accelerating (AHRQ) ACTION contract no. 290–2006–000–191, task order no. 8. American Institutes for Research, Texas A&M University School of Rural Public Health, and TMF Health Quality Institute, Rockville, MD. 2013.

86. Zimmerman S, Sloane PD, Bertrand R, et al. Successfully reducing antibiotic prescribing in nursing homes. *J Am Geriatr Soc* 2014; 62:907–912.

87. Schwartz DN, Abiad H, DeMarais PL, et al. An educational intervention to improve antimicrobial use in a hospital-based long-term care facility. *J Am Geriatr Soc* 2007; 55:1236–1242.

88. Monette J, Miller M, Monette M, et al. Effect of an educational intervention on optimizing antibiotic prescribing in long-term care facilities. *J Am Geriatr Soc* 2007; 55:1231–1235.

89. Pettersson E, Vernby A, Mölstad S, Lundborg CS. Can a multifaceted educational intervention targeting both nurses and physicians change the prescribing of antibiotics to nursing home residents? A cluster-randomized controlled trial. *J Antimicrob Chemother* 2011; 66:2659–2666.

90. Naughton BJ, Mylotte JM, Ramadan F, Karuza J, Priore RL. Antibiotic use, hospital admissions, and mortality before and after implementing guidelines for nursing home-acquired pneumonia. *J Am Geriatr Soc* 2001; 49:1020–1024.

91. Daneman N, Gruneir A, Bronskill SE, et al. Prolonged antibiotic treatment

in long-term care: role of the prescriber. *JAMA Intern Med* 2013; 173:673–682.

92. Fleet E, Gopal Rao G, Patel B, et al. Impact of implementation of a novel antimicrobial stewardship tool on antibiotic use in nursing homes: a prospective cluster-randomized control pilot study. *J Antimicrob Chemother* 2014; 69:2265–2273.

93. Barlam TF, Cosgrove SE, Abbo LM, et al. Implementing an antibiotic stewardship program: guidelines by the Infectious Disease Society of America and the Society for Healthcare Epidemiology of America. *Clin Infect Dis* 2016; 62:e51–77.

94. Centers for Disease Control and Prevention. Checklist for core elements of hospital antibiotic stewardship programs. 2012. (Accessed April 12, 2016, at www.cdc.gov/getsmart/healthcare/pdfs/checklist.pdf.)

95. Centers for Disease Control and Prevention. Checklist: the core elements of antibiotic stewardship for nursing homes. 2015. (Accessed April 12, 2016, at www.cdc.gov/longtermcare/pdfs/core-elements-antibiotic-stewardship-checklist.pdf.)

96. Saint S, Kowalski CP, Banaszak-Holl J, Forman J, Damschroder L, Krein SL. The importance of leadership in preventing healthcare-associated infection: results of a multisite qualitative study. *Infect Control Hosp Epidemiol* 2010; 31:901–907.

97. Dellefield ME, Kelly A, Schnelle JF. Quality assurance and performance improvement in nursing homes: using evidence-based protocols to observe nursing care processes in real time. *J Nurs Care Qual* 2013; 28:43–51.

98. Capitano B, Leshem O, Nightingale C, Nicolau D. Cost effect of managing methicillin-resistant *Staphylococcus aureus* in a long-term care facility. *J Am Geriatr Soc* 2003; 51:10–16.

99. Dubberke ER, Olsen MA. Burden of *Clostridium difficile* on the healthcare system. *Clin Infect Dis* 2012; 55(Suppl 2): S88–92.

100. The Pew Charitable Trusts. A Path to Better Antibiotic Stewardship in Inpatient Settings. 2016:1–45. (Accessed May 1, 2016, at www.pewtrusts.org/~/media/assets/2016/04/apathtobetterantibioticstewardshipininpatientsettings.pdf.)

101. Castle N. Measuring staff turnover in nursing homes. *Gerontologist* 2006; 46:210–219.

102. Pronovost PJ, Berenholtz SM, Needham DM. Translating evidence into practice: a model for large scale knowledge translation. *BMJ* 2008; 337:a1714.

103. Stone ND, Ashraf MS, Calder J, et al. Surveillance definitions of infections in long-term care facilities: revisiting the McGeer Criteria. *Infect Control Hosp Epidemiol* 2012; 33:965–977.

104. Fisch J, McNamara SE, Lansing BJ, Mody L. The 24-hour report as an effective monitoring and communication tool in infection prevention and control in nursing homes. *Am J Infect Control* 2014; 42:1112–1114.

105. Loeb M, Bentley DW, Bradley S, et al. Development of minimum criteria for the initiation of antibiotics in residents of long-term-care facilities: results of a consensus conference. *Infect Control Hosp Epidemiol* 2001; 22:120–124.

106. Mylotte JM. Antimicrobial stewardship in long-term care: metrics and risk adjustment. *J Am Med Dir Assoc* 2016; 17:672.e13–8.

107. Mody L, Krein SL, Saint S, et al. A targeted infection prevention intervention in nursing home residents with indwelling devices: a randomized clinical trial. *JAMA Intern Med* 2015; 175:714–723.

108. Davey P, Brown E, Fenelon L, et al. Interventions to improve antibiotic prescribing practices for hospital inpatients. *Cochrane Database Syst Rev* 2005; 19:CD003543.

109. Gerber JS, Prasad PA, Fiks AG, et al. Effect of an outpatient antimicrobial stewardship intervention on broad-spectrum antibiotic prescribing by primary care pediatricians:

a randomized trial. *JAMA* 2013; 309:2345–2352.

110. Gyssens IC, Blok WL, van den Broek PJ, Hekster YA, Van der Meer JW. Implementation of an educational program and an antibiotic order form to optimize quality of antimicrobial drug use in a department of internal medicine. *Eur J Clin Microbiol Infect Dis* 1997; 16:904–912.

111. Morgan DJ, Croft LD, Deloney V, et al. Choosing wisely in healthcare epidemiology and antimicrobial stewardship. *Infect Control Hosp Epidemiol* 2016; 37:755–760.

112. Phillips CD, Adepoju O, Stone N, et al. Asymptomatic bacteriuria, antibiotic use, and suspected urinary tract infections in four nursing homes. *BMC Geriatrics* 2012; 12:73.

113. Crnich CJ, Drinka P. Improving the management of urinary tract infections in nursing homes: it's time to stop the tail from wagging the dog. *Ann Long Term Care* 2014; 22:32–36.

114. Nace DA, Drinka PJ, Crnich CJ. Clinical uncertainties in the approach to long term care residents with possible urinary tract infection. *J Am Med Dir Assoc* 2014; 15:133–139.

115. Ducharme J, Neilson S, Ginn JL. Can urine cultures and reagent test strips be used to diagnose urinary tract infection in elderly emergency department patients without focal urinary symptoms? *CJEM* 2007; 9:87–92.

116. Arinzon Z, Peisakh A, Shuval I, Shabat S, Berner YN. Detection of urinary tract infection (UTI) in long-term care setting: is the multireagent strip an adequate diagnostic tool? *Arch Gerontol Geriatr* 2009; 48:227–231.

117. Furuno JP, Comer AC, Johnson JK, et al. Using antibiograms to improve antibiotic prescribing in skilled nursing facilities. *Infect Control Hosp Epidemiol* 2014; 35 Suppl 3:S56–61.

118. Wenisch JM, Equiluz-Bruck S, Fudel M, et al. Decreasing *Clostridium difficile* infections by an antimicrobial stewardship program that reduces moxifloxacin use. *Antimicrob Agents Chemother* 2014; 58:5079–5083.

119. Mehta JM, Haynes K, Wileyto EP, et al. Comparison of prior authorization and prospective audit with feedback for antimicrobial stewardship. *Infect Control Hosp Epidemiol* 2014; 35:1092–1099.

120. Ouslander JG, Lamb G, Tappen R, et al. Interventions to reduce hospitalizations from nursing homes: evaluation of the INTERACT II collaborative quality improvement project. *J Am Geriatr Soc* 2011; 59:745–753.

121. Linnebur SA, Fish DN, Ruscin JM, et al. Impact of a multidisciplinary intervention on antibiotic use for nursing home-acquired pneumonia. *Am J Geriatr Pharmacother* 2011; 9:442–450.e1.

122. Trautner BW, Grigoryan L, Petersen NJ, et al. An innovative and successful antimicrobial stewardship approach to asymptomatic bacteriuria. *JAMA Internal Medicine* 2015; 175:1120–1127.

123. Bushen JL, Mehta JM, Hamilton KW, et al. Impact of two different antimicrobial stewardship methods on frequency of streamlining antimicrobial agents in patients with bacteremia. *Infect Control Hosp Epidemiol* 2017; 38:89–95.

124. Meeker D, Linder JA, Fox CR, et al. Effect of behavioral interventions on inappropriate antibiotic prescribing among primary care practices: a randomized clinical trial. *JAMA* 2016; 315:562–570.

125. Jump RLP, Heath B, Crnich CJ, et al. Knowledge, beliefs, and confidence regarding infections and antimicrobial stewardship: a survey of Veterans Affairs providers who care for older adults. *Am J Infect Control* 2015; 43:298–300.

126. Heath B, Bernhardt J, Michalski TJ, et al. Results of a Veterans Affairs employee education program on antimicrobial stewardship for older adults. *Am J Infect Control* 2016; 44:349–351.

Chapter 13

Outpatient Antibiotic Stewardship

Larissa May and Matthew P. Kronman

Introduction

Outpatient antibiotic stewardship strategies consist of efforts to promote appropriate prescribing of antibiotics for non-hospitalized patients in office- and clinic-based practices as well as emergency department settings. While outpatient antibiotic stewardship programs may vary by size and scope and be instituted by a variety of stakeholders, their overall goal is to improve appropriate antibiotic prescribing consistent with evidence-based practices in order to foster patient safety, improve clinical outcomes, and potentially reduce the emergence and transmission of drug-resistant bacteria in the community.[1]

The need for outpatient antibiotic stewardship is urgent. US national estimates have shown that more than one out of every two people receives an antibiotic prescription annually, yet only approximately two-thirds of these antibiotics are considered appropriate.[2] Collectively, more than 250 million antibiotic courses were prescribed in US outpatient settings in 2011, and substantial regional variability in antibiotics prescribing rates exists, with prescribing highest in the South and lowest in the West.[3] The national Choosing Wisely Campaign seeks to improve patient care by disseminating educational materials to both healthcare providers and the general public about the appropriate choice of antibiotics. It has been adopted by a variety of professional societies including the American Academy of Family Physicians (AAFP) and the American College of Emergency Physicians (ACEP).[4] Recommendations exist for a number of different clinical syndromes and infections (Table 1). For example, ACEP recommends against antibiotic treatment of uncomplicated cutaneous abscess after successful incision and drainage in patients who have adequate medical follow-up.

Because acute respiratory tract infections predominate as the reason for which ambulatory patients are prescribed antibiotics inappropriately, most existing work to improve ambulatory antibiotic prescribing addresses these infections.[5] Several large studies have shown that over half of antibiotic prescriptions for acute respiratory infections among both children and adults in primary care, urgent care, and emergency departments (EDs) are unnecessary.[6–8]

There are a number of common respiratory tract infections for which antibiotics are not routinely indicated in the outpatient setting (Table 1). It is widely accepted that antibiotics are not indicated for acute bronchitis, nonspecific URIs, or viral pharyngitis because these clinical syndromes are most often caused by viruses that will not respond to antibiotic therapy.[9, 10] Antibiotics may be indicated for other conditions such as acute otitis media, sinusitis, and streptococcal pharyngitis, but some of these conditions can also be managed with only supportive care.[11–15]

Table 1 Typical Antibiotic Recommendations for Common Outpatient Infections

Conditions for Which Systemic Antibiotics Are Rarely Indicated		
Condition	**Antibiotic Recommendation**	**References**
Asymptomatic bacteriuria	None	Nicolle et al. [101]
Bronchitis, acute	None	Snow et al. [10], Harris et al. [127], Irwin et al.
Impetigo with few lesions	Topical therapy only	Stevens et al. [119]
Otitis externa, uncomplicated	Topical therapy only	Rosenfeld et al. [120]
Otitis media with effusion	None	Rosenfeld et al. [121]
Pharyngitis, viral	None	Shulman et al. [12], Dowell et al.
Upper respiratory infection (URI), uncomplicated	None	Harris et al., Dowell et al., Hersh et al. [9]
Conditions for which systemic antibiotics are sometimes indicated		
Condition	**Antibiotic recommendation**	**References**
Otitis media, acute	Amoxicillin	Lieberthal et al. [13)
Pharyngitis, streptococcal	Penicillin or amoxicillin	Shulman et al. [12]
Sinusitis	Amoxicillin or amoxicillin/ clavulanate	Rosenfeld et al. [15], Harris et al., Chow et al. [14]
Urinary Tract Infection	Nitrofurantoin or trimethoprim-sulfamethoxazole	Gupta et al., American Academy of Pediatrics guidelines [122, 123]
Cutaneous abscess	Trimethoprim-sulfamethoxazole, clindamycin	Talan et al., Infectious Diseases Society of America guidelines [124–126]

This chapter will address the many barriers to changing practices for outpatient antibiotic prescribing, including physician, patient, and environmental factors that vary by setting and site.[16] The chapter also proposes possible interventions to address these barriers and improve evidence-based antibiotic prescribing in the outpatient setting.

Antibiotic Stewardship in Outpatient Settings

In 2016 the CDC released a clinician and facility checklist for core measures for outpatient antibiotic stewardship, which includes the following elements: commitment to optimizing antibiotic prescribing and patient safety, action for policy and practice, tracking and reporting antibiotic prescribing practices, and providing educational resources and expertise to both clinicians and patients on antibiotic prescribing.[17]

Interventions for Patients in Outpatient Settings

Antibiotic prescribing decisions in the ambulatory setting are complex because they involve both clinician knowledge and empowerment to avoid inappropriate prescriptions. A study of over 300 graduating medical students at three US medical schools demonstrated that only half could answer knowledge-based questions on antibiotics correctly, suggesting that training about antibiotic formulations, spectra of activity, and indications for antibiotics among young trainees and prescribers may be suboptimal.[18]

A variety of interventions have been designed and implemented to improve antibiotic prescribing in outpatient community settings (Table 2). In systematic reviews of published studies, no single strategy to improve antibiotic prescribing dominates as outperforming the others.[19, 20] In this regard, different strategies or combinations of strategies may be needed for a given patient population, infection type, and available resources within the healthcare system.

Behavior and Communication Interventions

Specific communication strategies have been associated with patient and parent resistance to treatment plans.[21] Even when parents desire that antibiotics be prescribed for their children, they seldom express this interest directly.[22] When providers use positive treatment recommendations, outlining specific actions parents can take to make their children feel better, or when they employ contingency prescriptions that can be used if a patient worsens, parental satisfaction is improved.[22, 23] When providers use a negative framing approach, ruling out the need for antibiotics, this increases the rate at which parents question the treatment plan. This parental questioning in turn increases the provider's perception that parents want antibiotics and leads to providers prescribing antibiotics inappropriately.[24] The combination of positive and negative treatment recommendations appears best, reducing inappropriate antibiotic prescribing for acute respiratory tract infections by 85%, while still gleaning the highest visit ratings by parents (independent of whether or not antibiotics were prescribed.) [25]

Other behavioral strategies have been used with moderate success in reducing antibiotic use in adult patients in community settings. A multifaceted strategy including distribution of patient educational materials consisting of informational brochures in study offices, a public awareness media campaign, and focus groups with physicians along with provision of a treatment algorithm for upper respiratory infection found an 18% decrease in the rate of antibiotic prescribing during the intervention period, with significant reductions in macrolide use.[26] Another study evaluated the use of behavioral "nudging" on antibiotic prescribing in five outpatient primary care clinics. The intervention included posters featuring clinician photographs and signatures documenting a commitment to avoiding inappropriate antibiotic use, along with educational materials for patients. The intervention reduced inappropriate prescribing from 43% to 34% during the study period, while inappropriate prescribing increased by a similar amount in the control group.[27] This absolute reduction of almost 20% in inappropriate prescribing represents a very large effect for the extremely low-cost intervention implemented.

Table 2 Example Stewardship Interventions, By Type and Care Location

Intervention Type	Outpatient	Emergency Department	Resources and Notes
Academic detailing	Lectures and other engagement of providers by stewardship experts to encourage evidence-based prescribing Provision of information to prescribers and families	Lectures and other engagement of providers by stewardship experts to encourage evidence-based prescribing Provision of information to prescribers and families	Lectures have a relatively low resource cost but relatively modest effect One-on-one academic detailing is more resource intensive
Antibiograms	Not generally currently available; most clinics could refer to local hospital antibiograms	Development of condition-specific antibiograms (e.g., for patients discharged with UTI)	Requires intensive informatics resource and partnership with clinical laboratory
Clinician feedback and peer comparisons	Individualized prescribing reports for common conditions (e.g., otitis media)	Individualized prescribing reports for common conditions (e.g., pneumonia) Review of broad-spectrum agent use by the ED as a whole	Requires intensive informatics resources. Effect may wane if audit and feedback removed
Behavioral modification	Delayed antibiotic prescribing Signed commitment posters	Delayed antibiotic prescribing Signed commitment posters	Low cost but potentially high impact interventions
Clinical decision support	Integrated guidance for common conditions (e.g., UTI)	Integrated guidance for common conditions (e.g., skin and soft tissue infections)	Can be paper or electronic. Can be based on national guidelines or local consensus
Clinical guidelines	Adapt and evaluate compliance with national guidelines for common conditions (e.g., bronchitis, pharyngitis)	Adapt and evaluate compliance with national guidelines for common conditions (e.g., sepsis)	AAFP, AAP, ACEP, CDC, IDSA, SHEA*
Rapid diagnostic testing	Rapid streptococcal testing Rapid influenza testing	Rapid streptococcal testing Rapid influenza testing Rapid respiratory viral testing Rapid chlamydia and gonorrhea testing	Effective but can be costly. Often requires partnership with clinical laboratory

* AAFP: American Academy of Family Physicians; AAP: American Academy of Pediatrics; ACEP: American College of Emergency Physicians; CDC: Centers for Disease Control and Prevention; IDSA: Infectious Diseases Society of America; SHEA: The Society for Healthcare Epidemiology of America

Another useful strategy is delayed prescribing, in which a provider does not prescribe antibiotics at the time of the clinical encounter, but instead either provides a post-dated antibiotic prescription that can be filled on a later date or clarifies a relatively simple way for patients to obtain an antibiotic prescription if symptoms continue. For example, Little and colleagues performed an open, factorial, randomized trial of primary care practices in the United Kingdom, randomizing patients with acute URIs not determined to need immediate antibiotics to one of four delayed prescribing strategies [28] including (1) providing post-dated prescriptions; (2) requiring patients to re-contact the primary care office by telephone if symptoms continue, at which time an antibiotic prescription would be called into a pharmacy if needed; (3) requiring patients to return physically to the office to obtain a prescription if needed; or (4) giving patients a prescription at the time of the initial clinical encounter but requesting that they not fill it. The authors found that across these four intervention arms, 33%–39% of all subjects ended up obtaining antibiotic prescriptions in the two weeks after the initial encounter, compared with 26% in the group offered no antibiotics initially. Rates of adverse outcomes were equal among the groups. This study demonstrates that the simple act of delaying antibiotics may help avoid antibiotic prescribing for 60% or more of adults with URIs.

Beyond having robust knowledge of antibiotics, providers must face patient and parent expectations for antibiotics, which can present a major challenge for physician adherence to prescribing guidelines, specifically for URIs. While there is concern that patient satisfaction may be influenced by interventions to reduce inappropriate antibiotic prescribing, reduction in antibiotic use for acute bronchitis has not been found to decrease satisfaction.[29] Nonetheless, given the emphasis placed on patient satisfaction in many healthcare systems, concerns about decreased patient satisfaction due to withheld antibiotics may limit stewardship interventions in the outpatient setting. However, physicians are often unable to assess patient expectations regarding antibiotics accurately, and patient satisfaction is likely related to improved communication rather than a decision to prescribe antibiotics in many cases.[30] Potential solutions to improving appropriate antibiotic prescribing in community settings while addressing patient satisfaction include multifaceted approaches incorporating shared decision-making with patients.[31–33] One additional barrier in the outpatient setting is the fact that pharmacists are not routinely incorporated into the flow of day-to-day clinical activities, limiting the ability for pharmacists to be involved in many routine outpatient stewardship interventions.

Rapid Diagnostic Testing

While the majority of URIs have a viral etiology, accurate and rapid tests are not routinely available to exclude bacterial infection in the outpatient setting.[34] The one condition for which rapid diagnostic testing is routinely and widely available in the outpatient setting is streptococcal pharyngitis. Rapid streptococcal antigen testing should always be performed to establish the diagnosis of streptococcal pharyngitis in the setting of appropriate signs and symptoms (such as fever and sore throat in the absence of rhinorrhea and cough).[12] For other conditions, discriminating between viral and bacterial infections is problematic, such as for acute otitis media or sinusitis, where aspirates for microbiologic cultures are not practical for most patients. Furthermore, routine bacterial cultures, which take 24–48 hours to result, are not available in a timely fashion to guide empiric antibiotic selection. Rapid influenza tests have traditionally been plagued by low sensitivity and specificity, however newly approved single target tests as well as multiplex respiratory virus panels may provide more accurate information to clinicians, albeit not necessarily in a cost-effective manner, and these tests are not available in all outpatient locations.[35–38]

Newer serum markers such as procalcitonin may provide an important opportunity to reduce unnecessary antibiotic treatment in outpatients with lower respiratory tract infection who are at low risk of bacterial infection. An observational study of consecutive outpatients presenting to EDs and clinics with lower respiratory tract infections found that the use of a procalcitonin algorithm resulted in shorter durations of antibiotic therapy without increasing rates of adverse events.[39] A second randomized study evaluating the use of procalcitonin for antibiotic selection in low risk outpatients diagnosed with community-acquired pneumonia found that antibiotic prescription at admission, total antibiotic exposure and overall treatment duration decreased significantly for the arm with procalcitonin-guided treatment, without a difference in clinical outcomes at four weeks.[40]

Clinical Guidelines

The use of clinical practice guidelines may be helpful in minimizing both the unnecessary and inappropriate use of antibiotics contributing to antibiotic resistance.[41] Common barriers to provider practice change and adherence to evidence-based guidelines in a variety of settings include external factors such as lack of time, resources, and patient expectations. Furthermore, physician-specific internal factors, such as knowledge, attitudes, and beliefs about guideline recommendations, influence prescribing patterns and likely vary by setting and site.[17] However, clinical guidelines have been shown in some settings to improve practice. A randomized trial that provided clinical guidelines for common acute respiratory tract infections, urinary tract infections, and skin and soft tissue infections to ambulatory intervention practices demonstrated an almost 5% absolute reduction in antibiotic prescribing for acute respiratory tract infections other than pneumonia, and an almost 4% absolute reduction in broad-spectrum prescribing across all included conditions.[42]

Academic Detailing and Clinical Decision Support

Academic detailing represents a set of core principles, including assessing provider knowledge, focusing efforts on specific clinicians, utilizing active educational strategies for clinicians, highlighting and repeating essential messages, and using positive reinforcement. A prospective, non-randomized controlled trial of ambulatory practices related to antibiotic use demonstrated a reduction in inappropriate antibiotic prescribing for adults with acute bronchitis from 74% to 48% at the practice that received an academic detailing intervention consisting of household- and office-based education and clinician education about appropriate prescribing for bronchitis.[43] In another study, an intervention that included providers reflecting on their own antibiotic prescribing data, teaching techniques of motivational interviewing, and use of online educational scenarios, videos, and web forums was able to reduce overall absolute antibiotic prescribing by 4%.[44] Brief academic detailing visits with a clinical pharmacist to outline appropriate antibiotic selections for common infections have also been shown to improve first-line antibiotic prescribing.[45] Interventions targeting community education have been less successful in reducing inappropriate antibiotic use in pediatric patients.[46]

Clinical decision support may also assist with reducing inappropriate antibiotic prescribing and reducing the use of broad-spectrum antibiotics for the treatment of URIs.[47]

Clinical decision support systems (CDSS) can improve access to evidence-based practice guidelines; randomized trials in community settings have demonstrated a reduction in overall and inappropriate antibiotic use when these systems are utilized.[48–51] Cluster-randomized trials within outpatient practices have shown that use of either paper-based or computerized CDSS for acute respiratory tract infections can decrease overall antibiotic prescribing for these conditions. One trial reduced inappropriate antibiotic prescribing by 32% for those conditions in the intervention clinics and by only 5% in the control clinics. [52, 53] Barriers to CDSS, however, are interference with workflow and the need for integration with computerized physician order entry for most interventions.[54, 55] CDSS can, however, be implemented with printed, paper decision support materials; these materials have been shown to be as effective as computerized materials at reducing antibiotic prescribing for adults with acute bronchitis in a cluster-randomized trial.[56] A systematic review of CDSS to support antibiotic prescribing demonstrated success utilizing various techniques, but the overall influence of CDSS on clinical management is difficult to assess in clinical practice.[57]

Clinician Feedback and Reports on Antibiotic Prescribing Practices

Another intervention that has been used to improve antibiotic prescribing is providing individualized feedback on prescribing patterns, in which providers' prescribing data are summarized by the stewardship team and then returned to those providers so they can evaluate their prescribing habits critically and learn from the experience to improve future prescribing. In a randomized trial of outpatient pediatric practices, use of personalized feedback in addition to minimal academic detailing was shown to reduce broad-spectrum prescribing for acute respiratory tract infections by 13% overall, compared to a 7% overall reduction among control practices.[58] The intervention was also shown to reduce off-guideline prescribing. However, after the study intervention was completed, the beneficial effect of the intervention waned and practices returned to baseline levels of prescribing.[59] Furthermore, physicians who participated in the intervention and were subsequently interviewed by a medical anthropologist about the study expressed skepticism about the utility and accuracy of the feedback reports, and some participants admitted ignoring the reports altogether.[60] Others noted the substantial pressure they felt from parents to prescribe antibiotics. In this regard, personalized feedback reports alone may be insufficient to improve antibiotic prescribing over the long term and may not be sustainable without ongoing education and feedback.

Antibiotic Stewardship in the Emergency Department Setting

Introduction

According to the Surviving Sepsis campaign, the initial antibiotic prescribed in the ED for patients admitted with serious infections is arguably the most important dose the patient receives. This decision should be based not only on the suspected source of infection but also host factors and prior antibiotic exposure.[61, 62] Research demonstrates that antibiotic selection in the ED may affect downstream treatment in hospitalized patients.[63] The antibiotic choice made by the ED clinician thus has a significant influence on what therapy is continued in the inpatient setting, thereby representing an important opportunity for antibiotic stewardship and collaboration with other specialties. In addition to making the decision regarding first antibiotic dose for inpatients, ED clinicians play a vital role in obtaining relevant cultures prior to administration of antibiotics that allow for tailoring or discontinuation of antibiotic therapy during hospitalization or, for discharged patients, outpatient management of antibiotics.

Barriers

The ED provides an important opportunity for reducing inappropriate antibiotic use for non-antibiotic-responsive conditions, given that up to half of all antibiotic prescriptions are not necessary.[64–66] Particularly problematic is the excessive use of broad-spectrum antibiotics (e.g., fluoroquinolones) [67–69] despite availability of resources such as local antibiograms and guidelines to help guide targeted antibiotic selection.[70, 71] Inappropriate antibiotic use in the ED and other settings is an important patient safety issue. An estimated 142,500 ED visits each year are related to adverse events associated with systemic antibiotics, with nearly 80% due to allergic reactions.[72] The rate of adverse events due to antibiotic exposure is therefore about half that of adverse events due to medications considered "high-risk" such as warfarin, digoxin, or insulin, and is higher than the rate of adverse events seen with certain other anticoagulants such as aspirin and clopidogrel.

Antibiotic stewardship, or optimizing antibiotic utilization, reduces unnecessary antibiotic use in inpatient and outpatient settings, but is not typically practiced in the ED. Recently researchers have argued that stewardship activities should rightly expand into the ED setting.[73–76] However, not all interventions for hospitalized patients are appropriate for translation to the ED setting. EDs are at the interface between the community and inpatient settings and thus are particularly important venues for antibiotic stewardship, given the frequent prescription of antibiotics for both outpatients being discharged from the ED and patients being admitted to the hospital who are first seen in the ED. Nonetheless, given the fast-paced environment of the ED, where quick clinical decisions must often be made with limited diagnostic or historical information, stewardship interventions can be tailored to the ED in order to be effective.

Similar to many healthcare settings, decision-making among ED providers regarding antibiotic prescribing is a complex process.[77] Barriers to practice change are numerous, including prescribing to meet patient expectations, provider anxiety regarding diagnostic uncertainty, and limitations in diagnostic specimen collection and testing in the busy ED environment. There are a set of distinct challenges associated with providing systematic education and oversight for antibiotic stewardship in the ED setting. These include high rates of ED overcrowding,[78] rapid rate of patient turnover, the need for quick decision-making usually without consultation, and importantly the large and varied mix of providers who work in a shift-based scheduling format, with relative high rates of staff turnover versus other clinical settings.[79] Specific barriers to implementing other public health measures in the ED have been previously described and include perceived lack of efficacy, concerns regarding reimbursement and resource availability, and potential interference with ED operational efficiency.[80, 81] Further, medical liability concerns, including the failure to diagnose and treat [82] specific conditions as well as requirements to satisfy local or national externally-monitored quality measures are associated with overuse of antibiotics and other medications.[83] In addition, clinicians' desire to maintain patient satisfaction has been demonstrated to be an important factor in antibiotic prescribing practice in the

ED setting;[84] previous studies have shown that provision of antibiotic prescriptions is associated with increased satisfaction for ED visits for URIs,[85] and physicians are more likely to prescribe antibiotics if they perceive patients want them.[86]

A study of clinical decision-making around antibiotic prescribing in the ED showed that of 150 survey respondents, 76% agreed or strongly agreed that antibiotics are overused in the ED, while half believed they personally did not overprescribe. Interview analysis identified five important themes: (1) resource and environmental factors that affect care; (2) access to and quality of care received outside of the ED consult; (3) patient-provider relationships; (4) clinical inertia; and (5) local knowledge generation. Some of the most important factors identified included lack of access to accurate and rapid diagnostic tests, limited support for follow-up of patients, healthcare system factors such as lack of access to primary care and an inability to ensure adequate patient follow-up, concerns regarding psychosocial and socioeconomic factors that may impact patient care, risk factors such as patient comorbidities, lack of access to ED-specific guidelines, and a desire not to compromise patient satisfaction.[77]

In addition, provider concerns about length of stay and crowding in the ED might impact the decision for empiric antibiotics versus targeted testing and treatment (e.g., for streptococcal pharyngitis). An observational study revealed limited patient understanding of antibiotic use. Providers relied heavily upon diagnostics and provided limited education to patients. Most patients denied *a priori* expectations of being prescribed antibiotics,[77] suggesting that patient, provider, and healthcare system factors should be considered when designing interventions to improve antibiotic stewardship in the ED setting. Another study confirms that providers in the ED perceive environmental and patient-related factors as primary barriers to guideline adherence.[87]

Interventions

Few systematic efforts to date have been described to translate effective stewardship strategies to the ED setting. Implementation of validated clinical decision rules in the ED setting has yielded mixed findings.[88, 89] However, despite existing challenges, unique facilitators to successful practice change in the ED include staff interest in novel tools such as electronic CDSS,[90] availability of local microbiologic resistance patterns,[91] and ED providers' comfort assuming new roles and responsibilities.[92]

Interventions to address ED barriers to appropriate antibiotic prescribing have been borrowed from inpatient antibiotic stewardship programs and largely mirror the same themes as interventions in the outpatient setting. These include provision of pathways with education and resources, audit and feedback to the clinical care team, and process changes for the perceived lack of time.[93] A systematic review of interventions to improve quality of care concluded that educational outreach for appropriate prescribing, reminders, and multifaceted interventions targeting barriers to change are most effective for improving quality of care.[76, 94] Strategies that could impact a reduction in inappropriate antibiotic prescribing in the ED include clinician education, tailoring of national guidelines to the local ED setting, support by an ED pharmacist where available, audit and feedback, clinical decision support enhancements including electronic medical record order sets, rapid diagnostic testing, and ED antibiogram development (see Table 2).[95] Collaborative efforts between ED clinicians, pharmacists, microbiologists, primary care and infectious diseases colleagues are likely to be the most fruitful in yielding long-term successes.[96] Any intervention should include measurement of processes and specific outcomes. Interventions optimally include a comprehensive multidisciplinary antibiotic management strategy and outcome measures to track antimicrobial utilization and resistance patterns carefully.[97]

There have been a number of recently published successful interventions in the ED setting, for a variety of clinical problems including urinary tract infection, skin and soft tissue infection, and respiratory tract infection. For example, a multifaceted educational intervention for the treatment of uncomplicated UTIs which included implementation of local guidelines and an ED-specific antibiogram coupled with audit and feedback, led to a 38% improvement in adherence to treatment recommendations without a significant impact on patient outcomes; the greatest change resulted from targeting narrow-spectrum therapy.[98] Educating ED providers about local resistance patterns has been shown to improve antibiotic prescribing, with increased narrow-spectrum prescribing and decreased broad-spectrum prescribing for urinary tract infections.[99] Additionally, a randomized trial of children 2–12 years old with acute otitis media seen in the ED demonstrated that delayed prescribing practices (in which patients in the intervention arm were offered observation alone without antibiotics and instructed to follow-up for care if symptoms persisted) were associated with an almost 30% absolute reduction in antibiotic use for those in the intervention arm, with only 19% of those patients acquiring an antibiotic in the 7–10 days following the ED visit.[100] Notably, there was no difference in patient outcomes between the two arms, providing a reminder that delaying antibiotic prescribing can be safe for a number of patients with diseases classically considered ones in which antibiotic prescribing is always indicated, such as acute otitis media and sinusitis. Another way to reduce antibiotic prescribing in the ED setting is to improve education regarding clinical conditions that do not routinely require antibiotic therapy, such as acute bronchitis. Antibiotic stewardship is also important for other clinical conditions besides respiratory infections; for example, antibiotics are not routinely indicated for most patients with asymptomatic bacteriuria because antibiotic treatment of this condition is not associated with prevention of infection or other long-term adverse outcomes (Table 2).[101, 102]

Antibiograms

The Clinical and Laboratory Standards Institute (CLSI) [103] provides guidelines for antibiogram creation. While typically routine cumulative antibiograms represent an entire institution, enhanced antibiograms may be stratified by various parameters including patient location or population, including community susceptibility patterns. Reliance on institutional antibiograms, even for ED outpatients, remains problematic as culture-based data are biased toward more complicated patients and cases and pathogen susceptibilities may vary significantly across settings. For example, a study reviewing 3,140 cultures, including 1,417 from the ED, found that the frequencies of pathogens isolated in the ED and hospital were similar, with the exception of *Escherichia coli*, which was more commonly isolated in ED patients.[104] Another study found that for *E. coli*, ciprofloxacin non-susceptibility was significantly less common in isolates from ED patients with cystitis and pyelonephritis than in isolates from hospitalized patients. *E. coli* non-susceptibility to ciprofloxacin was also significantly less common in ED isolates from patients with uncomplicated UTIs than in isolates from all ED patients with clinician-ordered urine cultures. [105] In most clinical environments, ED-specific data are not available to guide clinical decision-making, particularly for patients being discharged home with uncomplicated infections. However, even where available, enhanced antibiograms (i.e., those stratified by unit, age, or disease type) have yet to be validated in the clinical setting as to whether they indeed assist clinicians in optimizing antibiotic choice and improving clinical outcomes. Outpatient antibiograms that are most likely to be useful would include information on isolates from those organisms seen most commonly in the outpatient setting. Specifically, these antibiotics could include resistance patterns for urinary pathogens (e.g., *E. coli*), *S. aureus* (for skin and soft tissue infections), and for *S. pneumoniae* (for acute otitis media, pneumonia, and sinusitis).

Clinical Decision Support

As seen in the community setting, CDSS can improve evidence-based practice, and randomized trials in ED community settings have demonstrated their contributions to reductions in overall and inappropriate antibiotic use.[75, 106] Integration of CDSS into a set of strategies aimed at organizational and individual change can be generalized into an implementation toolkit to improve care in other ambulatory settings.[107] However, implementing strategies tested in the ambulatory setting to the fast-paced, acute care ED setting, where patients are seen in single encounters, requires special consideration. For example, attention to interference with workflow, communication challenges with patients, and integration with existing commercial electronic medical records are factors that should be taken into account in designing programs. Multilevel implementation strategies targeting barriers to change are most effective for improving quality of care.[108] An antibiotic stewardship intervention that included implementation of an order set for uncomplicated UTI and a second phase of audit and feedback found that guideline adherence increased significantly for each intervention period (68%–82% respectively, from a baseline of 44%), with a reduction in fluoroquinolone use.[109]

Patient-Centered Strategies

Strategies to address concerns regarding patient access to care and follow-up post-ED visits could also reduce overuse of empiric prescribing and increase the likelihood of sending cultures on patients started on empiric antibiotic therapy. Telephone follow-up is already being conducted in many EDs for purposes of patient satisfaction, such as Press Ganey scores, and could be leveraged to decrease unnecessary use of antibiotics in the ED. For example, a culture follow-up program for blood and urine cultures for adults discharged home from the ED using computer decision support and pharmacist follow-up reduced repeat visits to the ED significantly, including for uninsured patients.[110] Dedicated clinical pharmacist-managed stewardship programs could also reduce the time to review positive cultures.[111]

Rapid Diagnostic Testing with Result Reporting during the ED Visit

Improving access to rapid diagnostics may also help guide targeted antibiotic selection and improve patient outcomes. There is a growing arsenal of rapid diagnostic tests that could have potential utility in the ED setting to improve antibiotic prescribing and patient outcomes.[112] Many of these tests are already or could be made available at or near the point-of-care, such as rapid streptococcal antigen tests and newly emerging rapid molecular tests (e.g., molecular-based screening for *Staphylococcus aureus* colonization and infection;

Clostridium difficile; viral respiratory pathogens including influenza, and *Streptococcus pneumoniae* among others; and rapid testing for pathogens causing gastrointestinal disease). These multiplex platforms for pathogen diagnosis can be expensive, however, and additional investigation is needed to understand how to employ these new tools in the most cost-effective manner.

Nonetheless, several recent ED studies demonstrate potential value to providing pathogen results during the ED visit. For example, there is very poor adherence to guidelines for antibiotic use in discharged patients with cutaneous abscesses, likely due to concerns for the virulence of methicillin-resistant *Staphylococcus aureus* (MRSA). Use of antibiotics active against community-acquired MRSA for outpatients diagnosed with cellulitis in the ED increased from 2007 to 2010; agents active against MRSA accounted for 68% of all antibiotics given to those with cellulitis, with >20% of patients receiving trimethoprim-sulfamethoxazole alone, even though this agent does not cover streptococcal species, an important cause of cellulitis.[113] Furthermore, a prospective, randomized controlled trial of 252 adults compared a rapid molecular test to standard of care culture-based testing in patients presenting with cutaneous abscess to two urban academic EDs. The trial found that methicillin-sensitive *Staphylococcus aureus* (MSSA)-positive patients receiving the rapid test were approximately 15% more likely to be prescribed beta-lactams appropriately than controls while MRSA-positive patients receiving the rapid test were about 22% more often prescribed appropriate anti-MRSA antibiotics. There were no significant differences between the two groups in one week or three month clinical outcomes. A second study evaluating the same assay in ED patients hospitalized with skin and soft tissue infections found no beneficial impact in these patients, suggesting that merely providing rapid molecular tests might not change clinical practice without an effective implementation strategy.[114]

A 2014 study using a US nationally-representative database evaluated the use of rapid influenza diagnostic testing in the ED.[115] The authors found that subjects diagnosed with influenza and in whom rapid influenza testing was performed, when compared with subjects diagnosed with influenza and in whom rapid influenza testing was not performed, were less likely to have other ancillary tests performed (45% vs. 53%), were less likely to receive antibiotics (11% vs. 23%), and were more likely to receive antivirals (56% vs. 19%).

A randomized study on the effect of a new, rapid molecular test for *Chlamydia trachomatis/Neisseria gonorrhoeae* diagnosis compared to standard care on clinical ED decision-making found a significant reduction in unnecessary antibiotic treatment for symptomatic patients receiving the rapid test. Test patients with negative results were nearly 40% less likely to receive empiric antibiotic treatment than control patients. Thirty-seven participants (53%) were contacted for follow-up 7–10 days post-discharge. Test patients were 77% less likely to report missed antibiotic doses. There were no significant differences in patient charges or health care utilization measures. Provision of rapid diagnostic testing to rule in or rule out *C. trachomatis* or *N. gonorrhoeae* during a patient's ED visit could shift the paradigm from overuse of empiric antibiotics to targeted treatment and notification, with important public health implications.

Finally, the capability of new rapid diagnostics to distinguish pathogens has been demonstrated to improve clinical decision-making and ensures rapid and appropriate initiation of antibiotic therapy in patients presenting with acute respiratory infections; this strategy helps eliminate antibiotic use in the case of viral pathogens, and reduces use of broad-spectrum agents when a narrow-spectrum option is available.[116, 117]

An intervention that included an ED clinical pathway, a kit for appropriate antibiotics, dosing for community-acquired pneumonia and ability to dispense preloaded medications in the ED resulted in improved antibiotic selection for pneumonia from 55% to 93% over a three-year study period.[118]

Conclusion

The outpatient setting, both ambulatory primary care and specialty offices as well as EDs, represents an important area for the development of ongoing antibiotic stewardship interventions. Research has demonstrated a number of different types of effective interventions, including academic detailing, provider commitments to appropriate antibiotic prescribing, CDSS and guidelines, antibiograms, and the use of rapid diagnostic tests. Since the vast majority of human antibiotic use in the United States occurs in the outpatient setting, antibiotic stewardship interventions must be tailored to the different needs of these outpatient settings.

Appendix A

List of Useful Resources

- The Society for Healthcare Epidemiology of America: www.shea-online.org/PriorityTopics/AntimicrobialStewardship.aspx
- The Centers for Disease Control and Prevention: www.cdc.gov/getsmart/community/improving-prescribing/outpatient-stewardship.html
- The Infectious Diseases Society of America: www.idsociety.org/IDSA_Practice_Guidelines/
- Alliance for the Prudent Use of Antibiotics: www.tufts.edu/med/apua/

References

1. Centers for Disease Control and Prevention. Outpatient Antibiotic Stewardship for Healthcare Professionals. Accessed November 6, 2017, at www.cdc.gov/getsmart/community/improving-prescribing/outpatient-stewardship.html

2. Fleming-Dutra KE, Hersh AL, Shapiro DJ, et al. Prevalence of inappropriate antibiotic prescriptions among us ambulatory care visits, 2010–2011. *JAMA* 2016; 315 (17):1864–1873.

3. Hicks LA, Bartoces MG, Roberts RM, et al. US outpatient antibiotic prescribing variation according to geography, patient population, and provider specialty in 2011. *Clin Infect Dis* 2015; 60(9):1308–1316.

4. Choosing Wisely, Continue the Conversation. Clinician Lists. Accessed November 6, 2017, at www.choosingwisely.org/clinician-lists/.

5. Hersh AL, Shapiro DJ, Pavia AT, Shah SS. Antibiotic prescribing in ambulatory pediatrics in the United States. *Pediatrics* 2011; 128(6):1053–1061.

6. Sharp AL, Klau MH, Keschner D, et al. Low-value care for acute sinusitis encounters: who's choosing wisely? *Am J Manage Care* 2015; 21(7):479–485.

7. Hersh AL, Shapiro DJ, Pavia AT, Shah SS. Antibiotic prescribing in ambulatory pediatrics in the United States. *Pediatrics* 2011; 128(6):1053–1061.

8. US Centers for Disease Control and Prevention. Antibiotic Resistance Threats in the United States, 2013. Accessed November 6, 2017, at www.cdc.gov/drugresistance/pdf/ar-threats-2013-508.pdf.

9. Hersh AL, Jackson MA, Hicks LA, American Academy of Pediatrics Committee on Infectious D. Principles of judicious antibiotic prescribing for upper respiratory tract infections in pediatrics. *Pediatrics* 2013; 132 (6):1146–1154.

10. Snow V, Mottur-Pilson C, Gonzales R, et al. Principles of appropriate antibiotic use for treatment of acute bronchitis in adults. *Ann Intern Med* 2001; 134 (6):518–520.

11. Wald ER, Applegate KE, Bordley C, et al. Clinical practice guideline for the diagnosis and management of acute bacterial sinusitis in children aged 1 to 18 years. *Pediatrics* 2013; 132(1):e262–280.

12. Shulman ST, Bisno AL, Clegg HW, et al. Clinical practice guideline for the diagnosis and management of group A streptococcal pharyngitis: 2012 update by the Infectious Diseases Society of America. *Clin Infect Dis* 2012; 55(10):e86–110

13. Lieberthal AS, Carroll AE, Chonmaitree T, et al. The diagnosis and management of acute otitis media. *Pediatrics* 2013; 131(3): e964–999.

14. Chow AW, Benninger MS, Brook I, et al. IDSA clinical practice guideline for acute bacterial rhinosinusitis in children and adults. *Clin Infect Dis* 2012; 54(8): e72–e112.

15. Rosenfeld RM, Piccirillo JF, Chandrasekhar SS, et al. Clinical practice guideline (update): adult sinusitis. *Otolaryngol Head Neck Surg* 2015; 152(Suppl 2):S1–39.

16. Cabana M, Rand C, Powe N, et al. Why don't physicians follow clinical practice guidelines? A framework for improvement. *JAMA* 1999; 282(15):1458–1465.

17. Sanchez GV, Fleming-Dutra KE, Roberts RM, Hicks LA. Core elements of outpatient antibiotic stewardship. *MMWR Recomm Rep* 2016; 65(6):1–12.

18. Abbo LM, Cosgrove SE, Pottinger PS, et al. Medical students' perceptions and knowledge about antimicrobial stewardship: how are we educating our future prescribers? *Clin Infect Dis* 2013; 57 (5):631–638.

19. Ranji SR, Steinman MA, Shojania KG, Gonzales R. Interventions to reduce unnecessary antibiotic prescribing: a systematic review and quantitative analysis. *Med Care* 2008; 46(8):847–862.

20. Arnold SR, Straus SE. Interventions to improve antibiotic prescribing practices in ambulatory care. *Cochrane Database Syst Rev* 2005; (4):CD003539.

21. Stivers T. Non-antibiotic treatment recommendations: delivery formats and implications for parent resistance. *Soc Sci Med* 2005; 60(5):949–964.

22. Mangione-Smith R, McGlynn EA, Elliott MN, McDonald L, Franz CE, Kravitz RL. Parent expectations for antibiotics, physician-parent communication, and satisfaction. *Arch Pediatr Adolesc Med* 2001; 155(7):800–806.

23. Mangione-Smith R, Zhou C, Robinson JD, Taylor JA, Elliott MN, Heritage J. Communication practices and antibiotic use for acute respiratory tract infections in children. *Ann Fam Med* 2015; 13 (3):221–227.

24. Mangione-Smith R, Elliott MN, Stivers T, McDonald LL, Heritage J. Ruling out the need for antibiotics: are we sending the right message? *Arch Pediatr Adolesc Med* 2006; 160(9):945–952.

25. Mangione-Smith R, Zhou C, Robinson JD, Taylor JA, Elliott MN, Heritage J. Communication practices and antibiotic use for acute respiratory tract infections in children. *Ann Fam Med* 2015; 13 (3):221–227.

26. Rubin, MA, Bateman, K, Alder, S, Donnelly, S, Stoddard, GJ, Samore, MH. A multifaceted intervention to improve antimicrobial prescribing for upper respiratory tract infections in a small rural community. *Clin Infect Dis* 2005; 40(4):546–553. doi:10.1086/427500.

27. Meeker D, Knight TK, Friedberg MW, et al. Nudging guideline-concordant antibiotic prescribing: a randomized clinical trial. *JAMA Internal Medicine* 2014; 174 (3):425–431. doi:10.1001/ jamainternmed.2013.14191.

28. Little P, Moore M, Kelly J, et al. Delayed antibiotic prescribing strategies for respiratory tract infections in primary care: pragmatic, factorial, randomised controlled trial. *BMJ* 2014; 348:g1606.

29. Gonzales, R, Steiner, JF, Maselli, J, Lum, A, Barrett, PH Jr. Impact of reducing antibiotic prescribing for acute bronchitis on patient satisfaction. *Effective Clinical Practice* 2001; 4(3):105–111.

30. Shapiro E. Injudicious antibiotic use: an unforeseen consequence of the emphasis on patient satisfaction? *Clin Ther* 2002; 24 (1):197–204.

31. Leblanc A, Légaré F, Labrecque M, et al. Feasibility of a randomised trial of a continuing medical education program in shared decision-making on the use of antibiotics for acute respiratory infections in primary care: the DECISION+ pilot trial. *Implement Sci* 2011; 6(Jan.):5.

32. Wanderer JP, Sandberg WS, Ehrenfeld JM. Real-time alerts and reminders using information systems. *Anesthesiol Clin* 2011; 29(3):389–96. doi: 10.1016/j. anclin.2011.05.003.

33. Waldron N, Dey I, Nagree Y, Xiao J, Flicker L. A multifaceted intervention to implement guideline care and improve quality of care for older people who present to the emergency department with falls. *BMC Geriatr* 2011; 11:6.

34. Gill JM, Fleischut P, Haas S, Pellini B, Crawford A, Nash DB. Use of antibiotics for adult upper respiratory infections in outpatient settings: a national ambulatory network study. *Fam Med* 2006; 38 (5):349–354.

35. Chartrand C, Leeflang MM, Minion J, Brewer T, Pai M. Accuracy of rapid influenza diagnostic tests: a meta-analysis. *Ann Intern Med* 2012; 156(7):500–511.

36. Dugas AF, Coleman S, Gaydos CA, Rothman RE, Frick KD. Cost-utility of rapid polymerase chain reaction-based influenza testing for high-risk emergency department patients. *Ann Emerg Med* 2013; 62(1):80–88.

37. Brittain-Long R, Westin J, Olofsson S, Lindh M, Andersson LM. Access to a polymerase chain reaction assay method targeting 13 respiratory viruses can reduce antibiotics: a randomised, controlled trial. *BMC Med* 2011; 9:44.

38. Green DA, Hitoaliaj L, Kotansky B, Campbell SM, Peaper DR. Clinical utility of on-demand multiplex respiratory pathogen testing among adult outpatients. *J Clin Microbiol* 2016; 54(12):2950–2955.

39. Albrich WC, Dusemund F, Bucher B, et al. Effectiveness and safety of procalcitonin-guided antibiotic therapy in lower respiratory tract infections in "real life": an international, multicenter poststudy survey (ProREAL). *Arch Intern Med* 2012; 172 (9):715–722. doi:10.1001/ archinternmed.2012.770.

40. Long W, Deng, X, Zhang Y, Lu G, Xie J, Tang J. Procalcitonin guidance for reduction of antibiotic use in low-risk outpatients with community-acquired pneumonia. *Respirology* 2011; 16:819–824. doi:10.1111/j.1440–1843.2011.01978.x

41. Field MJ, Lohr KN (Eds.). *Guidelines for Clinical Practice: From Development to Use.* Washington, DC: National Academy Press, 1992.

42. Jenkins TC, Irwin A, Coombs L, et al. Effects of clinical pathways for common outpatient infections on antibiotic prescribing. *American Journal of Medicine* 2013; 126(4):327–335:e312.

43. Gonzales R, Steiner JF, Lum A, Barrett PH, Jr. Decreasing antibiotic use in ambulatory practice: impact of a multidimensional intervention on the treatment of uncomplicated acute bronchitis in adults. *JAMA* 1999; 281(16):1512–1519.

44. Butler CC, Simpson SA, Dunstan F, et al. Effectiveness of multifaceted educational programme to reduce antibiotic dispensing in primary care: practice based randomised controlled trial. *BMJ* 2012; 344: d8173.

45. Ilett KF, Johnson S, Greenhill G, et al. Modification of general practitioner prescribing of antibiotics by use of a therapeutics adviser (academic detailer). *British Journal of Clinical Pharmacology* 2000; 49(2):168–173.

46. Finkelstein JA, Huang SS, Kleinman K, et al. Impact of a 16-community trial to promote judicious antibiotic use in Massachusetts. *Pediatrics* 2008; 121(1): e15–23.

47. Rattinger GB, Mullins CD, Zuckerman IH, et al. A sustainable strategy to prevent misuse of antibiotics for acute respiratory infections. *PLoS ONE.* 2012; 7(12):e51147. doi:10.1371/journal.pone.0051147.

48. Hermsen ED, VanSchooneveld TC, Sayles H, Rupp ME. Implementation of a clinical decision support system for antimicrobial stewardship. *Infect Control Hosp Epidemiol* 2012; 33(4):412–415. doi:10.1086/664762.

49. Septimus EJ, Owens RC. Need and potential of antimicrobial stewardship in community hospitals. *Clin Infect Dis* 2011; 53(Suppl 1):S8–14. doi:10.1093/cid/cir363.

50. Tannenbaum D, Doctor JN, Persell SD, et al. Nudging physician prescription decisions by partitioning the order set: results of a vignette-based study. *J Gen Intern Med.* 2015; 30(3):298–304. doi:10.1007/s11606-014-3051-2.

51. McNulty CAM. European Antibiotic Awareness Day 2012: general practitioners encouraged to TARGET antibiotics through guidance, education and tools. *J Antimicrob Chemother* 2012; 67 (11):2543–2546. doi:10.1093/jac/dks358.

52. Samore MH, Bateman K, Alder SC, et al. Clinical decision support and appropriateness of antimicrobial prescribing: a randomized trial. *JAMA* 2005; 294(18):2305–2314.

53. Gulliford MC, van Staa T, Dregan A, et al. Electronic health records for intervention research: a cluster randomized trial to reduce antibiotic prescribing in primary care (eCRT study). *Annals of Family Medicine* 2014; 12(4):344–351.

54. McIsaac WJ, Moineddin R, Ross S. Validation of a decision aid to assist physicians in reducing unnecessary antibiotic drug use for acute cystitis. *Arch Intern Med* 2007; 167(20):2201–2206.

55. Steurbaut K, Van Hoecke S, Colpaert K, et al. Use of web services for computerized medical decision support, including infection control and antibiotic management, in the intensive care unit. *J Telemed Telecare* 2010; 16 (1):25–29.

56. Gonzales R, Anderer T, McCulloch CE, et al. A cluster randomized trial of decision support strategies for reducing antibiotic use in acute bronchitis. *JAMA Internal Medicine* 2013; 173(4):267–273.

57. Shebl NA, Franklin BD, Barber N. Clinical decision support systems and antibiotic use. *Pharm World Sci* 2007; 29(4):342–349. Epub Apr 26, 2007.

58. Gerber JS, Prasad PA, Fiks AG, et al. Effect of an outpatient antimicrobial stewardship intervention on broad-spectrum antibiotic prescribing by primary care pediatricians: a randomized trial. *JAMA* 2013; 309 (22):2345–2352.

59. Gerber JS, Prasad PA, Fiks AG, et al. Durability of benefits of an outpatient antimicrobial stewardship intervention after discontinuation of audit and feedback. *JAMA* 2014; 312(23):2569–2570.

60. Szymczak JE, Feemster KA, Zaoutis TE, Gerber JS. Pediatrician perceptions of an outpatient antimicrobial stewardship intervention. *Infect Control Hosp Epidemiol* 2014; 35(Suppl 3):S69–78.

61. Dellinger RP, Levy MM, Carlet JM, et al. International Surviving Sepsis Campaign guidelines committee Surviving Sepsis Campaign: international guidelines for management of severe sepsis and septic shock, 2008. *Crit Care Med* 2008; 36 (1):296–327.

62. Menéndez R, Torres A, Reyes S, et al. Initial management of pneumonia and sepsis: factors associated with improved outcome. *Eur Respir J* 2012; 39 (1):156–162.

63. Kiyatkin D, Bessman E, McKenzie R. Impact of antibiotic choices made in the emergency department on appropriateness of antibiotic treatment of urinary tract infections in hospitalized patients. *J Hosp Med* 2015; 11(3):181–184.

64. Tamma P, Cosgrove SE. Antimicrobial stewardship. *Infect Dis Clin North Am* 2011; 25:245–260.

65. May L, Harter K, Yadav K, et al. Practice patterns and management strategies for purulent skin and soft-tissue infections in an urban academic ED. *Am J Emerg Med* 2012; 30(2):302–310. doi:10.1016/j.ajem.2010.11.033.

66. May L, Mullins P, Pines J. Demographic and treatment patterns for infections in ambulatory settings in the United States, 2006–2010. *Academic Emergency Medicine* 2014; 21(1):17–24. doi:10.1111/acem.12287.

67. Stuck AK, Täuber MG, Schabel M, Lehmann T, Suter H, Mühlemann K. Determinants of quinolone versus trimethoprim-sulfamethoxazole use for outpatient urinary tract infection. *Antimicrob Agents Chemother* 2012; 56 (3):1359–1363. doi:10.1128/AAC.05321–11.

68. Copp HL, Shapiro DJ, Hersh AL. National ambulatory antibiotic prescribing patterns for pediatric urinary tract infection, 1998–2007. *Pediatrics* 2011; 127 (6):1027–1033. doi:10.1542/peds.2010–3465.

69. Lautenbach E, Larosa LA, Kasbekar N, Peng HP, Maniglia RJ, Fishman NO. Fluoroquinolone utilization in the emergency departments of academic medical centers: prevalence of, and risk factors for, inappropriate use. *Arch Intern Med* 2003; 163(5):601–605. doi:10.1001/archinte.163.5.601.

70. Ducharme J, Neilson S, Ginn JL. Can urine cultures and reagent test strips be used to diagnose urinary tract infection in elderly emergency department patients without focal urinary symptoms? *CJEM* 2007; 9 (2):87–92.

71. Khawcharoenporn T, Vasoo S, Ward E, Singh K. High rates of quinolone resistance among urinary tract infections in the ED. *Am J Emerg Med.* 2012; 30(1):68–74. doi:10.1016/j.ajem.2010.09.030.

72. Shehab N, Patel PR, Srinivisan A, Budnitz DS. Emergency department visits for antibiotic-associated adverse events. *Clin Infect Dis* 2008; 47:735–743.

73. Mistry RD, Dayan PS, Kuppermann N. The battle against antimicrobial resistance: time for the emergency department to join the fight. *JAMA Pediatr* 2015; 169 (5):421–422.

74. File TM, Solomkin JS, Cosgrove SE. Strategies for improving antimicrobial use and the role of antimicrobial stewardship programs. *Clin Infect Dis* 2011; 53(Suppl 1):S15–22. doi:10.1093/cid/cir364.

75. Drekonja D, Filice G, Greer N, et al. *Antimicrobial Stewardship Programs in Outpatient Settings: A Systematic Review.* Washington, DC: Department of Veterans Affairs, 2014.

76. May L, Cosgrove S, L'Archeveque M, et al. A call to action for antimicrobial stewardship in the emergency department: approaches and strategies. *Ann Emerg Med* 2013; 62(1):69–77.e2.

77. May L, Gudger G, Armstrong P, et al. Multisite exploration of clinical decision making for antibiotic use by emergency medicine providers using quantitative and qualitative methods. *Infect Control Hosp Epidemiol* 2014; 35(9):1114–1125.

78 Bernstein SL, Aronsky D, Duseja R, et al. Society for academic emergency medicine, emergency department crowding task force. the effect of emergency department crowding on clinically oriented outcomes. *Acad Emerg Med.* 2009; 16(1):1–10.

79. Schafermeyer RW, Asplin BR. Hospital and emergency department crowding in the United States. *Emerg Med (Fremantle)* 2003; 15(1):22–27.

80. Delgado MK, Acosta CD, Ginde AA, et al. National survey of preventive health services in US emergency departments. *Ann Emerg Med* 2011; 57(2):104–108.e2.

81. Bernstein SL, Bernstein E, Boudreaux ED, et al. Public health considerations in knowledge translation in the emergency department. *Acad Emerg Med* 2007; 14 (11):1036–1041.

82. Studdert DM, Mello MM, Sage WM, et al. Defensive medicine among high-risk specialist physicians in a volatile malpractice environment. *JAMA* 2005; 293 (21):2609–2617.

83. Pines JM, Hollander JE, Lee H, Everett WW, Uscher-Pines L, Metlay JP. Emergency department operational changes in response to pay for performance and antibiotic timing in pneumonia. *Acad Emerg Med* 2007; 14:545–548.

84. Ong S, Moran GJ, Krishnadasan A, Talan DA. For the EMERGEncy ID NET Study Group. Antibiotic prescribing practices of emergency physicians and patient expectations for uncomplicated lacerations. *West J Emerg Med.* 2011; 12(4):375–380.

85. Stearns CR, Gonzales R, Camargo CA Jr, Maselli J, Metlay JP. Antibiotic prescriptions are associated with increased patient satisfaction with emergency department visits for acute respiratory tract infections. *Acad Emerg Med* 2009; 16 (10):934–941.

86. Ong S, Nakase J, Moran GJ, Karras DJ, Kuehnert MJ, Talan DA For the EMERGEncy ID NET Study Group. Antibiotic use for emergency department patients with upper respiratory infections: prescribing practices, patient expectations, and patient satisfaction. *Ann Emerg Med* 2007; 50:213–220.

87. Meurer WJ, Majersik JJ, Frederiksen SM, Kade AM, Sandretto AM, Scott PA. Provider perceptions of barriers to the emergency use of tPA for acute ischemic stroke: a qualitative study. *BMC Emerg Med* 2011; 11:5.

88. Stiell IG, Clement CM, Grimshaw JM, et al. A prospective cluster-randomized trial to implement the Canadian CT Head Rule in emergency departments. *CMAJ* 2010; 182 (14):1527–1532

89. Stiell IG, Clement CM, Grimshaw J, et al. Implementation of the Canadian C-Spine Rule: prospective 12 centre cluster randomised trial. *BMJ* 2009; 339:b4146. doi: 10.1136/bmj.b4146.

90. Gupta A, Ip IK, Raja AS, Andruchow JE, Sodickson A, Khorasani R. Effect of clinical decision support on documented guideline adherence for head CT in emergency department patients with mild traumatic brain injury. *J Am Med Inform Assoc* 2014; 21(e2):e347–351. doi:10.1136/amiajnl-2013-002536.

91. Hindler JF, Stelling J. Analysis and presentation of cumulative antibiograms: a new consensus guideline from the clinical and laboratory standards institute. *Clinical Infectious Diseases* 2007; 44(6): 867–873 doi:10.1086/511864.

92. Clement CM, Stiell IG, Davies B, OConnor A, et al. Perceived facilitators and barriers to clinical clearance of the cervical spine by emergency department nurses: a major step towards changing practice in the emergency department. *Int Emerg Nurs* 2011; 19(1):44–52.

93. Waldron N, Dey I, Nagree Y, Xiao J, Flicker L. A multifaceted intervention to implement guideline care and improve quality of care for older people who present to the emergency department with falls. *BMC Geriatr* 2011; 11:6.

94. Grimshaw JM, Shirran L, Thomas R, et al. Changing provider behavior: an overview of systematic reviews of interventions. *Med Care* 2001; 39(8 Suppl 2):II2–45.

95. May L, Cosgrove S, L'Archeveque M, et al. A call to action for antimicrobial stewardship in the emergency department: approaches and strategies. *Ann Emerg Med* 2013; 62(1):69–77.e2. doi:10.1016/j.annemergmed.2012.09.002.

96. Drew RH. Antimicrobial stewardship programs: how to start and steer a successful program. *Journal of Managed Care Pharmacy* 2009; 15(2): S18–S23.

97. Dellit TH, Owens RC, McGowan JE Jr, et al. Infectious Diseases Society of America; Society for Healthcare Epidemiology of America. Infectious Diseases Society of America and the Society for Healthcare Epidemiology of America guidelines for developing an institutional program to enhance antimicrobial stewardship. *Clin Infect Dis* 2007; 44 (2):159–177.

98. Percival K, Valenti K, Schmittling S, Strader B, Lopez R, Bergman S. Impact of an antimicrobial stewardship intervention on urinary tract infection treatment in the ED. *American Journal of Emergency Medicine* 2015; 33(9):1129–1133. doi:10.1016/j.ajem.2015.04.067.

99. Hudepohl NJ, Cunha CB, Mermel LA. Antibiotic prescribing for urinary tract infections in the emergency department based on local antibiotic resistance patterns: implications for antimicrobial stewardship. *Infect Control Hosp Epidemiol* 2016: 37(3):359–60.

100. Chao JH, Kunkov S, Reyes LB, Lichten S, Crain EF. Comparison of two approaches to observation therapy for acute otitis media in the emergency department. *Pediatrics* 2008; 121(5):e1352–1356.

101. Nicolle LE, Bradley S, Colgan R, Rice JC, Schaeffer A, Hooton TM. Infectious Diseases Society of America guidelines for the diagnosis and treatment of asymptomatic bacteriuria in adults. *Clin Infect Dis* 2005; 40(5):643–654.

102. Trinh TD, Klinker KP. Antimicrobial stewardship in the emergency department. *Infect Dis Ther* 2015; 4 (Suppl 1):39–50.

103. CLSI. *Analysis and Presentation of Cumulative Antimicrobial Susceptibility Test Data; Approved Guideline–Fourth Edition. CLSI document M39-A4.* Wayne, PA: Clinical and Laboratory Standards Institute, 2014.

104. Draper HM, Farland JB, Heidel RE, May LS, Suda KJ. Comparison of bacteria isolated from emergency department patients versus hospitalized patients. *Am J Health Syst Pharm* 2013; 70 (23):2124–2128.

105. Zatorski C, Jordan JA, Cosgrove SE, Zocchi M, May L. Comparison of antibiotic susceptibility of *Escherichia coli* in urinary isolates from an emergency department with other institutional susceptibility data. *Am J Health Syst Pharm* 2015; 72 (24):2176–2180.

106. Hermsen ED, VanSchooneveld TC, Sayles H, Rupp ME. Implementation of a clinical decision support system for antimicrobial stewardship. *Infect Control Hosp Epidemiol* 2012; 33(4):412–415. doi:10.1086/664762.

107. McNulty CAM. European Antibiotic Awareness Day 2012: general practitioners encouraged to TARGET antibiotics through guidance, education and tools.

J Antimicrob Chemother 2012; 67 (11):2543–2546. doi:10.1093/jac/dks358.

108. Powell BJ, McMillen JC, Proctor EK, et al. A compilation of strategies for implementing clinical innovations in health and mental health. *Med Care Res Rev* 2012; 69(2):123–157. doi:10.1177/1077558711430690.

109. Hecker, MT, Fox CJ, Son AH. Effect of a stewardship intervention on adherence to uncomplicated cystitis and pyelonephritis guidelines in an emergency department setting. *PLoS ONE* 2014; 9(2),e87899. http://doi.org/10.1371/journal.pone.0087899.

110. Dumkow L, Kenney R, Macdonald N, Carreno J, Malhotra M, Davis, S. Impact of a multidisciplinary culture follow-up program of antimicrobial therapy in the emergency department. *Infect Dis Ther* 2014; 3(1):45–53.

111. Baker SN, Acquisto NM, Ashley ED, Fairbanks RJ, Beamish, SE, Haas CE. Pharmacist-managed antimicrobial stewardship program for patients discharged from the emergency department. *Journal of Pharmacy Practice* 2012; 25(2):190–194. http://doi.org/10.1177/0897190011420160.

112. Tenover FC. Potential impact of rapid diagnostic tests on improving antimicrobial use. *Ann NY Acad Sci* 2010; 1213:70–80.

113. Pallin DJ, Camargo CA, Schuur JD. Skin infections and antibiotic stewardship: analysis of emergency department prescribing practices, 2007–2010. *Western Journal of Emergency Medicine* 2014; 15 (3):282–289. http://doi.org/10.5811/westjem.2013.8.18040.

114. Terp S, Krishnadasan A, Bowen W, et al. Introduction of rapid methicillin-resistant *staphylococcus aureus* polymerase chain reaction testing and antibiotic selection among hospitalized patients with purulent skin infections. *Clin Infect Dis* 2014; 58 (8):129–132. doi:10.1093/cid/ciu039.

115. Blaschke AJ, Shapiro DJ, Pavia AT, et al. A national study of the impact of rapid influenza testing on clinical care in the

emergency department. *J Pediatric Infect Dis Soc* 2014; 3(2):112–118.

116. Bauer KX, West JX, Balada-Llasat JM , et al. An antimicrobial stewardship program's impact with rapid polymerase chain reaction methicillin-resistant *staphylococcus aureus/S. aureus* blood culture test in patients with *S. aureus* bacteremia. *Clin Infect Dis* 2010 51 (9):1074–1080.

117. Brittain-Long R, Westin J, Olofsson S, Lindh M, Andersson LM. Access to a polymerase chain reaction assay method targeting 13 respiratory viruses can reduce antibiotics: a randomised, controlled trial. *BMC Med* 2011; 9:44.

118. Ostrowsky B, Sharma S, Defino M, et al. Antimicrobial stewardship and automated pharmacy technology improve antibiotic appropriateness for community-acquired pneumonia. *Infect Control Hosp Epidemiol* 2013; 34(6):566–572.

119. Stevens DL, Bisno AL, Chambers HF, et al. Practice guidelines for the diagnosis and management of skin and soft tissue infections: 2014 update by the Infectious Diseases Society of America. *Clin Infect Dis* 2014; 59(2):e10–52.

120. Rosenfeld RM, Schwartz SR, Cannon CR, et al. Clinical practice guideline: acute otitis externa. *Otolaryngology–Head and Neck Surgery* 2014; 150(Suppl 1):S1–24.

121. Rosenfeld RM, Shin JJ, Schwartz SR, et al. Clinical practice guideline: otitis media with effusion (update). *Otolaryngology–Head and Neck Surgery* 2016; 154(Suppl 1):S1–41.

122. Gupta K, Hooton TM, Naber KG, et al. International clinical practice guidelines for the treatment of acute uncomplicated cystitis and pyelonephritis in women: A 2010 update by the Infectious Diseases Society of America and the European Society for Microbiology and Infectious Diseases. *Clin Infect Dis* 2011; 52(5): e103–120.

123. Subcommittee on Urinary Tract Infection SCoQI, Roberts KB. Urinary tract infection: clinical practice guideline for the diagnosis and management of the initial UTI in febrile infants and children 2 to 24 months. *Pediatrics* 2011; 128(3):595–610.

124. Talan DA, Mower WR, Krishnadasan A, et al. Trimethoprim-sulfamethoxazole versus placebo for uncomplicated skin abscess. *N Engl J Med* 2016; 374 (9):823–832.

125. Talan DA, Lovecchio F, Abrahamian FM, et al. A randomized trial of clindamycin versus trimethoprim-sulfamethoxazole for uncomplicated wound infection. *Clin Infect Dis* 2016; 62 (12):1505–1513.

126. Stevens DL, Bisno AL, Chambers HF, et al. Infectious Diseases Society of America. Practice guidelines for the diagnosis and management of skin and soft tissue infections: 2014 update by the Infectious Diseases Society of America. *Clin Infect Dis* 2014; 59(2):e10–52.

127. Harris AM, Hicks LA, Qaseem A, High value care task force of the American College of P, for the Centers for Disease C, Prevention. Appropriate antibiotic use for acute respiratory tract infection in adults: Advice for high-value Care from the American College of Physicians and the Centers for Disease Control and Prevention. *Ann Int Med* 2016; 164(6):425–434.

Maintaining an Antibiotic Stewardship Program: Keeping Everyone Happy and Remaining Relevant

Marisa Holubar, B. Joseph Guglielmo, and Stan Deresinski

Maintaining support for an established antibiotic stewardship program (ASP) depends on the continuing provision of value to its stakeholders – patients, clinicians, society, and the sponsoring institution or healthcare organization and its administrators. That value must be continually communicated and demonstrated to these constituencies, in particular the institutional administration. In this chapter, we discuss how an ASP can remain relevant well after it has been in place.

Antibiotic Stewardship Beneficiaries

Despite its overall goal of optimization of clinical outcomes, the ASP and its activities are largely invisible to the patients and the public who are its beneficiaries[1] and may not always be apparent to healthcare administrators. The potential benefits to patients include safer, more effective therapy; shorter durations of hospitalization; reduced costs; and earlier hospital discharges. The benefits to the public and society in general include reduced medical costs and the slower emergence of drug-resistant organisms.

The results of ASP activities will become increasingly transparent to patients and other interested parties outside the institution as public reporting of their activities and outcomes becomes mandatory. In 2011, the Centers for Disease Control and Prevention (CDC) and National Healthcare Safety Network (NHSN) implemented antimicrobial use and antimicrobial resistance surveillance through electronic capture of data (i.e., eliminating the need for manual data entry). Participation by acute care hospitals and long-term acute care hospitals is currently optional, but it may become mandatory in the future.[3] In January 2017, The Joint Commission (TJC) included ASP assessments in surveys of hospitals and long-term care facilities.[2] Similarly, beginning November 2017, the Centers for Medicare and Medicaid requires antibiotic stewardship in long-term care facilities for reimbursement of healthcare costs.[3] ASPs will likely follow the path of infection prevention and control programs for which public reporting of programmatic outcome data is required. This information will be of interest, not only to patients, but also to third-party payers and regulatory and governmental agencies.

Institutional benefit accrues from a variety of factors, including a reduction in antibiotic acquisition costs, reduced patient complications, shortened hospital stays, reduced readmissions, improved transitions of care, and improved reputation in an increasingly competitive healthcare market.[4] These factors are becoming increasingly important as the health care system transitions from volume-based to value-based business models – with the ultimate goal being the provision of high-value care.[5, 6] These factors may be used by the institution's administration to assess their ASP's return on investment (ROI). Independent of non-financial benefits associated with the program, the ROI must also be expressed in monetary terms. Also of critical importance to healthcare facility administrators is the alignment of ASP goals with those of agencies such as TJC and the National Quality Forum.[7]

Administrators must be continually convinced of all the patient-centered, societal, and especially, institutional benefits of ASPs since it is they who ultimately decide to provide financial and other needed resources to sustain ASPs.

Maintaining Institutional Support

For healthcare providers, the notion of assessing the ASP based on ROI may seem too fiscally oriented to comfortably apply to patient care. Thus, it is better to consider the ASP in terms of value – and more specifically, *the value equation*, where value is defined as the achievement of best possible patient health outcomes, both in terms of quality and experience, at the lowest possible financial cost. This definition is based on a patient-centered model but value is in the eye of the beholder.[8] Benefits and value to other stakeholders, such as hospital administrators, must be demonstrated and must be aligned with the stakeholders' priorities.

Measurement and documentation of "high-value care" is critical given the rapidly evolving secular trends within US healthcare systems. These trends include demand for transparency, accountability and public reporting, increasing competition, greater patient interest in cost particularly as it impacts insurance deductibles and co-pays, and the rising prevalence of value-based payment, including bundled-payment models.[8] ASPs make critical contributions toward high-value care, requiring ongoing support along with programmatic development and growth.

Measuring Cost Savings

The success of ASPs has traditionally been measured by the reduction of antibiotic acquisition costs. However, relying on this approach is short sighted. Most successful stewardship programs demonstrate significant cost savings during the first years of a program's inception due to formulary changes, targeting "low-hanging fruit" (e.g., IV to PO conversion), and implementing core stewardship strategies including prior authorization and prospective audit and feedback. These dramatic results unfortunately may lead administrators to expect substantial cost savings year after year.

Programs must emphasize the importance of maintaining early gains through continued stewardship interventions. The University of Maryland Medical Center serves as a cautionary tale. Standiford et al. showed that their successful stewardship program achieved a 46% decrease in antibiotic expenditures/1,000 patient days over the course of seven years. Most cost savings were within the first three years. Hospital administration stopped support for the program believing the infectious disease consult team had equivalent stewardship expertise and could maintain the same results. However, within 2 years of discontinuing the program, antibiotic costs increased 32% resulting in an estimated $2 million increased expenditures.[9] Similarly, a cluster-randomized trial assessed the impact of stewardship interventions on community-based pediatric primary care practices. This interventional study demonstrated a 50% relative reduction in broad-spectrum antibiotic use.[10] After education about guideline-directed management of common infections, the intervention clinics received 1 year of feedback regarding their prescribing practices. Gerber et al. found that over the following 18 months when feedback was no longer provided, providers prescribed more broad-spectrum antibiotics over time and ultimately exceeded baseline rates.[11] These two studies demonstrate that continued stewardship interventions are necessary to sustain reductions in inappropriate antibiotic use.

One way to demonstrate the continued value of an ASP and mitigate the cost-savings plateau is to compare current utilization and antibiotic costs to those projected if the ASP had not been instituted. Beardsley et al. reported an annual cost-savings metric defined as the difference between the expected antibiotic expenditure (calculated on cost data for six months prior to ASP inception) and actual antibiotic expenditure normalized by patient day minus programmatic labor costs (primarily personnel salary.) Over an 11-year span, the average annual estimated cost savings was at least $920,000, with higher estimates depending upon the utilized inflation rate methodology.[12] When comparing utilization to projected figures, this program was able to demonstrate continued value through estimated cost savings. This financial benefit does not account for other cost savings such as reduced costs associated with hospitalization. Consequently, the savings are likely an underestimate of the true cost avoidance attributable to the stewardship program.

ASP interventions that continue to provide ongoing cost savings after implementation should be highlighted and included each year moving forward in the fiscal assessment of the ASP. One example of such a recurring savings is switching from the use of costly oral vancomycin tablets to the inexpensive intravenous solution for patients with *Clostridium difficile* infection (CDI). Depending on hospital size, this maneuver can result in annual savings of tens of thousands of dollars; those savings will occur each year until the standard for treatment is changed or the price differential between the two formulations narrows. Thus, it is critical to reinforce that the benefit is not limited to the year in which the change is made; rather the cost savings are ongoing.

Measuring Clinical Outcomes

In addition to measuring and reporting cost savings, programs should monitor the relevant clinical outcomes related to ASP interventions to demonstrate value. These outcomes include length of hospital stay, length of ICU stay, readmission rates, and mortality due to specific types of infection (e.g., pneumonia or skin and soft tissue infections.) These data can be parsed by ICD-10 codes; collaboration with the finance department is often necessary to obtain the relevant data. This collaboration may also allow programs to estimate the cost savings attributed to their interventions associated with shortening inpatient stays. It is also important to monitor balancing measures – ensuring an improvement in one area is not negatively impacting another area – to confirm that ASP interventions have not resulted in harm.[7]

Programs should also track whether antibiotic stewardship interventions have impacted the number of patients with infections due to multidrug-resistant organisms (e.g., methicillin-resistant *S. aureus*) or CDI. Such tracking results in a natural collaboration with the infection control department who already monitors many of these infections. Caution should be used when deciding to formally monitor drug-resistant infection or CDI rates as large numbers of patients receiving stewardship interventions may be needed to see differences in these outcomes and non-stewardship related interventions (i.e., infection control lapses) may contribute to their incidence.

Improving Safety

Patient safety is of critical concern to healthcare facilities. Evidence of ongoing contributions of the ASP to improve patient safety argues strongly for institutional support and maintenance of the program. As stated by the CDC "improving antibiotic use is a medication-safety and patient-safety issue" and ASPs play a critical and necessary role in these activities.[1] ASP surveillance activities identify opportunities for optimization and risk-reduction directly related to antibiotic use, as well as additional patient safety and quality issues. Tamma and colleagues have outlined a number of ASP issues relating to safety including reducing CDI, improving outpatient parenteral antibiotic therapy, systematizing therapeutic drug monitoring, ensuring appropriate surgical antibiotic prophylaxis, and managing drug interactions as well as antibiotic allergies (which account for almost one-fifth of emergency department visits for drug-related adverse events.)[13, 14]

Visibility

ASPs should report data regularly to administration, physician and pharmacy leaders, and quality improvement groups within the healthcare organization. This reporting allows for increased visibility of ASP interventions and successes, identification of other opportunities for antibiotic optimization, recruitment of physician and pharmacy champions, and forums for education. ASP members should regularly attend and participate in hospital committees such as the Pharmacy and Therapeutics committee, Infection Control Committee, and Medication Safety Committees and report ASP data at these meetings. Education of the clinical staff is an ongoing activity of an ASP, but probably even more important to its success is the continuing education of administrators to ensure their understanding of antibiotic stewardship and its associated value. Administrators need ongoing education regarding ASP activities that do not have immediate dollar savings but remain critical, such as slowing the emergence of antibiotic resistance by reducing antibiotic pressure. If the ASP's activities are not persistently "advertised," administrators are less likely to continue their support.

Role in Regulatory Compliance

Another important contribution of ASPs is its role in institutional compliance with accreditation and regulatory agency standards, as well as state and federal law. ASPs are also integral to preventing and managing specific infections, such as CDI, that are tracked by numerous health-quality organizations via healthcare scorecards used to benchmark hospitals. Although these outcomes are multifactorial and beyond the complete control of ASPs, they offer additional opportunities for programs to demonstrate value and relevance to their healthcare organization.

Performance Measures

The Healthcare Effectiveness Data and Information Set (HEDIS) is a standardized measurement tool used by more than 90% of America's health plans to measure performance on important aspects of care and service. Altogether, HEDIS consists of 81 measures across five domains of care. Because so many plans collect HEDIS data, and because the measures are specifically defined, HEDIS allows for a direct comparison of the performance of various health plans. Considering this broad utilization, benchmarking of HEDIS performance is commonplace. A poor HEDIS performance may result in reduced ability for a hospital to partner with payors and others; conversely, a strong HEDIS performance may increase opportunities for collaboration.

Specific to antibiotic stewardship, the National Committee for Quality Assurance (NCQA) has recommendations associated with the treatment of certain upper respiratory tract infections. It is well established that antibiotics play no role in the treatment of acute bronchitis. Consequently, one HEDIS measure states that antibiotic treatment be avoided in adults with acute bronchitis; this measure specifically documents the percentage of adults 18–64 years of age with a diagnosis of acute bronchitis who were not given an antibiotic prescription. This HEDIS measure provides ASPs with an opportunity to leverage benchmarked data for an outpatient stewardship target that is considered "low-hanging fruit." Improvement in these HEDIS scores (e.g., reduced numbers of acute bronchitis patients receiving antibiotics) may serve an important surrogate marker of the quality of an institution.

Accreditation Standards

Competent ASPs can influence accreditation status by improving compliance with TJC standards. According to the TJC's Antimicrobial Stewardship Standard, MM.09.01.01, which became effective on January 1, 2017, all critical access hospitals, hospitals, and nursing care centers are required to have antimicrobial stewardship programs. Noncompliance with TJC standards has substantial implications including loss of accreditation, financial penalties and costs, and unwanted notoriety associated with failure to meet these standards. By participating in or leading initiatives to address relevant TJC standards, ASPs can align with institutional priorities, improving visibility and demonstrating value. While no longer a required data collection, TJC previously created a number of standards associated with the appropriate treatment of community-acquired pneumonia (CAP). These standards included appropriate selection of empiric antibiotic therapy based upon the Infectious Diseases Society of America and American Thoracic Society Guidelines (IDSA-ATC) [15] and other published outcomes data. ASPs played a major role in ensuring that CAP therapy at their institution complied with TJC standards, for example, through active participation and creation of TJC-compliant CAP order sets. These order sets have been associated with significant reductions in in-hospital mortality, 30-day mortality, and direct costs as well as a significant increase in core measure compliance.[16] Clearly, ASPs that improve compliance with TJC standards add value to their institution.

ASPs can also sound the alarm when regulatory standards may result in unintended consequences. TJC took note of a study conducted by Houck et al. that evaluated Medicare patients older than 65 years who were hospitalized with CAP.[17] In this study, it was observed that antibiotic administration within four hours of arrival at the hospital was associated with reductions of in-hospital mortality, mortality within 30 days of admission, and length of stay exceeding the five-day median. In addition, the mean length of stay was found to be 0.4 days shorter with antibiotic administration within four hours when compared with later administration. Based upon the results of this study and others, TJC issued standard PN-5b, which required at least 90% of CAP patients receive antibiotics within four hours of presentation to the emergency department (ED). However, once this standard was implemented, due to difficulties in arriving at a diagnosis in such a short time period, antibiotics were often administered to patients without pneumonia. Fee and Weber reported that the time window for this standard was unrealistic.[18] They suggested a more realistic performance standard for antibiotic administration should be established and case definitions modified to include only patients with a final ED diagnosis for CAP or with objective clinical and radiographic evidence of pneumonia. Ultimately, TJC increased the required window of antibiotic administration to six hours, and this standard was endorsed by the National Quality Forum (NQF), the IDSA-ATS CAP guidelines committee, and the Technical Expert Panel for the Centers for Medicare and Medicaid Services (CMS) National Pneumonia Project. When involved in multi-disciplinary efforts to meet regulatory requirements, ASPs can serve as content experts and provide valuable input and assessment of standards to identify challenges in implementation and risks of unintended consequences.

In addition to requirements regarding the treatment of CAP, TJC and CMS also created a number of standards intended to prevent CAP by providing pneumococcal and influenza vaccinations for all at-risk patients. While not classically antibiotic stewardship, prevention of infections through vaccination contributes to the overarching goal of less antibiotic use. Participating in efforts like this provide ASPs opportunities to gain visibility and demonstrate value to the institution.

ASP can also play an important role in advocating for the appropriate use of antibiotics used for surgical prophylaxis by participating in their facility's Surgical Care Improvement Project (SCIP). The CDC checklist highlights surgical antibiotic prophylaxis as an important target for ASPs.[19] SCIP evolved from a national quality partnership of organizations interested in improving surgical care by significantly reducing surgical complications. The SCIP measures have been used by TJC and CMS as quality indicators. Many of these measures involve the appropriate selection and timing of surgical antibiotic prophylaxis. It is well established that the choice of antibiotic prophylaxis clearly influences the likelihood for postoperative surgical wound infection. Similarly, the timing of administration of the preoperative antibacterial dose strongly predicts the risk for wound infection. Lastly, for almost all elective surgical procedures, continuation of antibiotic prophylaxis, beyond preoperative and intraoperative administration, is not associated with improved outcomes and may increase the risk for superinfection and development of bacterial resistance. In light of these findings, TJC and CMS have developed SCIP measures that mandate appropriate selection of antibiotic, timing of the preoperative dose and restrictions on postoperative antibacterial administration. Hospital groups with higher SCIP compliance with antibiotic timing and appropriate antibiotic selection measures have significantly lower surgical site infections (SSI) rates. For example, Cataife et al. demonstrated that a 10% improvement in administering antibiotics within 1 hour before surgical incision led to a 5% decrease in SSI rates.[20] SCIP measures provided another opportunity for ASPs to improve patient outcomes as well as capitalize on an institutional priority.

State Requirements

In addition to the ASP's role in improving adherence with the above national regulatory standards and quality measures, state law may mandate the implementation and maintenance of antibiotic stewardship programs in the near future. In 2008, California passed a bill requiring general acute care hospitals develop a process for monitoring the judicious use of antibiotics and report results to appropriate quality improvement committee(s) at their institution. In September 2014, California Senate Bill 1311 further required hospitals to adopt and implement an antibiotic stewardship policy in accordance with guidelines established by federal government and professional organizations. This bill further requires a physician-supervised multidisciplinary antibiotic stewardship committee with at least one physician or pharmacist who has undergone specific training related to antibiotic steward-ship. Missouri has also passed similar legislation (Missouri Senate Bill 579) in June of 2016 requiring ASPs in both hospitals and ambulatory surgical centers. Despite the presence of ASP mandates, however, antibiotic stewards and ASP champions will need to continually make the case for adequate resources for their programs.

Federal Regulatory Requirements

The Obama Administration issued an Executive Order – Combating Antibiotic-Resistant Bacteria, in September 2014, instructing federal agencies to review existing regulations and propose new regulations or other actions to require hospitals to implement robust ASPs that adhere to best practices. In addition to the acute care setting, these federal agencies will also require implementation of ASPs in other settings, such as long-term care and ambula-tory care. By 2016, CMS issued a new rule requiring antibiotic stewardship programs in long-term care facilities.

Another federal initiative with implications for ASPs is the Hospital-Acquired Condi-tion (HAC) Reduction Program, estimated to save Medicare approximately $350 million each year. In close cooperation with the CDC, among others, the HAC Reduction Program uses NHSN metrics to measure the rate of central line-associated bloodstream infection (CLABSI), catheter-associated urinary tract infection (CAUTI), surgical site infection (elective colon surgery and abdominal hysterectomy), methicillin-resistant S. aureus infection, and CDI. Hospitals that are in the lowest-performing quartile for these metrics will receive lower payments from CMS. Early readmission for CAP is a disease state which CMS will not reimburse. Prevention of readmission for CAP represents an opportunity for antibiotic stewardship by improving appropriate choice and duration of antibiotic therapy.

In addition, as of 2008, CMS will not pay for conditions that cause the patient harm as a result of preventable errors associated with acute hospital care. The hospital cannot bill for any charges associated with any of these HACs. Most other third-party payors have also adopted this CMS policy. Some examples of errors relevant to ASPs include CAUTIs, CLABSIs, and mediastinitis. If ASPs are able to contribute to the reduction in incidence of these non-reimbursable infectious diseases-associated errors, they are adding substantial value to their healthcare institutions.

Scorecard Improvement

There are also initiatives relevant to ASPs that emphasize the reporting and benchmarking of CDI. For example, NHSN routinely evaluates the rate of laboratory-identified, hospital-onset CDI cases defined as C. difficile positive stool samples obtained on hospital day four or later. Public health departments monitor and report CDI rates as well.

In these reports, a CDI standardized infection ratio (SIR) is provided. The SIR is a risk-adjusted summary measure that compares the observed number of infections to the expected number of infections based on NHSN aggregate data. The SIR adjusts for certain factors, including affiliation with a medical school, hospital bed size, and the burden of community-onset CDI in patients admitted to the hospital. Benchmarking of CDI data among institutions results in adoption of best practices and widespread dissemination of hospital performance. In those instances in which antibiotic stewardship efforts reduce rates of CDI or result in a favorable scorecard, the ASP can be associated with considerable value to the healthcare institution.

In summary, compliance with accreditation and regulatory agencies' standards and improvement in healthcare scorecards are of clear value to healthcare institutions. Compliance with these standards has been documented to be associated with tangible objective benefits to patients and healthcare organizations. ASPs have a major role in optimizing performance.

Value for Front-Line Providers

Clinicians benefit from ASP activities as a result of oversight, provision of guidelines and pathways, as well as general assistance in their use of antibiotic agents with resultant improved efficiency and, ultimately, improvement in patient outcomes. It is important that ASP interventions, including audit and feedback, are well received by the majority of providers at an institution. Tracking success rates of interventions, broadcasting results, and seeking feedback from providers are important. It is also critical that ASP team members are seen as content experts, able to provide counsel regarding the use of new antibiotics and how to best manage infections caused by multidrug-resistant organisms. ASPs also regularly update local guidelines to reflect best practices and organize multi-disciplinary meetings so these guidelines are both evidence-based and practical.

Maintaining Effectiveness: Taking Care of the Team

Important to the maintenance of an effective ASP is the morale of team members who must feel that they are accomplishing matters of importance and they are valued and respected. ASP team members should be involved in the identification and development of solutions to problems, which should also be encouraged of the general clinical staff. ASP goals are often long term and difficult to fully achieve, resulting, on occasion, in a feeling of stagnation. In contrast, setting and achieving short-term goals provides an ongoing sense of accomplishment and each of these achievements should be acknowledged and publicized.

Conclusion

Many successful ASPs demonstrate significant cost savings during the first years of a program's inception due to formulary changes and targeting "low-hanging fruit." However, in order to maintain ongoing support and remain relevant and effective, ASPs should reorient its focus, and that of the administration's, toward providing maximal *value* to patients, clinicians, and administration. ASPs should be viewed as patient quality programs – having broad scope and reach among various initiatives. Programs should align the priorities of both the hospital administration and clinical staff, such as optimizing clinical outcomes and reducing length of stay, to target interventions accordingly. Demonstrating value will allow for expansion of the ASP's reach to additional environments, including the complete and broad range of outpatient settings such as dialysis clinics and outpatient surgical centers.

References

1. Centers for Disease Control and Prevention. Why Inpatient Stewardship? (Accessed March 14, 2016, at www.cdc.gov/getsmart/healthcare/inpatient-stewardship.html.)

2. Joint Commission. Proposed Standard for Antimicrobial Stewardship in AHC, CAH, HAP, NCC, and OBS. (Accessed March 14, 2016, at www.jointcommission.org/prepublication_standards_antimicrobial_stewardship_standard/.)

3. Centers for Disease Control and Prevention. NHSN AUR Module. (Accessed March 14 2016, at www.cdc.gov/nhsn/acute-care-hospital/aur/.)

4. Lynch JB. Promoting value through antimicrobial stewardship. *Health Financ Manage* 2016; 70(3):38–41.

5. Centers for Medicare and Medicaid Services. The hospital value-based purchasing program. (Accessed July 15, 2016, at www.cms.gov/Medicare/Quality-Initiatives-Patient-Assessment-Instruments/Value-Based-Programs/HVBP/Hospital-Value-Based-Purchasing.html.)

6. Conway PH. Value-driven health care: implications for hospitals and hospitalists. *J Hosp Med* 2009; 4(8):507–511.

7. Nagel JL, Stevenson JG, Eiland EH, Kaye KS. Demonstrating the value of antimicrobial stewardship programs to hospital administrators. *Clin Infect Dis* 2014; 59(Suppl 3):S146–153.

8. Scheurer D, Crabtree E, Cawley PJ, Lee TH. The value equation: enhancing patient outcomes while constraining costs. *Am J Med Sci* 2016; 351(1):44–51.

9. Standiford HC, Chan S, Tripoli M, Weekes E, Forrest GN. Antimicrobial stewardship at a large tertiary care academic medical center: cost analysis before, during, and after a 7-year program. *Infect Control Hosp Epidemiol* 2012; 33(4):338–345.

10. Gerber JS, Prasad PA, Fiks AG, et al. Effect of an outpatient antimicrobial stewardship intervention on broad-spectrum antibiotic prescribing by primary care pediatricians: a randomized trial. *JAMA* 2013; 309 (22):2345–2352.

11. Gerber JS, Prasad PA, Fiks AG, et al. Durability of benefits of an outpatient antimicrobial stewardship intervention after discontinuation of audit and feedback. *JAMA*. 2014; 312 (23):2569–2570.

12. Beardsley JR, Williamson JC, Johnson JW, Luther VP, Wrenn RH, Ohl CC. Show me the money: long-term financial impact of an antimicrobial stewardship program. *Infect Control Hosp Epidemiol* 2012; 33 (4):398–400.

13. Tamma PD, Holmes A, Ashley ED. Antimicrobial stewardship: another focus for patient safety? *Curr Opin Infect Dis* 2014; 27(4):348–355.

14. Shehab N, Patel PR, Srinivasan A, Budnitz DS. Emergency department visits for antibiotic-associated adverse events. *Clin Infect Dis* 2008; 47(6):735–743.

15. Mandell LA, Wunderink RG, Anzueto A, et al. Infectious Diseases Society of America/American Thoracic Society consensus guidelines on the management of community-acquired pneumonia in adults. *Clin Infect Dis* 2007; 44(Suppl 2) : S27–72.

16. Fleming NS, Ogola G, Ballard DJ. Implementing a standardized order set for community-acquired pneumonia: impact on mortality and cost. *Jt Comm J Qual Patient Saf* 2009; 35(8):414–421.

17. Houck PM, Bratzler DW, Nsa W, Ma A, Bartlett JG. Timing of antibiotic administration and outcomes for Medicare patients hospitalized with community-acquired pneumonia. *Arch Intern Med* 2004; 164(6):637–644.

18. Fee C, Weber EJ. Identification of 90% of patients ultimately diagnosed with community-acquired pneumonia within four hours of emergency department arrival may not be feasible. *Ann Emerg Med* 2007; 49(5):553–559.

19. Centers for Disease Control and Prevention. Core Elements of Hospital

Antibiotic Stewardship Programs. US Dep Health Human Services, 2014; 1–25. (Accessed March 30, 2016 at www.cdc.gov/getsmart/healthcare/implementation/core-elements.html.)

20. Cataife G, Weinberg DA, Wong HH, Kahn KL. The effect of Surgical Care Improvement Project (SCIP) compliance on surgical site infections (SSI). *Med Care* 2014; 52(2 Suppl 1):S66–73.

Chapter 15

Practical Antibiotic Stewardship
Implementing an Antibiotic Stewardship Program

Richard H. Drew and Rebekah W. Moehring

Introduction

A well-planned, well-executed antibiotic stewardship program (ASP) must carefully choose among evidence-based interventions and activities, and tailor them to an institution's needs, goals, available resources, and culture.[1–4] Once the elements of the program are identified, the ASP team must then determine how to best introduce them into their facility's practice and prescriber workflow. The objectives of this chapter are to describe the basic steps needed for implementation of an active antibiotic stewardship (AS) intervention, to discuss potential barriers that may be encountered, and to propose solutions to the most common of these problems utilizing a case-based approach.

General Approach to Implementing an Active AS Intervention

The following twelve steps are what we consider to be the basic process for implementing an active AS intervention (see Table 1). This outline should be considered a general guideline and not prescriptive, as individualized plans must be crafted based on the type of intervention and the specific healthcare setting. Also, such steps do not necessarily proceed sequentially. Some steps may occur simultaneously or repeatedly, as determined by the type of intervention, events that unfold, and the workflow of the group.

Step 1: Clearly Define the Problem and Rationale for the Proposed Intervention

AS interventions seek to address antibiotic-related safety, quality of care, and cost. The initial step in launching an active ASP initiative, therefore, is to identify the main goal and target for the intervention, or "driver."[5] The AS team must then determine what positive outcomes would be anticipated if implemented, and clearly define the rationale for instituting it into practice.

Step 2: Develop the Intervention

Development of the intervention should include a review of key internal data, comprehensive literature searches, guideline reviews, and discussion with peers who have prior experience with developing and implementing interventions. Institution-specific factors, including available resources and personnel, must be weighed. A proposed process for the interventions should then be developed collaboratively, with help from key stakeholders in the area targeted for the intervention. This step may be revised multiple times as more data and experiences are gained.

Table 1 Steps to Implementation of an ASP

1. Clearly define the problem and rationale for the proposed intervention.
2. Develop the intervention.
3. Determine the outcome(s) of interest and set reasonable goals.
4. Anticipate barriers and address them early.
5. Create a quality improvement or research study design and timeline based on projected numbers.
6. Finalize a written, formal proposal.
7. Gather institutional support.
8. Begin intervention period.
9. Refine the process and address any new barriers.
10. Collect data, perform data validity checks, and ensure the intervention is being delivered
11. Evaluate outcomes.
12. Share your experience.

Step 3: Determine the Outcome(s) of Interest and Set Reasonable Goals

Outcomes targeted for improvement as a result of the intervention can be patient- or facility-level. These outcomes may include clinical, economic, or humanistic outcomes. Examples of clinical outcomes include treatment outcomes or adverse events. Economic outcomes include length of stay or cost of antibiotics. Humanistic outcomes capture prescriber or patient preferences. In many cases, a cost analysis may be necessary to gain approval from administrative leaders. Reasonable goals for success of the intervention should be established using conservative estimates for feasibility and effectiveness.

Step 4: Anticipate Barriers and Address Them Early

After completing the initial drafts for implementation, anticipate potential barriers and develop a plan to address them (see Table 2). Barriers may include program-related costs, staff responsibilities, recruitment of key stakeholders, and competing institutional priorities. Reaching out to potential dissidents, recruitment of influential leaders, or development of intervention delivery methods that bypass the barriers are key to success.

Step 5: Create a Design for Quality Improvement or Research, including a Reasonable Timeline Based on Projected Numbers

While most AS interventions are conducted as quality improvement initiatives, a research study may be considered depending on the novelty of the intervention. In either case, design decisions should take into account the estimates for effectiveness and the number of patients potentially impacted. These estimates may come from the medical literature and facility-level data (e.g., antibiotic utilization data, number of admissions). We recommend lowering the estimates of effect if extracted from the medical literature in order to provide a conservative estimate for "real-world" application. A pilot study or tiered roll-in approach

Table 2 Antibiotic Stewardship Strategies: Barriers and Potential Solutions

Strategy	Barriers to Effective Implementation	Potential Solutions
Audit and feedback	Problems in identifying patients who are receiving suboptimal therapy	Use rules-based computer reports that combine pharmacy and microbiologic data to flag patients of interest Review targeted therapy or populations Review microbiologic data to identify targeted pathogens
	Difficulty communicating recommendations to providers	Time communication for greatest likelihood of impact (e.g., before rounds) Hold intermittent, regularly scheduled antibiotic rounds between the stewardship team and staff from services that heavily use antibiotics
	Lack of clarity in appropriate methods for providing feedback	Create forms for written communication in the medical record
	Medico-legal concerns about providing feedback in the medical record	Use approved policy delineating appropriate means of communicating recommendations Stick to approved interventions/programs/criteria Elevate complicated cases to consultation Strong pharmacist intervention independent of stewardship team Program review by risk management ID-MD intervention (vs. PharmD) Mandatory ID consults for select indications (e.g., *S. aureus* bacteremia)
Restriction and/or preauthorization	Perceived challenge to physician autonomy	Have an approved policy by the medical executive committee Grant time-restricted approvals (e.g., for 24–72 hours) to balance physicians' and stewardship concerns Regularly review the use of restricted agents to evaluate their continued restriction
	Integration of restriction policies into workflow	Use computerized physician order-entry systems to provide restriction guidelines Use dedicated pagers for restricted agents to minimize delays in authorization Establish clear procedures for authorization after hours
Prescriber education	Lack of knowledge about the role of stewardship programs	Present at grand rounds to explain AS and provide hospital-specific data

Table 2 (cont.)

Strategy	Barriers to Effective Implementation	Potential Solutions
Guideline implementation (see also Table 3)	Poor knowledge of, and adherence to, guidelines for antibiotic use	Disseminate information in printed pocket handbooks, internet, or intranet Integrate into antibiotic order-entry process Involve opinion leaders from multiple specialties in developing guidelines Provide needed flexibility in choice based on patient-specific factors (allergies, population, etc.)
Application of information technology.	Considerable investment of financial and human resources Inadequate IT resources	Emphasize its importance in patient safety and the potential to avoid substantial costs Identify and request reports from existing administrative, pharmacy, and microbiology databases
Intravenous-to-oral switch	Identification of eligible patients	On a daily basis, review patients receiving intravenous forms of highly bioavailable antibiotics (e.g., fluoroquinolones) Develop criteria to help clinicians determine candidacy for switch (e.g., body temperature, white blood cell count)
De-escalation or streamlining	Unwillingness of providers to de-escalate or streamline	Refer to studies that demonstrated safety of de-escalation or streamlining when resistant organisms were not identified
Optimization of antibiotic dose and frequency (including use of extended infusion)	Nursing concerns regarding prolonged administration due to increased potential for drug incompatibility and IV access	Create protocols for administration and list compatible drugs Provide nursing education about the benefits of extended infusions compared with standard infusions
Optimization of antibiotic dose and frequency (including use of extended infusion)	Nursing concerns regarding administration and drug incompatibility Availability of pharmacist with expertise to perform required dose adjustment	Create protocols for administration and list compatible drugs Provide nursing education about the benefits of extended compared with standard infusions. Create protocols for "pharmacist-to-dose" based on indication and organ function
Duration of therapy	Optimal duration of therapy unknown for many infections	Automatic ("hard stop") or "time outs" (usually 48 hours after start) for re-evaluation. Require documentation to justify continued therapy. Reminder messages

Table 2 (*cont.*)

Strategy	Barriers to Effective Implementation	Potential Solutions
	Excessive durations increase cost, adverse effects	Guideline (protocol) driven durations Indication- or drug-specific defaults with "opt out" for exceptions

Adapted from reference [51] with permission

may be useful in gaining feasibility data and experience before expanding the intervention to all targeted areas. Based on design decisions, a reasonable timeline should be developed to further plan for involvement of key stakeholders, requests for additional resources, and defining expectations.

Step 6:   Finalize a Written, Formal Proposal

A written plan that includes rationale, supporting evidence, a clear description of the intervention and process, expected outcomes, timeline, and plan for review and reassessment helps to communicate the intent and expectations for the intervention. Clearly defining the project is important for AS team members as well as collaborators and facility leaders.

Step 7:   Gather Institutional Support

Formal support and approval from facility-level committees or administrators establishes the authority to move forward with the intervention. This step allows the ASP to cite confirmed and documented support from the institutional leadership when barriers or conflicts are encountered during implementation. Additionally, presenting and gaining approval from the appropriate committees helps clearly define and communicate expectations from all stakeholders. These presentations also highlight the ongoing efforts of the ASP to influential leaders.

Step 8:   Begin Intervention

Initiation of the intervention should be timed appropriately to the availability of key data and support personnel. Data collection may be as challenging as the intervention activity itself. Starting with a small pilot project can provide the experience needed to work through conflicts or process problems before facility-wide expansions which may affect large numbers of prescribers and patients. Documentation of the process as well as outcomes should begin simultaneously in order to prove that the interventions were delivered as intended.

Step 9:   Refine the Process and Address Any New Barriers

Refinement or revision of the original plan for the intervention may be necessary depending on conflicts that occur. Need for permission for such modifications are dependent on the nature of the change and degree of regulatory and administrative oversight of the intervention.

Step 10: Collect Data, Perform Data Validity Checks, and Ensure the Intervention Is Being Delivered

Throughout the intervention period, situational changes may occur. Therefore, routine data validity and feasibility assessments should be incorporated into weekly or monthly team meetings to address any areas of conflict, mistakes, over-extended personnel, or data errors as they arise.

Step 11: Evaluate Outcomes

Patient- and facility-level outcomes should be analyzed and reviewed. Barriers and solutions to implementation are also critical to discuss as these data are interpreted. Only through thoughtful analyses can future plans be made to modify, maintain, ask for additional resources, expand, or discontinue the intervention.

Step 12: Share Your Experience

Interventional outcomes should be shared internally with the key stakeholders, collaborators, committees, and targeted prescribers. Single-center experiences are valuable and important to share externally so that other institutions, peers, and patients may benefit from the implementation process and lessons learned.

Case Studies in Implementing Stewardship Interventions

Case 1   A New ASP Implementing Formulary Restriction and Preauthorization

Case Introduction

Dr. J is one of four clinical pharmacists working at a 200-bed, suburban, community hospital named W Memorial Hospital (WMH). WMH has an 8-bed intensive care unit (ICU) and is primarily staffed by private practice physician groups. In her daily review of medication orders, Dr. J notes that expensive, broad-spectrum antibiotics are frequently used at her hospital and continued for long durations of therapy. This is consistent with quarterly reports from her pharmacy director indicating a large proportion of the pharmacy budget was dedicated to antibiotics. The hospital has maintained no restrictions on which drugs could be ordered (i.e., an "open formulary") for many years.

As part of her continuing education activities, Dr. J attended a conference and learned that several hospitals in her area have ASPs which performed active interventions. She learned that formulary restriction and preauthorization of targeted antibiotics can be an effective way to reduce cost and inappropriate antibiotic use. She recognizes an opportunity to improve this problem at her hospital. When she returns home, she reviews the Infectious Diseases Society of America (IDSA) and Society for Healthcare Epidemiology (SHEA) guidelines on antibiotic stewardship and available published studies regarding the impact of formulary restriction and preauthorization of targeted antibiotics. She then approaches her pharmacy director, who is impressed with both her initiative and background research. He reviews the institution's antibiotic expense data in more detail and observes the highest antibiotic costs based on a per-dose, acquisition-cost estimate includes doripenem, ceftaroline, linezolid, and daptomycin. The largest proportion of these drugs are prescribed in their ICU. Together they plan to present the idea of a restricted antibiotic formulary at the next quarterly Pharmacy and Therapeutics (P&T) committee meeting.

While Dr. J and her director agree that improving the appropriate use of targeted drugs and reducing excessive antibiotic costs are their major goals, they want to make sure that this is not achieved at the expense of quality patient care. They first speak with Dr. B, a well-respected, private practice infectious diseases (ID) physician, who provides consultations and has admitting privileges at WMH. He is immediately supportive of the idea and offers his advice and assistance. He had previously noted that his colleagues practicing in the ICU occasionally use new and costly drugs empirically and for prolonged durations. His review of the pharmacy data supports this observation. He anticipates that the ICU director, Dr. H., will be hesitant to accept a preauthorization policy because of concerns that this might lead to delays in ill patients receiving necessary antibiotic therapy.

Discussion

Antibiotic restriction and preauthorization is a core strategy for AS.[1] Formulary restriction may be the initial approach used in settings where formal financial support for an ASP has not yet been established, such as small, community hospitals.[6, 7] Thus, this intervention can often be the starting point for introducing the concepts of AS and the important principle that antibiotic prescribing decisions require clear rationale and justification for use. This is a challenge, especially in settings where prescribers have never previously faced a challenge to their antibiotic prescribing patterns.

Loss of autonomy is a well-known concern from prescribers subjected to preauthorization. [8, 9] There are several methods to address this concern. Gaining approval for the preauthorization policy from facility administrators, committees, and physician leaders are essential first steps.[10] The approval and support from hospital administrators often provides the necessary credibility and authority to proceed, even when there are critics. Efforts to educate and approach prescribers with informal discussions or formal presentations allow development of their understanding of the rationale for AS and their inclusion into the implementation process. During these educational interactions, the addition of facility-level data demonstrating need for stewardship delivered in an academic, educational, or informational format can be persuasive, especially if also accompanied by external comparative data from similar institutions. Recruiting the support of influential members of targeted physician groups, a "physician champion," is very helpful in convincing peers that the activity is a necessary part of quality patient care. Despite these efforts, some prescribers may not fully accept or agree with a preauthorization policy. In our experience, these individuals will eventually be outnumbered in settings of high administrative support and agreement from other influential clinicians.

Obtaining adequate resources to support AS activities is a significant as well as the most commonly cited barrier to preauthorization implementation.[9, 11, 12] This limitation is especially true in small, community or rural hospital settings with competing interests for limited resources.[3, 6, 13, 14] Traditionally, preauthorization requires a phone and pager-based system with approval granted by an ID physician, ID-trained pharmacist, or dedicated microbiology consultant.[15] Ideally, the individuals answering the calls should be compensated for the time and effort required. In addition to these personnel requirements, an important decision regarding implementation of preauthorization includes determining the time needed to perform approvals. Determining how many drug approval calls per day are expected can be estimated by evaluating antibiotic utilization data. However, uncontrollable factors such as an influx or clusters of drug-resistant infections, seasonality, and changing patient case mix may all affect antibiotic use independently.[16, 17] Practice and disease are dynamic over time; therefore, initial estimates of time and personnel requirements may not remain accurate as time passes. Thus, reassessments of the work-load burden and plans for documenting work-load are needed not only at the beginning of the intervention but routinely as practice continues.

The level of expertise of the personnel granting drug approvals should be considered. Although specialists in ID are the most qualified to answer questions about antibiotic management, experts are not available in all practice settings. Clinical pharmacists following approved guidelines and with ID physician or ID-trained pharmacist oversight may be equally effective if properly supported [18] or if criteria for the use of targeted agent(s) are free from subjective judgment. Likewise, hospitalists can also effectively serve the goals of the ASP.[19, 20] Attending physicians or ID pharmacists would generally be preferred over ID fellows for providing pre-approval.[21] Ultimately, availability of experts and financial support for the activity will determine who can perform this task.

ASPs have utilized multiple different models of implementing preauthorization to address the barrier of finite resources. One solution is to limit the need for authorization only to requests not meeting pre-approval criteria or indications. However, many settings do not yet require routine documentation of antibiotic indication at the time of order entry, making validation of compliance with indication-specific criteria difficult.[3] Even if documentation of indication is integrated into the order-entry process, the clinician may select an inaccurate indication that meets pre-approval criteria in order to facilitate rapid drug delivery. Another solution is to provide limited personnel hours for preauthorization and allow an unapproved dose or two overnight until the AS team returns in the morning and can review all overnight orders. When this approach was used, researchers found that prescribers were more likely to order restricted drugs in the hour after pre-approval pager coverage ended compared with the hour before.[22] Also, these antibiotics were more likely to be inconsistent with guideline recommendations. Despite this phenomenon, we believe that limited hours for AS activities are better than none. The majority of antibiotic decision-making occurs during daylight hours and would be subject to the preauthorization activity even though the effect of the intervention may be blunted by a few overnight doses. Other potential solutions to overcoming resource limitations are to use information technology, internet-based approvals, or order entry-based solutions which require documentation and/or certification of compliance with preauthorization criteria.[23–26]

Case Continued

Dr. J, Dr. B, and the WMH pharmacy director decide to do a bit more exploring before addressing the P&T committee with a proposal. First, Dr. B meets with Dr. H one-on-one to approach the idea of antibiotic stewardship and discuss use of the high-cost antibiotics. Dr. B invites Dr. H to be a key partner in developing institutional criteria and guidelines for use of the antibiotics. Dr. H is happy to be involved as he considers himself knowledgeable in the area due to his experience as the ICU director.

The pharmacy director approaches the Chief Executive Officer (CEO) of the hospital with the idea of supporting dedicated pharmacist time for antibiotic stewardship. The CEO is interested, but unfortunately, the hospital budget has recently taken a large setback and the timing for the request is not ideal. He suggests that a cost analysis and estimate of savings would be necessary before he can consider financial support. He is, however, interested in cost savings that could be accomplished with streamlining the formulary. He suggests that a P&T Formulary Review Subcommittee be formed to avoid duplicative antibiotics. The pharmacy director and the chair of P&T Committee select a multidisciplinary group of individuals to be represented on the new antibiotic formulary subcommittee. This subcommittee is able to define local criteria for optimal and appropriate use for each drug, which ultimately requires P&T Committee approval. Dr. J works with the two physicians to perform complete medication use evaluations (MUE) on the drugs targeted for preauthorization based on these approved criteria.

Since there is no individual financially-supported by the hospital to conduct antibiotic stewardship, the group has to determine who will be responsible for approving the four targeted antibiotics. According to information gathered from the MUEs, this would be approximately 2–5 prescriptions per day. Due to the low volume and clear guidance from the newly-developed institutional criteria, the group proposes that the drug-approval process be decentralized and performed by a staff pharmacist. Dr. H expresses concern that gaining a phone approval when pharmacy staffing was low overnight may take too much time, especially when septic patients are admitted to the ICU. Thus, the group compromises and identifies hours of approval only during daytime and evening shifts, with overnight prescriptions reviewed for appropriateness and continuation during the following morning shift. Also, the group decides that the prescriber should check off the indication from a list of P&T-approved diagnoses when placing the computer order. That way the pharmacist will review the order and medical record for documentation of the appropriate indication, which will reduce the time needed for the phone call. Also, this would allow some application of the criteria during night shifts when no calls will occur.

Discussion

An important barrier to address is concern about interruption in workflow and time constraints associated with preauthorization.[8] Since prescribers' time is filled with the demands of patient care, documentation, and administrative requirements, it is difficult to add yet another disruption to their working day. However, the requirement for additional effort on the part of the prescriber for restricted medications may encourage the prescriber to choose the path of least resistance and opt for a different antibiotic when the clinical situation does not absolutely demand use of the restricted drug. That being said, the goal of preauthorization is to provide a moment for thinking and weighing options, not for battling against logistical headaches. Thus, the challenge to the AS team is to provide a streamlined process for preauthorization. Truly, if the ASP fails to address this concern, each hurdle a clinician must jump to care for their patients could perpetuate a negative impression that prescriber and patient care interests are not valued. One way to address this concern early is to have a front-line staff member collaborate with the group in developing a practical and achievable process that integrates well into daily workflows.

A worrisome potential consequence of a poorly executed preauthorization process is delay in receipt of important antibiotics to septic patients. Incidents that significantly delay necessary drugs for sick patients must be avoided or the overall intent and goals of optimizing antibiotic therapy are nullified. Thus, in addition to the main outcomes of interest that show that the preauthorization intervention works to improve appropriateness of prescribing, potential negative patient outcomes must also be tracked and remedied if they occur. An active effort to understand other points of view, combined with a commitment to reviewing and improving the practice, is recommended to address negative impressions that stem from these incidents. Indeed, successfully working through conflicts solidifies good relationships which are key to building reputation and rapport between the AS team and prescribers.

Despite the abundant evidence of cost savings attained through ASP interventions, a common challenge for new ASPs is to have an initial proposal for financial support declined. The key for prospective ASPs is to use published data to develop a clear proposal with

Case 1 (*cont.*)

estimates of institution-specific cost savings. If the first request for funding is declined, gathering more information about cost savings and documenting support from other individuals in the institution will help make subsequent proposals more convincing.

Case Resolution

After several discussions and drafts, Dr. J writes a formal proposal which includes a timeline to perform reviews of the impact of the intervention. Information on the number of approval calls, conflicts between prescribers and pharmacy, delayed doses, documentation of the indication, accuracy of the documented indication, and initiation of restricted drugs during night shifts is also collected. A feasibility report will be presented to P&T at 3 and 6 months after implementation. A full evaluation of patient and facility-level outcomes will be presented a year after implementation. The effect on appropriateness of use per institutional criteria is the main outcome of interest, with additional cost, antibiotic use data, and negative patient events as secondary outcomes.

Drs. B and H present the proposal to P&T and the executive medical staff committee for official approval. They also provide educational presentations at several medical staff meetings so prescribers understand the new process. During the first few weeks of implementation, Dr. B is available to review the restricted drug approvals with the pharmacists on a daily basis just before his rounds. If there are any conflicts or confusion, he takes a moment to speak with the prescriber about it individually. Dr. J works with the information technologists to adjust the order-entry process, and she educates the staff pharmacists.

Dr. J, Dr. B, and the pharmacy director plan to use the experience of implementing the drug-approval process and cost analysis to develop a clear business case for an ASP. They also plan to engage the newly formed subcommittee members to write formal letters of support for the proposed ASP. They hope this additional data will be helpful in convincing the CEO that a fully supported ASP is a wise investment for WMH.

Case 2 Established Hospital-Based ASP Wishing to Implement New Rapid Diagnostic Test for MRSA Bloodstream Infections

Case Introduction

Dr. Q is an ID physician and medical director of an ASP established five years ago at B University Medical Center (BUMC), a 620-bed acute care, academic-affiliated hospital. The program employs 1.5 full-time equivalents (FTEs) of ID PharmD time to conduct ASP activities, including post-prescription review of targeted antibiotics, IV-to-PO conversion, de-escalation, and approval of restricted antibiotics. Based on a monthly report of antibiotic utilization data received from the pharmacy, Dr. Q. and his staff discuss concerns for escalating the empiric use of vancomycin therapy for suspected methicillin-resistant *Staphylococcus aureus* (MRSA) infections. The drug is often continued as part of combination therapy even when no MRSA is isolated. The team wishes to promote the early use of beta-lactams such as nafcillin or cefazolin in settings where a methicillin-susceptible *S. aureus* (MSSA) is identified. Also, the AS team expresses concerns over the additional therapeutic drug monitoring required for vancomycin as well as concerns regarding the development of resistance if vancomycin is overused. Two patients at the BUMC dialysis center have developed vancomycin-intermediate *S. aureus* (VISA) infections over the last year, and this is very concerning to the infection control representative on the AS committee. Finally, the microbiology lab director, Dr. S. reports an increasing percentage of MRSA with vancomycin MICs of 2mcg/ml.

Case 2 *(cont.)*

Dr. Q is aware of the availability of new rapid diagnostic tests for identification of resistant Gram-positive infections, including MRSA. He begins discussions with Dr. S regarding the potential role and feasibility of, acquiring such tests at BUMC.

Discussion

The need for early appropriate antibiotic therapy often necessitates the initial empiric use of broad-spectrum antibiotics, especially in patients with serious or life-threatening infections. De-escalation of antibiotic therapy is an active AS strategy focused on decreasing the spectrum or stopping antibiotics used for initial empiric therapy following the availability of information from diagnostic tests and patient response.[27] However, the appropriate choice of both empiric and targeted therapies is significantly impacted by diagnostic uncertainty and diagnostic delays. Failure to obtain appropriate samples for culture contributes to this problem. Also, delays inherent in culture-based diagnostics often impact pathogen identification and susceptibility information. Therefore, the use of biomarkers and rapid diagnostics is a promising intervention to facilitate the selection of focused therapy.[28–35]

Similar to gaining support for personnel and technical needs, ASPs may be called upon to assist in the justification of support for laboratory or other diagnostic resources. These discussions generally include an evaluation of needed laboratory space, personnel, training and validation procedures, reagent costs, sample collection requirements, the projected volume of tests, sensitivity, specificity, and the urgency and feasibility of gaining rapid test results. In general, acquisition of such tests represents a significant capital investment for the clinical microbiology laboratory. While availability of such tests can improve antibiotic use when coupled with active ASPs,[36, 37] concerns regarding "cost shifting" from antibiotics to diagnostics must be addressed. Additional concerns have been raised regarding the reimbursement of such high-cost tests from third-party payers. Questions regarding the potential misuse or misinterpretation of test results combined with the expense, has prompted some institutions to develop guidelines or restrictions on test ordering. Finally, the availability of newer technologies under development may cause many laboratories to delay their request for such resources until those technologies are US Food and Drug Administration (FDA) approved and available.

Case Continued

Drs. Q and S meet to discuss whether to implement new diagnostic tests to facilitate treatment of infectious illnesses. Dr. S states that some clinicians express interest in obtaining tests for procalcitonin concentrations to assess the need for continued antibiotic therapies. Others like Dr. Q are more interested in the use of rapid molecular diagnostics, especially those that can differentiate MRSA from MSSA, and coagulase-negative staphylococci (CoNS) in blood specimens. They identify three products currently approved by the FDA, all with sensitivity and specificity exceeding 90%. Dr. S also explains that additional technology such as other polymerase-chain reaction (PCR) tests for other organisms, as well as matrix-assisted laser desorption ionization time-of-flight mass spectroscopy (MALDI-TOF MS), are also being investigated.[35]

Discussion

Ideally, quality patient care should outweigh the concern over shifting direct costs. Additional indirect cost savings, such as successful patient outcomes and reduced length of stay, would theoretically balance the costs of new tests. However, convincing administrators may require robust and complicated economic analyses, which is often beyond the scope or ability of AS team members or their microbiology colleagues.

Case 2 (*cont.*)

Perhaps the strongest support for the acquisition of additional diagnostic resources comes from cost-effectiveness studies. Outcomes such as time to effective therapy or length of therapy can be compared in the setting of a new diagnostic tool relative to the existing "standard of care." However, there are challenges inherent in cost-effectiveness evaluations of novel diagnostics for IDs.[38] Benefits of improved diagnostics are often difficult to quantify because the larger costs are driven by poor treatment decisions resulting from lack of information and uncertainty rather than the costs of the test itself.[38] There are currently few published studies evaluating the impact of rapid MRSA molecular testing on patient-level outcome and cost-effectiveness measures.[39–41]

Case Resolution

Drs. Q. and S. further evaluate the potential role of rapid diagnostic testing for MRSA in the blood of patients at BUMC. They obtain pharmacy data regarding the frequency and duration of inpatient vancomycin use. An MUE conducted one year prior provides data regarding the variety of indications for vancomycin use at BUMC. They also contact colleagues at other academic institutions with comparable patient populations to understand their experiences with molecular tests. Finally, Dr. S queries the microbiology laboratory data on the frequency of negative blood cultures as well as the prevalence of CoNS, MRSA, and MSSA. Based on these data, Drs. Q and S enlist the help of a Masters of Business Administration student at the university to conduct a crude economic modeling analysis. Their model estimates a mean reduction of 1.7 days of vancomycin therapy per patient. Among the assumptions in the analysis is the availability of the MRSA rapid testing 16 hours per day, 5 days per week with a turnaround time not to exceed 4 hours. However, the model is unable to provide reasonable estimates for proposed reductions in length of stay, vancomycin-associated adverse events, vancomycin monitoring, or declining vancomycin susceptibility. The potential savings in reductions in antibiotic volume alone would not offset annual expenses related to test acquisition and conduct.

Because the team is unable to demonstrate cost savings associated with the request, the proposal is revised to emphasize the potential enhancements to the quality of patient care by reducing time delays to appropriate antibiotic therapy, along with reductions in unnecessary vancomycin use and monitoring. The proposal is supplemented by a discussion between Dr. Q. and the hospital administrator regarding a recent patient with staphylococcal bacteremia whose delay to appropriate antibiotic therapy of approximately three days would have been reduced to a few hours if optimal testing methods were available.

Case 3 A Long-Term Care Facility Wishing to Implement Institutional Guidelines and Order Sets for Diagnosis and Treatment of Urinary Tract Infections (UTIs)

Introduction

Dr. B is a geriatrics specialist and medical director at Lake Pines, a 150-bed long-term care facility (LTCF) consisting of a five-bed chronic ventilator unit, 30-bed physical rehabilitation unit and a nursing home. Computerized physician order entry (CPOE) is not yet available in the facility. He expresses concern over the management of UTIs and asymptomatic bacteriuria at the facility after he receives a report from the local referral hospital that several patients transferred from his facility are infected with extended-spectrum beta-lactamase (ESBL)-producing *E.coli*. During a monthly patient care conference, Dr. B begins a discussion with Dr. O, an ID specialist who provides consultation to the facility, regarding the formation and use of guidelines for providers in the management of UTIs. He believes that the time is right

Case 3 (*cont.*)

for UTI treatment guidelines based on recent successful local initiatives to limit the use of urinary catheters.

Discussion

The high rate of both utilization and inappropriate use of antibiotics in long-term care facilities has been well-documented.[42, 43] This has been most notable for inappropriate antibiotic therapy in patients with suspected UTIs which can then lead to the emergence of antibiotic-resistant bacterial infections or *C. difficile* infections.[44] However, the promotion of appropriate antibiotic use at LTCFs is a special challenge. Despite their high frequency of antibiotic use, ASPs practicing active patient interventions are rarely found in these settings. Therefore, institution-specific guidelines have often been proposed in such settings as an initial step to promote appropriate antibiotic use in the absence of active AS initiatives. The impact of treatment guidelines for IDs is often questioned. Barriers to successful implementation include awareness of the guidelines, perceived loss of prescribing autonomy, perceptions of inflexibility, and lack of immediate access to the guidelines at the time of prescribing (Table 3).

Table 3 Development of Local Antibiotic Guidelines: Barriers and Solutions

Barriers
- Clinicians unaware of local guidelines
- Perceived loss of prescribing privileges or autonomy
- Vocal opinion leader may influence others' practice
- May be controversial (despite "consensus" and approval from local authorities)
- May be perceived as inflexible and poorly applicable to the providers' patient population (e.g., "My patients are sicker")
- May not be accessible at time of prescription
- Require local modifications and time to develop
- Require frequent updates
- Prescriber adherence is variable
- Distribution poses a logistical challenge
- Prescriber lacks belief in value of local guidelines

Solutions
- Antibiotic care bundles and order sets that include local guidelines
- Educate staff regarding availability and location
- Customize to local environment and patient population to maximize applicability
- Design triggers for updates:
  - Key studies publication
  - National guidelines publication
  - Antibiogram revisions
  - Formulary changes

- Obtain Pharmacy and Therapeutic or other hospital level committee review and approval
- Gain input from key opinion leaders
- Make available in chart, local intranet, and/or Computerized Prescription Order Entry
- Provide options addressing allergies
- Complete an assessment of adherence and feed back to prescribers
- Distribute via the internet
- Acquire data on antibiotic practices from peer-institutions with similar patient populations

Case 3 *(cont.)*

Case Continued

In the absence of a formal infrastructure to create antibiotic use guidelines for the institution, Dr. B obtains a copy of the UTI care bundle currently utilized by the area's acute care referral hospital. He also obtains reports from both the infection control practitioner of that hospital and the microbiology laboratory used by the facility to identify susceptibility patterns of bacteria isolated from the facility's patients. Dr. B adjusts the guidelines from the acute care hospital to more accurately target the microbiology data obtained from the LTCF. He then presents a draft of the proposed guidelines to a meeting of the medical staff. Two medical staff members express concern about the potential for low acceptance and utilization of the guidelines because of the current paper-based method of diagnostic, laboratory, and medication ordering in the facility. Dr. B requests a report from the pharmacy regarding current antibiotic utilization in patients with UTIs, but they are unable to provide an indication for the antibiotics used by the facility's patients.

Discussion

Formulation of facility-specific guidelines should first get input and "buy in" from key stakeholders and prescribers. Whenever possible, institution-specific guidelines should be based on national guidelines and evidence-based standards but modified to incorporate local formulary agents and microbiology data. Guidelines should be reviewed by the responsible committees and involve local opinion leaders to increase their validity and acceptance. They should be readily available at the time of prescribing to facilitate their use. Finally, they should be reviewed on a regular basis to keep them current to evolving published evidence and national guideline updates.

Case Resolution

After much debate, the medical staff agree to approve the antibiotic treatment guidelines as part of a UTI bundle. After presentation at the next staff meeting, a copy of the bundle is provided as part of a laminated section divider in the order section of the patient medical record. The guidelines also appear in the facility's intranet website after being announced to prescribers via an email. Additionally, a paper order set worksheet is designed to include checkboxes for commonly ordered diagnostics and prompts to evaluate the patient for symptoms. The guidelines provide institution-specific recommendations for empiric treatments with appropriate dosing for weight and renal function. Also included are standardized nursing instructions for specimen collection and Foley catheter change for ease of prescriber ordering. The nursing staff help prompt prescribers to review the guidelines and use the order set whenever possible.

Dr. B. contacts the representative of the medical staff in charge of quality assurance and requests that the order set guidelines serve as criteria for an audit in 6 months to assess compliance. The quality officer requests clarification of the endpoints of interest: process measures such as guideline compliance or outcome measures such as rates of patients with multidrug-resistant pathogens. Dr. B indicates that guideline compliance defined as guideline-concordant antibiotic choice and duration would be the best indication of the impact of the bundle. They plan to report back to the medical staff after the six-month review.

Case 4 An Outpatient Practice Introducing Delayed Prescription for
Acute Respiratory Infections

Introduction

Dr. C is a family physician who interacts with the inpatient AS team through audit and feedback activities at the local community hospital where he holds admitting privileges.

Case 4 (*cont.*)

As he learned ways to improve his use of antibiotics for hospitalized patients, he also becomes interested in investigating ways to avoid antibiotic exposures in the patients he and his partners see in their outpatient family practice. First, he speaks with the hospital antibiotic stewardship pharmacist, Anna. He explains that the majority of the prescriptions he writes for his outpatients are for upper respiratory infections including pharyngitis and sinusitis, otitis media, community-acquired pneumonia, and UTIs. She asks him to reflect on logistical or personnel resources that may help with patient-centered AS strategies in his outpatient practice. He immediately thinks of Karen, the clinic nurse who he's been working with for over 10 years. She knows all of his patients personally and is excellent at providing patient education and phone follow-up. Dr. C has limited time with his patients due to strict scheduling requirements and his periodic need to care for inpatients. Anna asks Dr. C if he has considered avoidance of antibiotic prescribing for acute respiratory tract infections. Dr. C is worried about this approach because he does not want to have conflicts with his patients who he perceives would be frustrated if they came for a visit and did not receive a prescription. Anna then asks if Dr. C has considered using a delayed prescribing strategy.

Discussion

Antibiotics for upper respiratory tract infections (URIs) comprise the greatest proportion of outpatient antibiotic prescriptions. A recent study examining US ambulatory care visits reported that approximately one-half of antibiotic prescriptions for URIs were inappropriate.[45] Delayed prescribing for uncomplicated upper respiratory infections is a strategy that has been in use for over ten years for low risk patients likely to have acute viral infections or when it is unclear whether the patient has a bacterial or viral pathogen at the time of clinical evaluation.[46] This practice is widely employed in outpatient settings in Europe, but its frequency of use in the United States is unknown.[47] There are several ways to operationalize delayed prescribing: writing a post-dated prescription, requiring the patient to re-contact the clinic if symptoms do not improve, or providing a prescription and instructing the patient to fill only if symptoms do not improve after a predetermined time.[48] Although initial trial data indicated that delayed prescription might result in worse symptom control than immediate-use antibiotics,[48] this has not been demonstrated in other reports.[46, 49–52] Thus, implementation should be determined based on what matches the physician, patient, and clinic practice characteristics and preferences.

Case Continued

Anna provides Dr. C with some published literature on delayed prescribing as well as references on the CDC website. He discusses the possibility of employing delayed prescription strategies with Karen. They agree that many patients who frequent the practice would not take well to a no prescription strategy but that a post-dated prescription or re-contact strategy is possible. Dr. C is most interested in maintaining high levels of patient satisfaction in addition to reducing antibiotic use among his patients. He and Karen agree that she will provide phone follow-ups for a sample of patients who receive a post-dated prescription over the first month to gauge their satisfaction and collect information about prescriptions being filled.

To his surprise, Dr. C encounters only a few patients who immediately reject the idea of a delayed prescription. In fact, he is pleased at the positive responses and the satisfaction expressed in their working doctor-patient relationship as well as their appreciation of his trust in allowing them to be in charge of their own medical decision-making. Dr. C wonders if there

Case 4 (*cont.*)

are other non-obtrusive ways to inform his patients about the importance of avoiding antibiotics when not necessary.

During the first month, Dr. C enters the delayed date for filling the prescription in the comments of the electronic prescription. However, Karen receives several calls from retail pharmacies confused about the comments. One of his patients calls stating that he had tried to fill the prescription after leaving the office and the pharmacy would not fill it due to the post-dating comments.

Discussion

Patient selection and patient education are key components of employing delayed prescription strategies.[49, 51] In general, this strategy is best used when the infection does not appear to be severe and the possibility of viral pathogens causing the infection is high. Further, appropriate patient selection should target patients who can understand and follow instructions, be receptive to education, and reliably return to collect the prescription or contact the clinic if symptoms are worsening or unresolved. Reinforcing verbal instructions with written materials often helps to clearly solidify instructions and education for delayed prescribing. Also, receipt of tangible materials seems to help increase the perception that the provider is "doing something" for the presenting complaint which may increase satisfaction with care. Further, studies of delayed prescriptions have revealed that beliefs about antibiotics were stronger in groups of patients given immediate prescriptions compared with those receiving delayed prescription strategies.[46, 49] Thus, engaging patients to wait and re-evaluate their symptoms, may help them develop a healthy understanding of the limited role of antibiotics in future episodes of upper respiratory infections.

Case Resolution

Based on these experiences, Dr. C and Karen agree that in addition to Dr. C explaining the process, Karen will follow up during the exit interview and provide a handout with written instructions informing patients about the process for filling a post-dated prescription. Patients are also told they can use this handout to assist with communication with retail pharmacists about the delayed prescription process. In the short-term, she also provides a follow-up call three days after the clinic visit to make sure there are no outstanding questions and to determine if the patient intended on filling the prescription.

Upon review of the number of antibiotic prescriptions filled, patient satisfaction surveys, and anecdotal experiences, Karen and Dr. C determine that their strategy has been successfully deployed. Patients who receive delayed prescriptions maintain a high satisfaction score and fill their prescriptions in approximately a third of cases. Dr. C takes this information back to his partners to discuss and encourage incorporating a delayed prescription strategy into their practices as well.

Conclusion

Above, we proposed twelve steps to implement active AS initiatives and provided illustrative cases regarding their use. We also identified common barriers to successful implementation and provide potential solutions to these barriers. While the specific challenges to implementation of ASPs vary between institutions, these common barriers can often be anticipated early in the design phases of the program. They are often overcome with careful planning and effective communication of program goals and methods.

References

1. Barlam TF, Cosgrove SE, Abbo LM et al. Implementing an antibiotic stewardship program: guidelines by the Infectious Diseases Society of America and the Society for Healthcare Epidemiology of America. *Clin Infect Dis* 2016; 62(10):e51–77.

2. Pollack LA, Srinivasan A. Core elements of hospital antibiotic stewardship programs from the Centers for Disease Control and Prevention. *Clin Infect Dis* 2014; 59(Suppl 3):S97–100.

3. Pollack LA, van Santen KL, Weiner LM, Dudeck MA, Edwards JR, Srinivasan A. Antibiotic stewardship programs in U.S. acute care hospitals: findings from the 2014 National Healthcare Safety Network Annual Hospital Survey. *Clin Infect Dis* 2016; 63(4):443–9.

4. Moehring RW, Anderson DJ. Antimicrobial stewardship as part of the infection prevention effort. *Curr Infect Dis Rep* 2012; 14(6):592–600.

5. Centers for Disease Control and Prevention and Institute for Healthcare Improvement. Antibiotic Stewardship Driver Diagram and Change Package, 2012. (Accessed Feb 7, 2016, at www.cdc.gov/getsmart/ healthcare/pdfs/antibiotic_stewardship_ change_package.pdf.)

6. Ohl CA, Dodds AE. Antimicrobial stewardship programs in community hospitals: the evidence base and case studies. *Clin Infect Dis* 2011; 53(Suppl 1): S23–28.

7. Goff DA, Bauer KA, Reed EE, Stevenson KB, Taylor JJ, West JE. Is the "low-hanging fruit" worth picking for antimicrobial stewardship programs? *Clin Infect Dis* 2012; 55(4):587–592.

8. Seemungal IA, Bruno CJ. Attitudes of housestaff toward a prior-authorization-based antibiotic stewardship program. *Infect Control Hosp Epidemiol* 2012; 33 (4):429–431.

9. Drew RH. Antimicrobial stewardship programs: how to start and steer a successful program. *J Manag Care Pharm* 2009; 15(Suppl 2): S18–23.

10. Bal AM, Gould IM. Antibiotic stewardship: overcoming implementation barriers. *Curr Opin Infect Dis* 2011; 24(4):357–362.

11. Johannsson B, Beekmann SE, Srinivasan A, Hersh AL, Laxminarayan R, Polgreen PM . Improving antimicrobial stewardship: the evolution of programmatic strategies and barriers. *Infect Control Hosp Epidemiol* 2011; 32(4):367–374.

12. Doron S, Boucher HW. Antibiotics for skin infections: new study design and a step toward shorter course therapy. *JAMA* 2013; 309(6):609–611.

13. Curcio D. Antibiotic stewardship: the "real world" when resources are limited. *Infect Control Hosp Epidemiol* 2010; 31 (6):666–668.

14. Yam P, Fales D, Jemison J, Gillum M, Bernstein M. Implementation of an antimicrobial stewardship program in a rural hospital. *Am J Health Syst Pharm* 2012; 69(13):1142–1148.

15. Dellit TH, Owens RC, McGowan JE Jr et al. Infectious Diseases Society of America and the Society for Healthcare Epidemiology of America guidelines for developing an institutional program to enhance antimicrobial stewardship. *Clin Infect Dis* 2007; 44(2):159–177.

16. McGowan JE. Antimicrobial stewardship–the state of the art in 2011: focus on outcome and methods. *Infect Control Hosp Epidemiol* 2012; 33(4):331–337.

17. Ibrahim OM, Polk R. Benchmarking antimicrobial drug use in hospitals. *Expert Rev Anti Infect Ther* 2012; 10 (4):445–457.

18. DiazGranados CA, Abd TT. Participation of clinical pharmacists without specialized infectious diseases training in antimicrobial stewardship. *Am J Health Syst Pharm* 2011; 68(18):1691–1692.

19. Rohde JM, Jacobsen D, Rosenberg DJ. Role of the hospitalist in antimicrobial stewardship: a review of work completed and description of a multisite collaborative. *Clin Ther* 2013; 35(6):751–757.

20. Srinivasan A. Engaging hospitalists in antimicrobial stewardship: the CDC

perspective. *J Hosp Med* 2011; 6(Suppl 1): S31–3.

21. Linkin DR, Paris S, Fishman NO, Metlay JP, Lautenbach E. Inaccurate communications in telephone calls to an antimicrobial stewardship program. *Infect Control Hosp Epidemiol* 2006; 27(7): 688–694.

22. LaRosa LA., Fishman NO, Lautenbach E, Koppel RJ, Morales KH, Linkin DR. Evaluation of antimicrobial therapy orders circumventing an antimicrobial stewardship program: investigating the strategy of "stealth dosing." *Infect Control Hosp Epidemiol* 2007; 28(5):551–556.

23. Buising KL, Thursky KA, Robertson MB, et al. Electronic antibiotic stewardship–reduced consumption of broad-spectrum antibiotics using a computerized antimicrobial approval system in a hospital setting. *J Antimicrob Chemother* 2008; 62 (3):608–616.

24. Sick AC, Lehmann CU, Tamma PD, Lee CK, Agwu AL. Sustained savings from a longitudinal cost analysis of an internet-based preapproval antimicrobial stewardship program. *Infect Control Hosp Epidemiol* 2013; 34(6):573–580.

25. Agwu AL, Lee CK, Jain SK et al. A World Wide Web-based antimicrobial stewardship program improves efficiency, communication, and user satisfaction and reduces cost in a tertiary care pediatric medical center. *Clin Infect Dis* 2008; 47 (6):747–753.

26. Cha YY, Lin TY, Huang CT et al. Implementation and outcomes of a hospital-wide computerised antimicrobial stewardship programme in a large medical centre in Taiwan. *Int J Antimicrob Agents* 2011; 38(6):486–492.

27. Kaye KS. Antimicrobial de-escalation strategies in hospitalized patients with pneumonia, intra-abdominal infections, and bacteremia. *J Hosp Med* 2012; 7 (Suppl):S13–21.

28. Dusemund F, Bucher B, Meyer S, et al. Influence of procalcitonin on decision to start antibiotic treatment in patients with a lower respiratory tract infection: insight

from the observational multicentric ProREAL surveillance. *Eur J Clin Microbiol Infect Dis* 2013; 32(1):51–60.

29. Bauer KA, West JE, Balada-Llasat JM, Pancholi P, Stevenson KB, Goff DA. An antimicrobial stewardship program's impact with rapid polymerase chain reaction methicillin-resistant *Staphylococcus aureus/S. aureus* blood culture test in patients with *S. aureus* bacteremia. *Clin Infect Dis* 2010; 51 (9):1074–1080.

30. Goff DA, Jankowski C, Tenover FC. Using rapid diagnostic tests to optimize antimicrobial selection in antimicrobial stewardship programs. *Pharmacother* 2012; 32(8):677–687.

31. Perez KK, Olsen RJ, Musick WL, et al. Integrating rapid pathogen identification and antimicrobial stewardship significantly decreases hospital costs. *Arch Pathol Lab Med* 2013;137(9):1247–1254.

32. Pulido MR García-Quintanilla M, Martín-Peña R, Cisneros JM, McConnell MJ. Progress on the development of rapid methods for antimicrobial susceptibility testing. *J Antimicrob Chemother* 2013; 68 (12):2710–2717.

33. Povoa P, Salluh JI. Biomarker-guided antibiotic therapy in adult critically ill patients: a critical review. *Ann Intensive Care* 2012; 2(1):1–9.

34. Wong JR, Bauer KA, Mangino JE, Goff DA. Antimicrobial stewardship pharmacist interventions for coagulase-negative staphylococci positive blood cultures using rapid polymerase chain reaction. *Ann Pharmacother* 2012; 46 (11):1484–1490.

35. Afshari A., Schrenzel J, Ieven M, Harbarth S. Bench-to-bedside review: rapid molecular diagnostics for bloodstream infection – a new frontier? *Crit Care* 2012; 16(3):222.

36. Clerc O, Prod'hom G, Vogne C, Bizzini A, Calandra T, Greub G Impact of matrix-assisted laser desorption ionization time-of-flight mass spectrometry on the clinical management of patients with Gram-negative bacteremia: a prospective

observational study. *Clin Infect Dis* 2013; 56 (8):1101–1107.

37. Lodes U, Bohmeier B, Lippert H, König B, Meyer F. PCR-based rapid sepsis diagnosis effectively guides clinical treatment in patients with new onset of SIRS. *Langenbecks Arch Surg* 2012; 397 (3):447–455.

38. Andrews JR Lawn SD, Dowdy DW, Walensky RP. Challenges in evaluating the cost-effectiveness of new diagnostic tests for HIV-associated Tuberculosis. *Clin Infect Dis* 2013; 57(7):1021–1026.

39. Geiger K, Brown J. Rapid testing for methicillin-resistant *Staphylococcus aureus*: implications for antimicrobial stewardship. *Am J Health Syst Pharm* 2013; 70 (4):335–342.

40. Brown J, Paladino JA. Impact of rapid methicillin-resistant *Staphylococcus aureus* polymerase chain reaction testing on mortality and cost effectiveness in hospitalized patients with bacteraemia: a decision model. *Pharmacoeconomics* 2010; 28(7):567–575.

41. Hübner C, Hübner NO, Kramer A, Fleßa S. Cost-analysis of PCR-guided pre-emptive antibiotic treatment of *Staphylococcus aureus* infections: an analytic decision model. *Eur J Clinl Microbiol Infect Dis* 2012; 31(11):3065–3072.

42. Jump RL, Olds DM, Seifi N et al. Effective antimicrobial stewardship in a long-term care facility through an infectious disease consultation service: keeping a lid on antibiotic use. *Infect Control Hosp Epidemiol* 2012; 33(12): 1185–1192.

43. Peron EP, Hirsch AA, Jury LA, Jump RL, Donskey CJ. Another setting for stewardship: high rate of unnecessary antimicrobial use in a veterans affairs long-term care facility. *J Am Geriatr Soc* 2013; 61 (2):289–90.

44. Rotjanapan P, Dosa D, Thomas KS. Potentially inappropriate treatment of urinary tract infections in two Rhode Island nursing homes. *Arch Intern Med* 2011; 171(5):438–443.

45. Fleming-Dutra KE, , Hersh AL, Shapiro DJ et al. Prevalence of inappropriate antibiotic prescriptions among US ambulatory care visits, 2010–2011. *JAMA* 2016; 315 (17):1864–1873.

46. de la Poza Abad M, Mas Dalmau G, Moreno Bakedano M et al. Prescription strategies in acute uncomplicated respiratory infections: a randomized clinical trial. *JAMA Intern Med* 2016; 176 (1):21–29.

47. McCullough AR, Glasziou PP, Delayed Antibiotic Prescribing Strategies–Time to Implement? *JAMA Intern Med* 2016; 176 (1):29–30.

48. Spurling GK, Del Mar CB, Dooley L, Foxlee R, Farley R. Delayed antibiotics for symptoms and complications of respiratory infections. *Cochrane Database Syst Rev* 2017; 9:cd004417.

49. Little P, Moore M, Kelly J et al. Delayed antibiotic prescribing strategies for respiratory tract infections in primary care: pragmatic, factorial, randomised controlled trial. *BMJ* 2014; 348:g1606.

50. Worrall G , Kettle A, Graham W, Hutchinson J. Postdated versus usual delayed antibiotic prescriptions in primary care: reduction in antibiotic use for acute respiratory infections? *Can Fam Physician* 2010; 56(10):1032–1036.

51. Drew RH, White R, MacDougall C et al. Insights from the Society of Infectious Diseases Pharmacists on antimicrobial stewardship guidelines from the Infectious Diseases Society of America and the Society for Healthcare Epidemiology of America. *Pharmacother* 2009; 29(5):593–607.

Index